prohealthsys

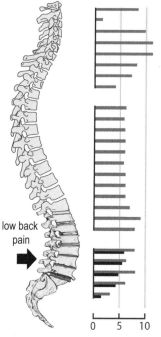

low back pain

0   5   10

Introduction · Head & Neck · Knee · Assessment · Shoulder & Arm · Leg, Ankle & Foot · SI & Pelvis · Elbow · Functional Rehab · L-Spine · Wrist & Hand · Appendix

Congratulations on making the best investment of your life - your own education. Mobilization of the **~456 joints** in the body is among **the most gratifying of treatments available**. Often with instant results, you will help people **move better, breath deeper, stand taller** and have an overall improved sense of well being - you will provide increased function for all aspects of their life (work, play, sex and sport). **This text bridges the gap between academics and practical application.** Information sources include: original research articles with cutting-edge information, 100s of cadaver dissections & decades of evidence based, multidisciplinary clinical experience. We also demo with different sized practitioners to show variation in biomechanics and gender application (5ft/100lbs female vs. 6ft/170lbs male).

Countless hours of research & design were spent to develop the content & format of this text. To help ensure gender equity, 'his' & 'her' are used interchangeably throughout the text. The ☺ symbol signifies a section containing humor, laughter is recommended but optional ☺.

The book's size allows for easy transport and storage. Chapters are marked with soft tabs, icons & the start of each chapter provides a detailed table of contents for that section. The paper used is uncoated to allow you to **write your own notes** directly on the pages. If you require your book coil bound take it to your local print shop, have the spine cut and coil bound. This text is supported by numerous student, clinician & instructor **resources, videos, quizzes & patient handouts on our website** (including palpation, muscle testing, assessment, special tests and treatment video). **Remember movement = health and motion is life.** - Dr. Nikita Vizniak

For instructors
- *Simplify your instruction technique*
- *PowerPoint presentations & syllabi*
- *Regional quizzes & grading rubrics*
- *Follow-up evidence based physical assessment & orthopathology texts*

For students
- *Execute the steps of ...*
- *and joint-play includin...*
- *position, contact, tissu...*
- *Chapter **quizzes & fin...***
- ***Video** of ROM, special tests & mobilizations*

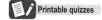 Printable quizzes   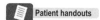 Patient handouts   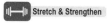 Stretch & Strengthen   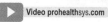 Video prohealthsys.com

As health care providers, our fundamental professional goal is to accurately and **efficiently assess and offer treatment options** for our patients. Part of the pattern recognition process requires an understanding of the basic tissues injured and setting the conditions required to promote optimal healing and health; to encourage the body to heal itself (no doctor or therapist actually heals anything - it is done on the cellular level - we just help set the stage).

It is crucial to realize that our role is to help **facilitate the body's natural healing** abilities. The most powerful therapeutic benefit any clinician has to offer is the ability to give their patients the confidence to realize that they CAN get better. Across all conditions, the sooner a person returns to regular activity the better!

In most outpatient encounters, assessment & treatment progression from **least to most invasive is optimal.** Remember your basic anatomy & physiology education and try to ensure treatments are simple and easy to follow for maximum compliance (**MED - minimal effective dose**).

Use your clinical prediction rules with **multiple source of evidence to support your findings and rationale for treatment.** Simply put, after 1000s of patients, xrays, MRIs and cadaver dissections, there is an overwhelming amount of **anatomical variation** in the size and shape of the body (muscle, bone, ligament, fascia) for simple static exams to be accurate (see x-ray of C5 SP below) - combine assessment with history, palpation, ROM and special tests for more accurate evaluation of the tissue and patient as a whole. **Treat the patient, not pictures of their anatomy.**

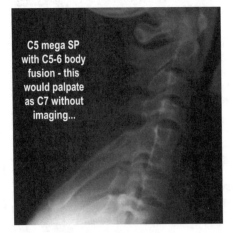

C5 mega SP with C5-6 body fusion - this would palpate as C7 without imaging...

For manual treatment there are 3 main options

1. **Mobilize** (ROM, stretch, massage, IASTM etc.)
2. **Stabilize** (exercise (contracture), brace, etc.)
3. **Leave it alone** (prevent further injury & work on compensation - set conditions for optimal healing)

Follow the 7 principles of medicine:

1. **First Do No Harm** (*Primum Non Nocere*) - choose assessment/treatment options that are safe & effective, to increase health & decrease harmful side effects (**progress from least to most invasive in assessment & treatment**).

2. **The Healing Power of Nature** (*Vis Medicatrix Naturae*) - work to restore & support the powerful & inherent healing abilities of the physical, mental & emotional to prevent further disease from occurring ('Stimulate the Vis').

3. **Identify & Treat the Causes** (*Tolle Causam*) - The primary goal is to treat the underlying cause of disease, not treat or mask the symptoms of the dysfunction (avoid treatments that only treat symptoms, find the cause & treat the specific tissue damaged!) - **Assessment is Therapeutic**

4. **Doctor as Teacher** (*Docere*) - Educate & support patients on personal health management; be part of a team that empowers patients to take responsibility for their own health & work together to find solutions both in clinic and at home/work.

5. **Treat the Whole Person** (*Tolle Totum*) - holistic treatment recognizes the body as an integrated whole; **treat the patient, not the disease**. Address the nutritional status, lifestyle, family history, physical, mental, emotional, genetic, environmental & social factors in a person's life. Also realize the limitation of your practice scope and ability; create a strong network of professionals you can refer to for co-management (attend to patient comfort).

6. **Disease Prevention & Health Promotion** (*Praeventio*)- applies to all of the principles in a proactive form of disease prevention & health promotion (optimal health maintenance & prevention are still the best medicine).

7. **Follow the evidence.** (*Nullius in verba*) 'take nobody's word for it' - is an expression used by the Royal Society of London for Improving Natural Knowledge to withstand the domination of authority and to verify all statements with facts determined by experiment. Use multiple sources and follow the science not authority!

If you use joint mobilizations on a regular basis I would strongly encourage you to enroll in Brazilian Jujitsu (BJJ). Aside from the amazing cardiovascular HIIT fitness and self confidence it provides, many of the positions and submissions require detailed biomechanical ability to effectively take joints to end ranges using lever advantage. It also **teaches smaller practitioners better joint vector methodology and allows larger body types to develop more finesse in motion**. As it was designed, BJJ favors technique over size and can make very small practitioners surprisingly powerful. The practice has truly been a humbling experience and improved both the way I move my own body, and how I perform and teach joint mobilizations.

> Joints should NOT be viewed as simple articulations between bones, rather joints should be viewed as dynamic organs (*joint organs*). Joint organs consist of bones, cartilage, ligaments, capsules, adipose, neurovascular and musculotendinous structures that have significant effects on the entire kinetic chain and overall health. When joint organs are combined with the neuromuscular system that acts on them, they make up the largest organ system of the body.

The table below shows age specific findings in *asymptomatic* patients. ***Treat the patient as they present, not pictures of their anatomy,*** that may not even be the cause of the ailment. It is surprising how many clinicians and educators are unable to differentiate the sources of **joint sounds** and their potential cause - see page 26 to help you with that process (joint articular sounds). Remember the graph of **knowledge and expertise** below ☺.

I would like to thank all of the individuals and organizations involved in the creation and review of this text. In addition, I would also like to thank the readers of this book, readers like you, for making my passion such a huge success. I invite any and all suggestions in support of continuing to improve and expand this text and our other resources.

Lastly, one of my favorite quotes for inspiration:

'People will forget what you said and the things you did, but they will never forget how you make them feel.' *Dr. Maya Angelou*

I hope you make people feel amazing, and look forward to hearing from you or meeting you at our CE seminars.

Thank you for your time,

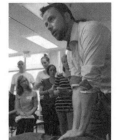

Dr. Nikita Vizniak
nik@prohealthsys.com

Age specific findings in asymptomatic patients

Finding	Age (yrs)						
	20	30	40	50	60	70	80
Facet degen.	4%	9%	18%	32%	50%	69%	83%
Disc degeneration	37%	52%	68%	80%	88%	93%	96%
Disc height loss	24%	34%	45%	56%	67%	76%	84%
Disc bulge	30%	40%	50%	60%	69%	77%	84%
Disc protrusion	29%	31%	33%	36%	38%	40%	43%
Annular fissures	19%	20%	22%	23%	25%	27%	29%
Spondylolisthesis	3%	5%	8%	14%	23%	35%	50%

W. Brinjikji, P.H. Luetmer, B. Comstock, B.W. Bresnahan, L.E. Chen, R.A. Deyo, S. Halabi, J.A. Turner, A.L. Avins, K. James, J.T. Wald, D.F. Kallmes and J.G. Jarvik. **Systematic Literature Review of Imaging Features of Spinal Degeneration in Asymptomatic Populations.** American Journal of Neuroradiology April 2015, 36 (4) 811-816; DOI: https://doi.org/10.3174/ajnr.A4173

Dong Sun, Peng LiuEmail author, Jie Cheng, Zikun Ma, Jingpei Liu and Tingzheng Qin. **Correlation between intervertebral disc degeneration, paraspinal muscle atrophy, and lumbar facet joints degeneration in patients with lumbar disc herniation.** BMC Musculoskeletal DisordersBMC series – open, inclusive and trusted 2017 18:167. https://doi.org/10.1186/s12891-017-1522-4

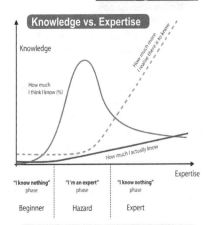

Knowledge vs. Expertise

Knowledge

How much I think I know (%)

How much more I realize there is to know

How much I actually know

Expertise

"I know nothing" phase — "I'm an expert" phase — "I know nothing" phase

Beginner | Hazard | Expert

Where are you on the graph above?

"If you're not assessing, you just guessing." Clinical Prediction Rules (CPRs) are designed to **improve clinical decision making** & assist in differential diagnosis, prognosis & treatment planning. CPRs provide practitioners with **powerful diagnostic information** from the history and physical examination that may serve as an accurate decision-making surrogate for more expensive diagnostic tests.[1] In most cases a good history & exam are **more diagnostic than MRI.**[2] Combined multiple diagnostic tests with **critical thinking** and clinical understanding of *dis-ease* processes to improve accuracy & treatment effectiveness.

1. Childs J and Cleland J. (2006). Development and Application of Clinical Prediction Rules to improve decision making in Physical Therapist Practice. PHYS THER. 2006. Jan;86(1):122-131. Web. 13 Aug 2014
2. McGurk B, King W, Govind J, Lowry J, Bogduk N. Safety, efficacy, and cost effectiveness of evidence based guidelines for the management of acute low back pain in primary care. Spine 2001;26:2615-2622

Carpal Tunnel Syndrome

- *Purpose:* identify patients who likely have carpal tunnel syndrome based on specific patient characteristics
- *Rule:*
    - Shaking hands for symptom relief
    - Wrist-ratio index greater than .67
    - Symptom Severity Scale score greater than 1.9
    - Reduced median sensory field of digit 1
    - Age greater than 45 years
- *Sensitivity:* 0.98 (3+ variables), 0.77 (4+ variables), 0.18 (5 variables)
- *Specificity:* 0.54 (3+ variables), 0.83 (4+ variables), 0.99 (5 variables)
- *Positive Predictive Value:* 52% (3+ variables), 70% (4+ variables), 90% (5 variables)

Wainner RS, et al. Development of a clinical prediction rule for the diagnosis of carpal tunnel syndrome. Arch Phys Med Rehabil. 2005; 86(4): 609-18.

Others available prohealthsys.com

- **Ottawa Ankle Rules, Ottawa Knee Rules**
- **Canadian Cervical Spine Rules**
- **Pittsburgh Knee Rules**
- **Subacromial Impingement**
- **Rotator Cuff Pathology**
- **Meniscal Pathology**
- **Stabilization for Low Back Pain**
- **Mechanical Traction for Low Back Pain**
- **Thoracic Manipulation for Neck Pain**

Manipulation in Low Back Pain

- *Purpose:* To identify patients with low back pain who likely will improve with spinal manipulation.
- *Rule:*
    - Duration of symptoms less than 16 days
    - At least one hip with greater than 35° of internal rotation
    - Lumbar hypomobility
    - No symptoms distal to the knee
- *Sensitivity:* 0.94 (3 variables), 0.69 (4 variables)
- *Specificity:* 0.62 (2 variables), 0.97 (3 variables), **1.00 (4 variables)**
- *Positive Likelihood Ratio:* 2.6 (2 variables), 24.4 (3 variables), **infinite (4 variables)**
- *Positive Predictive Value:* 68% (3 variables), 95% (4 variables)

1. Childs JD, et al. A clinical prediction rule to identify patients with low back pain most likely to benefit from spinal manipulation: a validation study. Ann Intern Med. 2004; 141(12): 920-8.

2. Cleland JA, et al. The Use of a Lumbar Spine Manipulation Technique by Physical Therapists in Patients Who Satisfy a Clinical Prediction Rule: A Case Series. J Orthop Sports Phys Ther. 2006; 36(4): 209–214.

3. Flynn T, et al. A clinical prediction rule for classifying patients with low back pain who demonstrate short-term improvement with spinal manipulation. Spine. 2002; 27(24): 2835-43.

- **Cervical Manipulation for Neck Pain**
- **Mechanical Traction for Neck Pain**
- **Cervicothoracic Manipulation for Shoulder Pain**
- **Manipulation for Patellofemoral Pain Syndrome**
- **Orthotics for Patellofemoral Pain Syndrome**
- **Taping for Patellofemoral Pain Syndrome**
- **Hip Mobilization for Knee Osteoarthritis**

- **Use basic clinical prediction rules and cluster findings to help ensure appropriate assessment and diagnosis** (including specific tissues damage - bone, muscle, ligament, nerve, joint, fascia, viscera). This must be done to ensure the correct management recommendations are given
- **Follow HIP-MNRS with every patient encounter to avoid errors in differential diagnosis - History, Inspection, Palpation, Motion, Neurovascular, Referred pain & Special tests** (to help rule in or out conditions and better direct treatment)
- **Clinicians performing exams must realize that no one sign is of absolute significance in isolation, each individual finding should be evaluated only in context of other evidence based clustered findings, clinical prediction rules & the patient as a whole**
- **Visit prohealthsys.com for more detailed information on all Clinical Prediction Rules (CPRs)**

 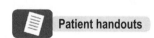

Evidence-Informed Medicine (EIM) is the conscientious use of *current best evidence* in making decisions about the assessment & care of individual patients[1]. All healthcare providers must realize that EIM alone is not enough for effective utilization of best practices & must be integrated with the following fundamental abilities to make **evidence informed** clinical decisions:

- A detailed understanding of pathoanatomy & expertise in performing a history, examination & condition management (including referrals)

- Understanding of the patient's family, personal & social history & the community in which they live

- Developing a relationship with the patient formed by mutual respect & an understanding of their desires, beliefs & values to help create a functional context for therapeutic decision-making

An evidence-informed medicine approach helps to promote life-long learning & liberates clinicians from a reliance on tradition, which further permits the critical evaluation of both conventional & alternative therapies on an even playing field. EIM puts the patient at the center of care by emphasizing outcome markers that matter directly to patients such as pain, activities of daily living, quality of life & even cost (financial & personal).

Why use Evidence-Informed Medicine?

It provides a solid foundation for evaluation of new evidence from the literature, critical appraisal of existing practices, & the effective use of clinical information gathered from patients.

Perhaps the most direct change due to EIM is the potential improvement in clinical efficiency, which results in reduced healthcare costs by improving both assessment & treatment, as well as a net increase in earning potential for its providers as they are better able to competently see more patients in a given time period.

Evidence Informed Practice Model

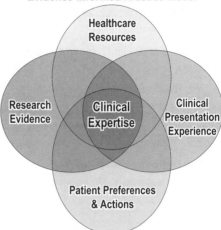

Hierarchy of Evidence

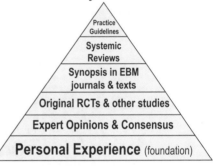

Gathering information?

To be useful, *information must be relevant to everyday practice, valid, easy to obtain & low cost. Knowing where to look for answers to clinical questions is an important skill.* Most clinicians gather information from a wide variety of sources;

1. Straus SE, et al. Evidence Based Medicine How to practice and Teach it. 4th Edition. Churchill Livingstone: Edinburgh, 2011.

Information source	Relevance	Validity	Work	Cost	Usefulness
Evidence-based textbook/website	High	High	Low	Low	High
Systematic review (evidence-based)	High	High	Low	High	High
Asking colleagues	High	Mod	Low	Low	High-mod
Practice guidelines (evidence-based)	Mod	High	Low	Low	High-mod
Practice guidelines (consensus)	Mod	Mod	Low	Low	Mod
Original journal articles	Low	High	Very High	High	Low

prohealthsys trusted EIM resources are relevant to everyday practice, valid, easy to obtain & low cost

1. **Address primary concerns** (not complaints) with **global assessment** (physical, mental, emotion)

2. **Identify, discuss and remove obstacles** to cure

3. **Treat the cause** of the disease, address the symptoms

4. **Activate** and **support the 'Vis'** (body's innate ability to heal)

5. **Re-establish homeostasis by** strengthening weak systems and organs

6. **Use specific local treatments**, for specific local problems

7. **Progress** from **least to most invasive** treatments with a focus on **minimal effective dose**

8. **Re-evaluate regularly** and work with a healthcare team of experts, including the patient

9. **Follow the evidence** (use multiple evidence-based findings and outcome markers for assessment and treatment progression)

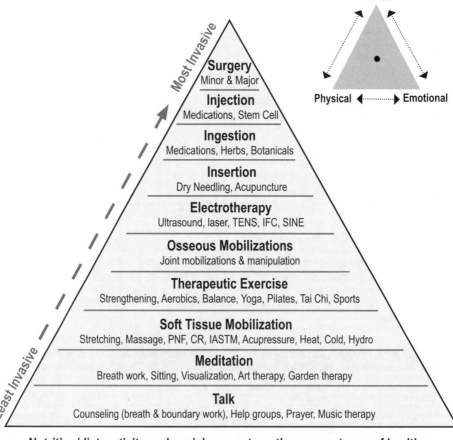

Most Invasive

Surgery
Minor & Major

Injection
Medications, Stem Cell

Ingestion
Medications, Herbs, Botanicals

Insertion
Dry Needling, Acupuncture

Electrotherapy
Ultrasound, laser, TENS, IFC, SINE

Osseous Mobilizations
Joint mobilizations & manipulation

Therapeutic Exercise
Strengthening, Aerobics, Balance, Yoga, Pilates, Tai Chi, Sports

Soft Tissue Mobilization
Stretching, Massage, PNF, CR, IASTM, Acupressure, Heat, Cold, Hydro

Meditation
Breath work, Sitting, Visualization, Art therapy, Garden therapy

Talk
Counseling (breath & boundary work), Help groups, Prayer, Music therapy

Least Invasive

Mental

Physical ◄·············► Emotional

Nutrition/diet, activity and social support are the cornerstones of health.

This is not a complete list & individual practitioners may offer a variety of therapeutic interventions depending upon the local scope of practice & practitioner educational level, experience and preference.

US = ultrasound (therapeutic), TENS = transcutaneous electrical neuromuscular stimulation, MENS = microcurrent, IFC = interferrential current, CR = contract-relax, PNF = proprioceptive neuromuscular facilitation, IASTM = instrument-assisted soft tissue mobilization

Fear Avoidance Model

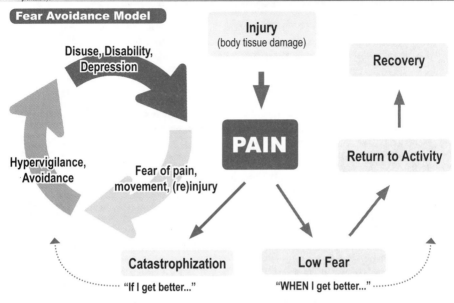

Injury
(body tissue damage)

Recovery

PAIN

Return to Activity

Disuse, Disability, **Depression**

Hypervigilance, Avoidance

Fear of pain, movement, (re)injury

Catastrophization
"If I get better..."

Low Fear
"WHEN I get better..."

Catastrophization, avoidance & fear of future injury creates a cycle for the development of chronic pain
Research & personal experience show that the best chance for recovery is a return to normal ADLs ASAP
It is important to have this conversation with patients for their own understanding & healing

**Below are the basic prognostic indicators that should always be considered
when deciding on the priorities & direction of a selected treatment protocol**

Factors that SLOW healing

- **Depression, poor sleep habits**
- Increased age, malnourishment
- Low blood supply to damage tissue
- Poor aerobic level & lack of exercise
- Smoking, alcoholism
- Prolonged immobilization/rigid fixation
- Corticosteroids/ NSAIDs
- Diabetes, high cholesterol
- Excessive soft tissue gap (complete tear)
- Excessive motion or stress or repeat injury (chronic injury)

Factors that IMPROVE healing

- **Laughter, positive mood & good sleep habits**
- **Love, community & social support**
- Younger age & **adequate nutrition (food is medicine)**
- **Good blood supply** (nutrient/waste exchange)
- Healthy **aerobic fitness**, activity & **movement**
- Vitamin A, D, E, K, Mg, Mn, Zn, Ca, water, antioxidants (free radicle elimination)
- Soft tissue/joint mobilization, massage & IASTM
- Electrotherapeutics (microcurrent, laser, ultrasound)
- Surgical gap closure & acupuncture/needling
- **Confidence in future wellness & health care provider's ability (positive expectations)**

**'The most powerful therapeutic intervention is the patient's belief in future wellness and
confidence in their healthcare team's ability to help them achieve it.'**
- Dr. Nikita Vizniak

'laughter is the best medicine, but a good tonic can help' ☺

Wound & Hemostasis (bleeding)
- If superficial wound consider topical antimicrobials - *Calendula*, polysporin
- Avoid medications, botanicals, vitamins & minerals that affect clotting & prolong bleeding time - consider liquid Band-Aid (developed by US military)

1. Acute Inflammation (after injury, hematoma formation)
- Usually 1-2 days, may last up to 5 days (depends on tissue & severity of injury)
- Cardinal Signs (SHARP) - Swelling, Heat, A loss of function, Redness, & Pain (chemical irritation & nerve pressure) - may not reach peak until 5-7 days post injury
- Consider: Vitamin A, increase protein intake, bromelain
    - Vitamin C enhances neutrophil migration & lymphocyte transformation

Clinical Objectives: relieve pain; prevent further injury, promote circulation; maintain muscle tone & PFROM; reduce effects of ischemia, address psychosocial issues

2. Post Acute Repair/ Proliferation (scar tissue formation)

- May last from 48 hours up to 6+ weeks
- Involves synthesis & deposition of collagen; macrophages/phagocytes remove cell debris, erythrocytes, & fibrin clot
- Collagen is not oriented in direction of tensile strength & quality is inferior to original
- Nutritional support (see specific tissues)
    - Increase vitamin C & *Centella asiatica* - promotes type 1 collagen synthesis
    - Glucosamine - for GAG synthesis & hyaluronic acid production
    - Zinc, Mn, Mg, Ca for protein synthesis, DNA synthesis & cell division

Clinical Objectives: prevent early adhesions; orient repair tissue along line of tension; relieve pain; maintain normal muscle tone; maintain normal ROM, reduce edema, PFROM & exercise to return to normal activity ASAP, address psychosocial issues to prevent transition to chronic condition

3. Remodelling (fibroblastic activity & fibrosis)
- May last from 3 weeks to 12+ months
- Collagen is remodeled to increase the functional capabilities of the tissue in the direction of stresses imposed upon it (PFROM/stretching help re-establish strength)
    - New collagen forms which increases tensile strength of wounds
    - Scar tissue is ~80% as strong as original tissue & residual fibrosis is common

Clinical Objectives: maintain nutrition, proper alignment of repair collagen; increase elasticity of scar tissue; reduce fibrotic adhesions; relieve muscle spasms; increase strength; increase range of motion; normalize joint & muscle activity, address psychosocial issues, prevent chronicity & permanent impairment

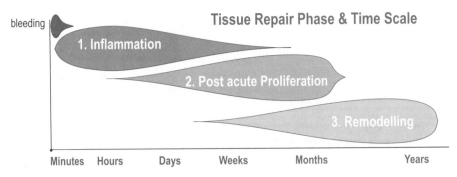

Tissue Repair Phase & Time Scale

bleeding

1. Inflammation

2. Post acute Proliferation

3. Remodelling

Minutes Hours Days Weeks Months Years

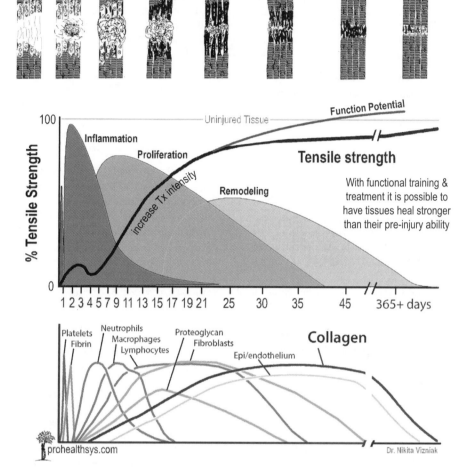

Bleeding	Inflammation	Proliferation	Remodeling
Coagulation to start homeostasis	Immune infiltration Debris reabsorption Pathogen killing	Fibroblast proliferation (collagen synthesis) Scar formation (contracture) Angiogenesis & neurogenesis	Scar maturation ECM remodeling Apoptosis
Weak Bandage tissue	Temporary thin tissue	Stronger tighter tissue	Restored final tissue

ECM = extracellular matrix - which remodels along lines of stress

Realize the graphic representations above are influenced by a number of factors including severity of injury, tissue type, pre-existing cofactors, nutrition, age, genetics, activity level and treatment options given & patient compliance.

Treatment plans must be specifically tailored for each individual patient; the **general rule is to follow the therapeutic order (least to most invasive)** with increasing levels of difficulty as tolerated by the patient. Numerous factors can influence progression through treatment (severity of injury, age, diet, aerobic fitness, general health, mind set to name a few). Phases overlap greatly & may relapse depending on patient healing ability, rest period & activity level. The number one factor in the development of a chronic injury is a return to full activity TOO HARD, TOO SOON!

Acute phase (~1-5 days)
- **Main goals:** relieve pain, prevent muscle atrophy without exacerbation, re-establish pain-free ROM & normalize biomechanical function - inflammation is a normal process in healing
- Pain free motion is key - **the sooner you move the better the outcome will be**

Good pain vs Bad Pain with Motion
Educate the patient that good pain challenges the tissue and you can breath through it ('joyful discomfort'). **Bad pain is sharp or stops your breath.** Pain should be respected but challenged.

PRICE (protection, rest, ice, compression, elevation); use **METH** later on (Move, Exercise, Traction, Heat)
- **Protect** - DO NOT re-injure damaged tissue (possible chronic condition & delayed healing)
- **Rest** - short term cessation of use (1-2 days max)
  - Continued excessive activity may cause further injury, delay healing & increase pain
- **Ice** (1-2 days maximum after injury)
  - Indicated if there is **concern for a compartment syndrome** (excessive swelling)
- **METH** (contraindicated in compartment syndrome)
  - Most patients will respond well to heat and movement as a therapy (see table below)

- When pain has decreased begin pain-free gentle PROM & active-assistive range of motion
- Even with mild grade 1 injury that may feel better after a few days, it is usually recommended that rehabilitation program is completed to avoid re-injury or development of a chronic condition

Post-acute phase (~2 days to 6 wks)
- **Main goals:** normalize ROM & biomechanics, perform symptom-free daily activities, & improve neuromuscular control & muscle strength
- **Warm up prior to activity**
- Key goal is restoring integrity & strength of dynamic & static stabilizers of region
- Isometrics progress to concentric exercises, then to eccentric exercises, & finally to activity/sport-specific exercises to potentially reverse degenerative changes
  - When performing strengthening exercises, it is safer to start out with low tension, followed by a gradual increase in force (avoids flare-ups)
- Tx includes AROM & mild strengthening activities
  - Aquatic therapy is helpful in encouraging activity with decreased weight bearing
  - Pain-free submaximal isometric exercises
  - Ultrasound & TENS may decrease pain
  - IASTM to promote tissue growth & healing
- Ice may decrease pain/inflammation post activity

RICE vs METH Comparison

Parameter	RICE (rest, ice, compress, elevate)	METH (movement, exercise, traction, heat)
Blood flow	Decreased	Increased
Collagen formation	Slowed	Encouraged
Healing time	Lengthened	Shortened
Range of motion	Decreased	Increased

Psychology, nutrition & sleep (recovery) are critical to healing. Short term use of natural analgesics are of benefit (bromelain, trypsin, and papain) - reduce viscosity of the extracellular fluid to increase nutrient exchange and decrease painful swelling of soft-tissue injuries but do not stop the natural inflammatory reactions that lead to healing (note corticosteroids can actually slow healing) - **Food is Medicine** Generally, treatments that increase local blood flow, neural stimulation & provide nutrient building blocks improve healing

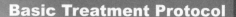

Remodeling phase (3 wks -12+ months)

- **Main goals:** maintain a high level of ability, prevent tissue contracture & reoccurrence of injury, maintain normal biomechanical function
- IASTM is one of the best ways to reduce scar tissue formation & promote healing
- Patient should be able to perform isometric exercises at 100% effort without pain
- Begin unilaterally with weights, using low weight & higher repetitions to monitor form & technique; slowly increase the weight as tolerated as long as pain/inflammation is not increased afterwards
- <u>DO NOT</u> increase weight or intensity too rapidly, may lead to a chronic injury (**10% per week max**)
- Once concentric strengthening is tolerated at a normal level, patient may begin eccentric strengthening (puts most strain on muscle), supervised exercising & slow progression of weight is recommended
- If patient experiences pain or stiffness, then decrease weight or intensity to a tolerable level
- **When affected side is within 10% of unaffected side, consider advancing to a more challenging work or sport specific activities**
- **Warm up & post activity stretching are essential**; address other regions of compensation (posture, restriction, imbalance, job ergonomics)

Functional stage (2 weeks to 6 months)

- Patient should have a normal gait pattern & can begin fast walking
  - When patient can ambulate for 20-30 minutes at fast speed without pain or stiffness, short periods of jogging can be added to fast walking
  - Sprinting may be added, 15 min of jog is OK
- Eventually, more activity/sport-specific exercises
- During later stages, plyometric exercises may be used to increase speed & power during training
  - Low intensity exercises may be used initially (eg, jumping rope), followed by higher-level

Elite athletes & the general population can use similar protocols. The higher the patient's ability prior to injury the faster they can progress through treatment and the faster the recovery.

DO NOT become a victim of pressure from coaches, parents or the patient themselves, maintain your professional demeanor & stick to your recommended treatment for the long-term benefit of the patient (athletes are more than their sport)

Be **SMART** when setting goals - make them
- □ **Specific**
- □ **Measurable**
- □ **Attainable**
- □ **Realistic**
- □ **Timed** (completion date)

exercises as tolerated (eg, side jumping over a low object, jumping on & off a box)
- Higher intensity exercises are associated with a higher rate of injury & should be performed with supervision

Return to play/work (3 weeks - 6 months)

- Isometric strength & flexibility testing should be done prior to return to ensure no subtle deficits are present that lead to recurrent or chronic injury
- Clinician must impress upon patient the importance of mild stretching & warm-up prior to activities to prevent re-injury
- Less than 5 weeks are needed before return to play for patients with
  - Superficial muscle injury or
  - Muscle injury that involves a small cross-section of muscle
  - Mild ligament injury
- In patients whose injury was due to poor biomechanics, address underlying causes
- Patient should be supervised during stretching & exercise in order to assess poor technique & correct it
- Conditioning & proper techniques are important for certain athletes due to improper biomechanics which may result in tissue fatigue & damage
- Flexibility & strengthening exercises continue after returning to activity/sport to prevent recurrence
- **The importance of mental training/toughness & visualization cannot be over stated**

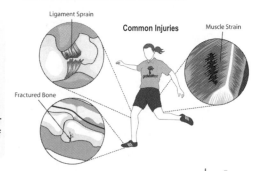
Ligament Sprain | Common Injuries | Muscle Strain | Fractured Bone

The most powerful therapeutic option any clinician has is the ability to give their patient's the confidence to realize they can get better. A positive mind set & the belief of future wellness is the single most important factor in healing for most out-patient health care encounters.

Phase	~Time Course	Clinical Objective
1 Acute*	2-3 days (up to ~7 days)	• **Reduce pain; PRICE or METH as indicated** • Emergency referral if required, prevent excess swelling/ischemia • Basic PFROM & activity as tolerated • Address psychosocial concerns (anxiety, depression)
2 Post Acute	2 days - 6 weeks	• Pain reduction, prevent early scar tissue adhesions • Begin orienting repair tissue along line of tension • Maintain normal muscle tone, ROM & functional capacity • Basic stretch, strength, functional & proprioceptive retraining
3 Chronic*	3 weeks - 12 month or more	• Proper alignment of repair collagen & myofascial tissue • Increase elasticity of scar tissue (increase ROM & strength) • Reduce fibrotic adhesions, relieve muscle spasms • Advanced stretch, strength, functional & proprioceptive retraining • Address psychosocial concerns (somatization, depression, etc.)

*Chronic recurrent episodes have acute flare-ups; PFROM = Pain Free Range of Motion, METH = Movement, Exercise, Traction, Heat

Select Treatment Guidelines

Modality	Phase	~Duration
Cold therapy		
Cryotherapy	1, 2	5-20 min
Ice Massage	1, 2	2-5 min
Heat Superficial		
Infrared heat light	2, 3	10-20 min
Hot packs	2, 3	10-20 min
Paraffin	2, 3	7-10 dips (10 min)
Hydrotherapy	2, 3	10-30 min
Laser	1, 2, 3	sec - minutes
Heat Deep		
Continuous US	2, 3	5-10 min
Pulsed US	2, 3	2-8 min
Diathermy	2, 3	5-30 min
Electrical		
MENS (subsensory)	1, 2, 3	none established
IFC (sensory)	1, 2, 3	10-30 min
TENS	1, 2, 3	10-30 min
Muscle stimulator	2, 3	10-30 min
Motor stimulation	2, 3	2-10 min

Modality	Phase	~Duration
Mechanical		
Bed Rest	1	0-2 days
Massage & IASTM	1, 2, 3	5-45 min
Mobilization/manip.	1, 2, 3	1-20 min
Traction (in-office)	1, 2, 3	1-20 min
Flexion-distraction	1, 2, 3	1-15 min
Ext. compression	1, 2, 3	1-15 min
Exercise (in-office)		
Passive	1, 2, 3	5-30 min
Active (gym, yoga)	1, 2, 3	15-90 min
ADLs (back school)	1, 2, 3	10-30 min
PNF/CR	2, 3	5-10 min
Bracing	1, 2	short duration
Work Hardening	3	2-8 hours
Acupuncture **Dry needling/IMS**	1, 2, 3	by technique
Nutrition/Herbal **Medications/Prolo**	1, 2, 3 1	entire treatment short duration
Surgery	1, 3	emergency or last resort

Specific treatment régimes must be tailored to the individual patient presentation.
In most cases, medication use should be short term (long-term use can result in chemical dependency & mask important signs & symptoms). Surgical intervention should be offered only in emergency injuries or as a last resort when conservative treatments have failed (surgery is not a guaranteed cure).

prohealthsys

Contents

Learning Objectives

After completing this chapter, students will be able to:

1. Discuss the history and education levels of various practitioners performing joint mobilizations

2. Differentiate regional ROM and joint classification based on anatomy and physiology

3. Explain osteokinematic and arthrokinematic movements related to slide, spin and roll

4. Build a mental construct of joint innervation, mechanoreceptors and cartilage loads

5. Discuss joint lever types, mechanical advantage and disadvantage

6. Summarize clinician contact points, grades of mobilization 1-5 with end-play/end feel

7. Differentiate sounds - cavitation, crepitus, snap clunk & discuss the physiology of joint cavitation

8. Recognize indications, contraindications and force vector (line of drive) application and tissue pulls for mobilizations

9. Identify evidence for effectiveness of joint mobilization and common side effects

10. Perform a basic joint mobilization set-up and practice drills

11. Identify and self analyze common foundational errors in technique that can limit performance

Introduction

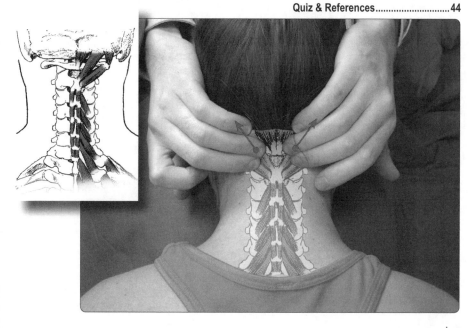

The human body is designed to move.

For 1,000's of years, that's exactly what we did. With urbanization & technological advances (cars, TV, computers, tractors) physical activity levels have been steadily dropping. As technology does more of the heavy lifting, people become increasingly sedentary. The impact our sedentary lifestyles (in office, school or home) may be one of the most unanticipated health threats of our modern time (sitting disease). Graph on the right shows the average ADLs for most urban dwellers in north America (source: BLS & NIH)

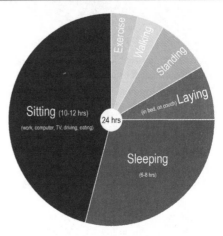

Sitting disease - *metabolic syndrome & ill-effects of an overly sedentary lifestyle*

Did you know? Physical Inactivity is the 4th leading cause of mortality in North America...

- **Prolonged sedentary time is independently associated with negative health outcomes regardless of physical activity!** - even if you engage in the doctor-recommended 150 minutes of moderate to vigorous activity per week, you are still subject to the negative impact of too much sitting.

- **Low intensity, 'non-exercise' activities like standing and walking are much more important than most realize.** Low level activities play a crucial metabolic role and account for more of our daily energy expenditure than moderate-to-high intensity activities if they are done over a long enough period of time

With **simple lifestyle changes** we can make big changes and reduce the risks. Research shows that if we choose to stand up, move more and sit less, we can experience a many benefits to our health, minds and bodies. On the most basic level, **alternate sitting and standing every 30 minutes for optimal health**.

Benefits if we sit less, stand up and move more.

1. **Bone/joint health** - require regular movement to maintain strength – low-level activity helps improve your bone health to reduce the risk of osteoporosis (rates are on the rise)

2. **Muscles** - position changes enlists large muscle groups the neurvous system. Unused, weak muscles leave joints unstable and prone to injury and chronic pain. Sitting makes hips tight, which can affect posture, balance &

ROM. Gluteal muscles weaken from lack of use ('dormant butt syndrome' or 'gluteal amnesia') becoming soft and undefined from lack of use.

3. **Reduced cancer risk** - Studies have linked prolonged sitting to a greater risk for colon, breast and endometrial cancers; regular movement increase antioxidant levels. Those who are physically active have a 40% decrease in cancer mortality.

4. **Brain power** - standing delivers more oxygen and nutrients to the brain through improved blood flow. Physical activity enhances neurogenesis in regions of the brain associated with critical thinking. Research shows in the classroom how that movement strengthens learning and improves memory and retrieval

5. **Improved Mood** - Sitting for 6+ hours during the workday puts you at a higher risk for anxiety and depression. In several studies, 100% of workers and students reported positive effects on mood states and productivity after reducing sitting time.

6. There are many, many more...

- Smith L, Hamer M, Ucci M, et al. Weekday and weekend patterns of objectively measured sitting, standing, and stepping in a sample of office-based workers: the active buildings study. BMC Public Health. 2015;15:9.
- Aggio D, Wallace K, Boreham N, Shankar A, Steptoe A, Hamer M. Objectively Measured Daily Physical Activity and Postural Changes as Related to Positive and Negative Affect Using Ambulatory Monitoring Assessments. Psychosomatic Medicine. 2017;79(7):792-797. doi:10.1097/PSY.0000000000000485.
- The pandemic of physical inactivity: global action for public health. Kohl HW 3rd, Craig CL, Lambert EV, Inoue S, Alkandari JR, Leetongin G, Kahlmeier S, Lancet Physical Activity Series Working Group. Lancet. 2012 Jul 21; 380(9838):294-305.

Disease is stagnation, motion is the potion

Neolithic period (~7000 BCE)
- The origin of physical medicine have existed since the beginning of man (massage, mobilization, body work). It is natural for people to massage & manipulate an aching muscle or limb; most people have twisted their back and shoulders to relieve muscle tightness & stiffness
- Massage was part of the culture of coastal inhabitants of the Mediterranean races, India, up the Pacific coast of China, and of the inhabitants along the coast of Mexico and Peru.
- The practice of massage, mobilization & bone-setting are too closely linked to assume that those who practiced massage did not apply pressure to the joints; especially when the joints seemed to be 'out of place' or less flexible.

3000 BCE Egypt - *Edwin Smith* Surgical Papyrus is the oldest known example of medical literature
- Contains 48 systematically arranged case histories, beginning with injuries of the head and proceeding downward to the thorax and spine, where the document unfortunately breaks off
- Each presentation of a case is divided into title, examination, diagnosis, and treatment.
- *Case Forty-Eight:* Instructions concerning a sprain of a vertebra [in] his spinal column
  - ***Examination:*** *If thou examinest [a man having] a sprain in a vertebra of his spinal column, thou shouldst say to him: "Extend now thy two legs (and) contract them both (again)." When he extends them both he contracts them both immediately because of the pain, the cause is in the vertebra of his spinal column in which he suffers.*
  - ***Diagnosis:*** *Thou shouldst say concerning him: "One having a sprain in a vertebra of his spinal column. An ailment which I will treat."*
  - ***Treatment:*** *Thou shouldst place him prostrate on his back; thou shouldst make for him....*

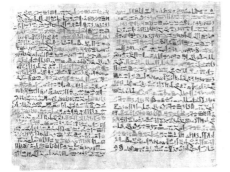

1700 BCE - Chinese document of *Tui Na*, a branch of TCM devoted to manual physical techniques - *Gua sha* - instrument assisted soft tissue mobilization (IASTM)

460-375 BCE: *Hippocrates* - "the father of medicine"
- Recommended simple measures such as rest, sunlight, exercise & diet
- Wrote three works on the bones/joints: ***On Fractures; On the Articulations***; and ***On Setting Joints by Leverage***
- In treatment of spinal curvatures, he recommended that the patient be placed face-down upon a bench "covered with robes, or any thing else which is soft, but does not yield much," with straps placed under the arm pits and across the chest, and around the knees and ankles, so that traction ("extension") could be applied from both ends of the bench while the correction was being made... the physician, or some person who is strong, and not uninstructed, should apply the palm of one hand to the hump, and then, having laid the other hand upon the former, he should make pressure, attending whether this force should be applied directly downward, or toward the head, or toward the hips. This method of applying force is particularly safe; and it is also safe for a person to sit upon the hump while the extension is made, and raising himself up, to let himself fall again upon the patient."
- Quote: "*Get knowledge of the spine, for this is the requisite for many diseases.*"

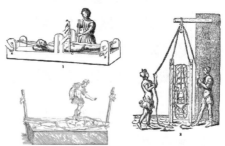

100-200 AD: *Claudius Galen*, gave the first correct anatomical description of the spinal column and its articulations. He divided the spinal column into cervical, thoracic, and lumbar regions, designating the correct number of vertebrae.

continued on next page...

1600 AD: *bonesetting* was a practice commonly used

in the homes of England in the 1600-1700s
- *Friar Moulton* (order of St. Augustine), wrote a book *Compleat Bonesetter*
- *Hernando Cortez* invaded Mexico, Aztec doctors were "concerting the bones," or manipulating the joints, as an essential requirement of the more qualified doctor's duties

1867 AD: *Sir James Paget,* a famous surgeon and authority on bone diseases in the 19th century, was one of the first qualified practitioners who observed that there was actually value in many of the manipulations performed by the bonesetter; in a lecture entitled "Cases That Bonesetters Cure," published in the British Medical Journal, January 5, 1867, he stated:

- *"Few of you are likely to practice without having a bone-setter for a rival; and if he can cure a case which you have failed to cure, his fortune may be made and yours marred....* **Learn to imitate what is good and avoid what is bad in the practice of bone-setters."**

1874 - Osteopathic
- *Andrew Taylor Still,* organized the art of bone-setting into an independent professional practice that attempted to uniformly treat disease
- The original basis of osteopathy was based on the belief that misplaced or maladjusted joints interfered with the nerve and blood supply, causing disease, and that it was only necessary to manipulate the joints to cure this disease
- In the US the first college was opened in 1892; in 1968 osteopathy was amalgamated by the American Medical Association (AMA)

1895 – Chiropractic
- *D.D. Palmer*, announces "discovery" of chiropractic (Greek "cheir-" referring to the hand + "praktos", done = Done by hands)
- First college was opened in 1896

1902 – Naturopathic
- *Benedict Lust,* begins using term "naturopathic"

2015 - Under grad students & Dr. Nikita Vizniak
- Accurately count all joints of the body (456 +/- anatomical variation) - most anatomy instructors and clinicians do not know how many joints are in the body... don't believe it? - ask one ☺ - see page 72

Total Educational Hours

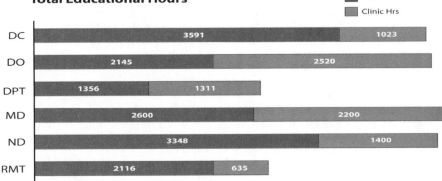

	Academic Hrs	Clinic Hrs
DC	3591	1023
DO	2145	2520
DPT	1356	1311
MD	2600	2200
ND	3348	1400
RMT	2116	635

Comparison of DC, DO, MD, ND, PT, RMT listed in alphabetical order. Data was collected from university academic calendars among the top ranked programs in North America. More details of specific hours of anatomy, physiology, orthopedics, diagnostic imaging, exercise rehab., soft tissue mobilization, manipulation, nutrition & botanicals, pharmacology & surgery hours are available on our website (this data is updated every year on our website - search: *professional comparison*)

Caution: avoid having negative attitudes due to preconceived notions and prejudice based on ignorance and lack of understanding of other practice types and techniques.

If one specific technique was truly 'the best' then all practitioners would be using it.

prohealthsys

Comparison of DC, DO, DPT, MD, ND, PT, RMT. Professions are listed in alphabetical order. Data was collected from academic calendars among the top ranked programs in North America.

DC - Chiropractic – University of Western States, DO – Touro Osteopathic, MD – Yale Medical, DPT - Doctor of Physical Therapy – University of Southern California, ND - Naturopathic - Bastyr University, RMT - Massage Therapist - WCCMT (Canada)

Charts are provided for basic comparison and core educational priorities by each profession. Please recognize that while education plays a role in practice style, the charts below do not take into consideration post graduate education, practice preference, personal experience or clinical specialization. - Other programs may vary, the information is **100% evidence based** from institutional academic calendars and can be easily independently verified...

Anatomy Education Hours

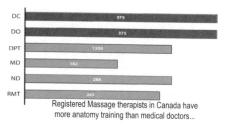

Registered Massage therapists in Canada have more anatomy training than medical doctors...

Physiology Education Hours

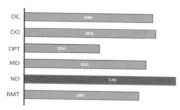

Diagnostic Imaging Hours

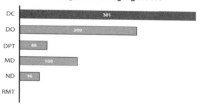

Orthopaedics Eductional Hours

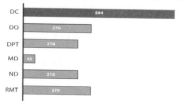

Soft Tissue Mobilization Educational Hours

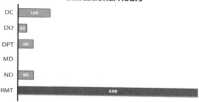

Rehab & Exercise Educational Hours

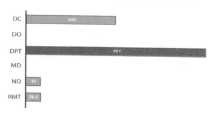

Osseous Mobes Education Hours

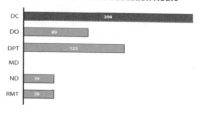

Osseous Manipulation Education Hours

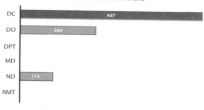

prohealthsys

Introduction

Arthrology - study of joints; **Kinesiology** - study of movement

Joint - a joint is the location at which **two bones make contact** & are constructed to allow movement. Joints are usually named for the two bones that make them up (e.g. sternoclavicular joint). It is important to note that a **joint really should be thought of as an organ unit consisting of many parts including bone, cartilage, fascia, ligaments, muscles, blood vessels and nerves** (with pain and sensory receptors).

Without a joint cavity - Fibrous joints

	Type	Definition (example)
Synarthrosis (immovable)	Suture	Two bones grow together, with only a thin layer of fibrous periosteum between (sutures of the skull)
	Cartilagenous (synchondrosis)	Temporary joint with cartilage that is later converted to bone (between diaphysis & epiphysis of long bones = growth plates)
	Gomphosis	Cone shaped peg fits firmly into a socket (root of the teeth into the mandible & maxilla)
Amphiarthrosis (slightly moveable)	Syndesmosis	Slight motion permitted by meager elasticity of ligaments between two bones (superior & inferior tibiofibular joints)
	Fibrocartilaginous (symphysis)	Bones are separated by a fibrocartilaginous disc, whose fibers join the bones. Motion is only allowed by deformation of the disc (between bodies of vertebrae, symphysis pubis)

With a Joint Cavity - Synovial joints

	Type (technical name)	Definition (examples)
Diarthrosis (moveable)	Gliding (plane joint)	**Uni-axial.** Allows gliding or twisting (intercarpal/intertarsal joints, vertebrae zygapophyseal joint)
	Hinge joint (ginglymus)	**Uni-axial.** a concave surface glides around a convex surface allowing flexion and extension (elbow joint - humeroulnar joint)
	Pivot joint (trochoid)	**Uni-axial.** Rotation around a vertical or long axis is allowed (atlantoaxial joint, proximal radioulnar joint)
	Condyloid (ellipsoid)	**Bi-axial.** Condyle or ovoid articular surface with an elliptical cavity to permit flexion, extension, adduction, abduction and circumduction, but no axial rotation (wrist, 2nd to 5th metacarpophalangeal joints)
	Saddle joint	**Bi-axial.** Both joints have saddle-shaped surfaces (reciprocally concave-convex) fitted into each other. Allows flexion, extension, abduction, adduction, circumduction (CMC joint of thumb)
	Ball & socket (spheroid)	**Poly-axial.** Spheroid ball and sockets allows flexion, extension, abduction, adduction, true circumduction, and rotation on long axis (shoulder and hip joints)

Regular motion and activity without injury are crucial to ensure optimal joint health

When cartilage & joints break down it is termed *degenerative joint disease (DJD)* or *Osteoarthritis*

Crepitus = repeatable clicking/ grinding sensation in a joint

Cavitation = 'popping' of a joint (air bubbles form in joint)

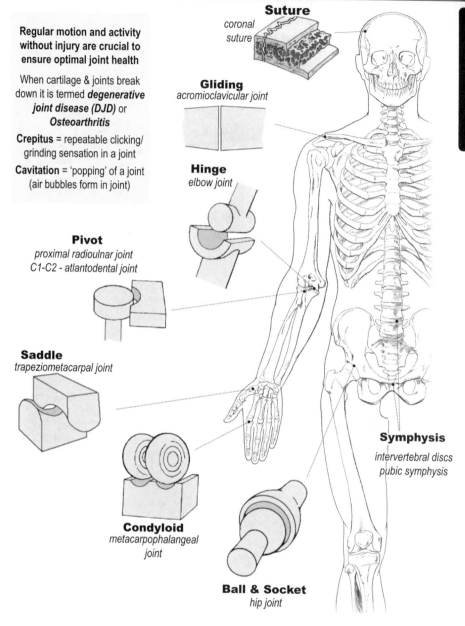

Suture

coronal suture

Gliding
acromioclavicular joint

Hinge
elbow joint

Pivot
proximal radioulnar joint
C1-C2 - atlantodental joint

Saddle
trapeziometacarpal joint

Symphysis
intervertebral discs
pubic symphysis

Condyloid
metacarpophalangeal joint

Ball & Socket
hip joint

Subluxation (world health organization): "A lesion or dysfunction in a joint or motion segment in which alignment, movement integrity and/or physiological function are altered, although contact between joint surfaces remains intact. It is essentially a functional entity, which may influence biomechanical and neural integrity."

Luxation = dislocation - **Subluxation** = partial dislocation

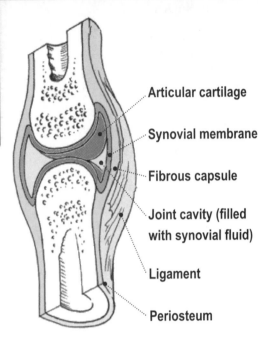

- Articular cartilage
- Synovial membrane
- Fibrous capsule
- Joint cavity (filled with synovial fluid)
- Ligament
- Periosteum

Right shoulder (glenohumeral) joint showing subacromial & subdeltoid bursae (note joint space is larger than normal)

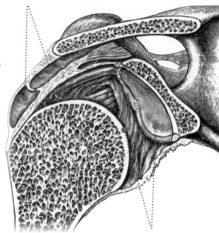

Hyaline Cartilage (lining humerus & scapula in the shoulder joint)

Articular (hyalin) Cartilage
- **Reduce friction**
- **Absorb shock** (muscle and bone absorb more)
- Note: some joints also contain *fibrocartilage* to decrease wear (eg. meniscus of the knee, SC joints, TMJ, TFC of wrist)

Synovial Membrane
- Lining the capsule from inside
- Secretes synovial fluid
- Synovial fluid brings nutrients to articular cartilage

Fibrous (articular) capsule
- Surrounds joint
- Thickenings in fibrous capsule called intrinsic ligaments

Ligaments
- Connect and stabilize bone to bone
- Extrinsic ligaments
  - Extracapsular ligaments outside joint capsule (eg. LCL of the knee)
  - Intracapsular ligaments are within capsule (eg. ACL of the knee)

Synovial fluid
- Thick (egg-like consistency), stringy liquid found in the cavities of synovial joints
- During normal movements, the synovial fluid held within the cartilage is squeezed out mechanically (weeping lubrication) to maintain a layer of fluid on the cartilage surface & circulate nutrients

Synovial fluid 3 main functions
- **Nutrient exchange for cartilage**
- **Reduces friction (lubrication)**
- **Shock absorption during movement**

Bursa
- Small fluid-filled sac located at the point where muscles, tendons or ligaments slide across bone
- Bursae reduce friction between two moving surfaces (between fascia)
- Bursae are filled with synovial fluid
- Bursae are also found between bone & skin (eg. subcutaneous olecranon bursa)
- Bursa is Latin for purse, which is what a bursa resembles when inflamed (bursitis) - please note bursitis is NOT a diagnosis but a symptom

Motion is the action or process of moving or of changing place or position; movement. The **shape and congruency of articulating joint surfaces determine the movements** permitted at various joints.

Body Planes and Motion

Coronal (X) Plane
- Divides body front & back sections
- *Actions:* Abduction, Adduction, Lateral Flexion

Sagittal (Y) Plane
- Divides body left and right
- *Actions:* Flexion, Extension, Plantar Flexion, Dorsiflexion

Transverse (Z) Plane
- Divides body upper and lower
- *Actions:* Rotation, Pronation, Supination, Spinal Rotation

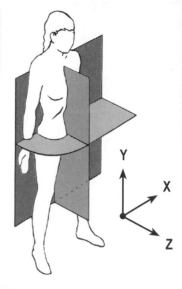

Angular Motion (example elbow flexion)

- Motion that occurs around a fixed or relatively fixed axis

- All points adjacent to the joint will follow the arc of a circle

- The center of the circle or arc is the axis of the joint (axis of rotation)

- **Speed at distal points is faster than that at the proximal points**

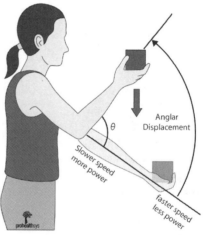

Anglar Displacement

Slower speed more power

faster speed less power

θ

Degrees of Freedom (DOF) - describes the number of planes in which a joint moves

- 1 plane (unixial) – 1 DOF (elbow)
- 2 planes (biaxial) – 2 DOF (radiocarpal joint)
- 3 planes (polyaxial) – 3 DOF (hip/shoulder)

Kinetic Chains

- Several segments connected by several joints
- **Open kinetic chain** - body part moves freely in space (eg. waving hello or picking up a weight)
- **Closed kinetic chain** - body moves around planted limb (eg. sitting in a chair - squat, push-up or chin-up)

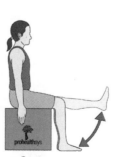

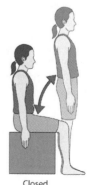

Open Kinematic Chain

Closed Kinematic Chain

Newton's Laws of Motion

Law of Equilibrium - *every object persists to remain in a state of equilibrium unless it is acted upon by other forces*

Law of Mass & Acceleration - *acceleration (A) of an object is proportionate to the force (F) imposed on it and inversely proportionate to it's mass; (M)*

- **F = MA** $(A = F/M)$

- More force is developed with more mass or moving faster

- When a muscle contracts, it shortens and produces the same amount of force at its origin and insertion. Thus, either one or both segments may move.

Law of Action & Reaction - *for every action force there is an equal and opposite reaction force*

Mechanical Advantage

Describes how functional a lever is; based on a simple equation:

$$\text{Mech.Ad.} = \frac{\text{Force Arm (FA)}}{\text{Load Arm (LA)}}$$

The **greater the FA** (effort arm distance from axis to effort force), **the less force required to overcome resistance**.

Muscle attaching farther from the joint will produce the most force, muscles closer to a joint develop less force. Also, longer limbs require stronger muscle effort to generate the same force as short limbs (why smaller weight lifter are 'stronger' as a percent of body weight)

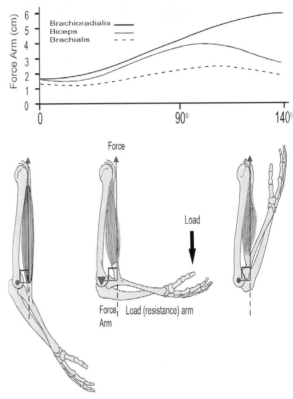

As the elbow flexes, the cross bridging of the muscle reaches maximum strength at the mid range. This is further amplified by longer force arms across the joint giving better mechanical advantage over the mid range

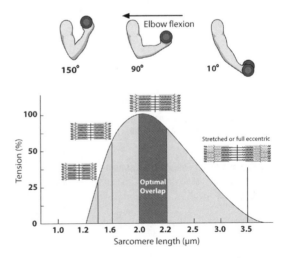

1st Class Lever

Can produce mechanical advantage or disadvantage depending on location of force (effort) & resistance (load)

Eg. neck extension

If force (muscle contraction) is further from fulcrum than load, then a strong load can be moved

Resistance (load): head on vertebral column weight of skull

Fulcrum: is joint between skull & atlas (C0-C1)

Force (effort): posterior neck muscles (trap, splenius)

Average speed & mobility

2nd Class Lever

Mechanical advantage

Load is closer to fulcrum

Sacrifice of speed for force

Eg. Raising up on your toes

Load: body weight

Fulcrum: ball of foot

Force (effort): is contraction of calf muscles which pull heel up off of floor

Slow & strong

proTip: use shorter levers to lower your effort as a clinician (stand closer to the patient)

3rd Class Lever

Mechanical disadvantage

Force (muscle) is closer to fulcrum

Eg. Flexor muscles at elbow

Load: weight in hand

Fulcrum: elbow joint

Force: contraction of biceps/ brachialis muscle

Most common lever in body,

Fast & weak

Small amount of muscle contraction will move a body segment over a great distance

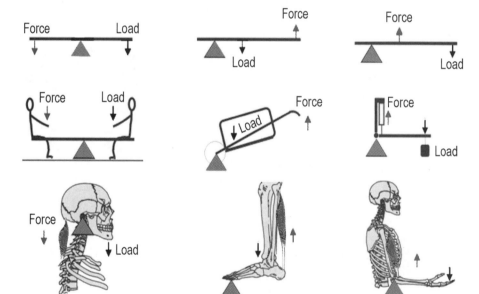

------------ How does this apply in practice? ------------

Standing close to patients requires less force/effort to move and improved biomechanical advantage will help reduce injury risk to clinician and the patient - this is a practice of experienced clinicians - **Clinicians save their bodies by using shorter resistance arms & body weight against long patient limbs for better mechanical advantage**

Introduction

Kinetics - study of forces that produce movement - forces can stop or modify the motion of the body and there is a constant changing force as the body moves (can be developed from gravity, muscles, external resistance, friction). Bones and joints need regular stress to be healthy and strong

- **Compression** - pushes an object to make it shorter and thicker. When you stand, **gravity** is 'pushing down' on your body while the reaction force of the floor is 'pushing up'. When the muscles contract they pull on the tendons at both ends, which stretch a little (tendons are under tensile stress but cause compression forces at the bone and joints)

- **Tension (pull/stretch)** - occurs when two forces pull on an object in opposite directions to stretch it and make it longer and thinner. The primary load a muscle experiences is a tension.

- **Shear** - parallel forces in opposite directions. Occurs every time you take a step and the leg takes all your weight creating a shear stress in the pelvis because the ground is pushing up on one side of body through the supporting leg while gravity is pushing down on the unsupported side.

- **Torsion (twisting)** - rotational forces moving in opposite direction. When you plant your foot and twist to change direction to bones & joints of the lower body are twisted between the ground and upper body motion

- **Bending** - forces in parallel direction around a fulcrum or pivot point (this is commonly how bones are fractured)

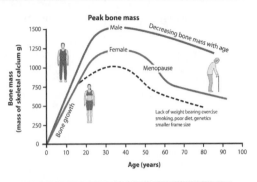

A common malpractice issues for practitioners using joint mobilizations revolves around fractures (usually rib fractures) secondary to osteoporosis. Modify treatment and be aware of the risk factors:

- **Age** (bone density peaks around age 30)
- **Gender** (women < 50 yrs 4x risk than men)
- **Family history**
- **Bone structure & weight** (small thin women)
- **Ethnicity** (Asian & Caucasian)
- **Medications** (steroids, prednisone)
- **Smoking, sedentary lifestyle**

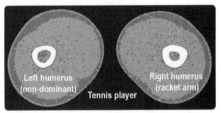

MRI of dominant vs non dominant humerus of tennis player ~20-30% difference between arms. Bones and joints experience huge forces during movement (olympic triple jumper's heels hit the ground, with ~15x their body weight)

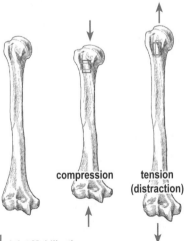

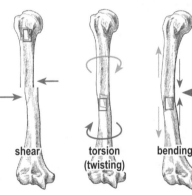

compression | tension (distraction) | shear | torsion (twisting) | bending

Functions of Articular Cartilage

- Distributes joint loads over a wide area, decreasing the stresses sustained by the contacting joint surfaces
- Allows relative movement of the opposing joint surfaces with minimal friction and wear
- Provides a friction-reducing, weight-bearing surface with a friction coefficient of 0.0025 (~10x more slippery than ice on ice)
- Works best at pressure range of 2-11 MPa
  - One leg stance 6.7 MPa
  - Light Jogging 7.7 MPa
  - Stair climbing 10 MPa

Hyaline cartilage is thickest on the distal femur, tibia and patella (2-4 mm). The material properties of articular cartilage depend on its extracellular matrix, but the existence and maintenance of the matrix depends on the chondrocytes.

Proteoglycans (PGs) are negatively charged proteins that give cartilage compressive stiffness (negative charges make the molecules extremely hydrophilic, causing water to be trapped inside the matrix).

The **collagen fibers** are like biological ropes that give tensile strength, but easily fold in compression.

The interaction between proteoglycan and collagen causes there to be a "balance of forces" within the cartilage.

When cartilage is compressed water and solutes are squeezed out until repulsive forces from PGs balance the load applied (**creep = slow deformation**). On removal of load, PGs rehydrate restoring shape of cartilage. The load-unload cycle is important for...
- Exchange of proteins in extracellular matrix
- Nutrient exchange, waste removal
- Intercellular signaling & matrix remodeling

As cartilage is compressed, its permeability decreases. When a joint is loaded, most of the fluid that crosses the articular surface comes from the cartilage closest to the joint surface. Under increasing load, fluid flow will decrease because of the decrease in permeability that accompanies compression.

Moderate running training has positive effects on cartilage (thicker, stiffer and higher PG concentration). Cartilage from older individuals fails at a lower stress than younger people, and **immobilization or strenuous training causes softening and thinning of articular cartilage** (up to 20% thinner with immobilization after 6 wks)

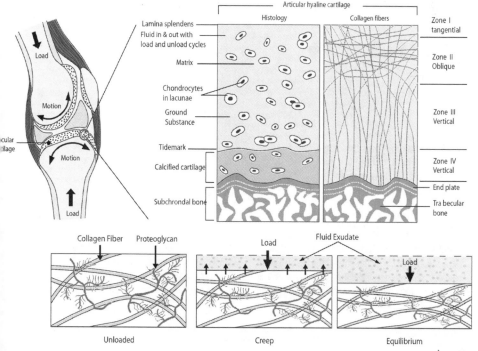

Osteokinematics (*osteo* - bone, *kinematics* - movements): refers to movements of body parts in anatomical planes (eg. flexion, extension, abduction, rotation, elevation) - **motion you see**

Arthrokinematics (*arthro* - joint, *kinematics* - movements): refers to movements that occur inside the joint, or between articular surfaces (eg. **roll, slide & spin** - any combination of these movements can occur in the same joint at the same time) - **motion you feel**

Arthrokinematic movements

Roll: one articular surface rolls on another. (eg. tibia rolls on femur as knee flexes or extends)

Slide (glide): one articular surface slides on another (eg. carpals slide as the wrist flexes)

Spin: bone moves but the mechanical axis remains stationary. (eg. humerus rotates (spins) during lateral rotation of the shoulder)

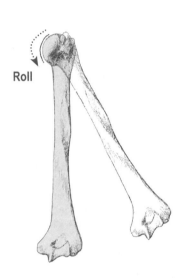

Roll

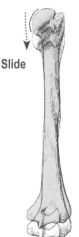

Slide

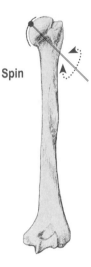

Spin

Pure Spin & Pure Roll

Pure Slide

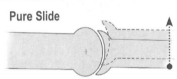

Pure slide motions can cause impingement of both the joint capsule & articular surfaces

Pure Roll

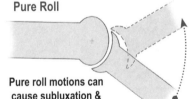

Pure roll motions can cause subluxation & dislocation

For most joints of the body the movements of **roll and slide are coupled motions** and because these motions occur at the same time less articular cartilage is needed to allow motion, and less wear on the articular surfaces occurs.

Understanding of this concept is crucial in clinical treatment decision making for the restoration of limited joint mobility. Roll, slide & spin motion restrictions can often be corrected with passive ROM type procedures (joint play, stretching)

Grade 5 mobilizations (manip) techniques are better suited to restore slide movement restrictions, but can also be used for roll & spin issues.

Arthrokinematic
(motion you feel)

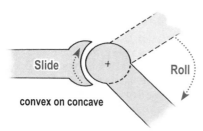

concave on convex

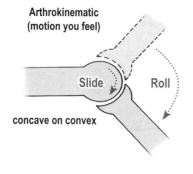

convex on concave

Osteokinematic
(motion you see)

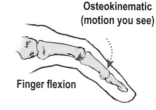

Finger flexion

Shoulder adduction

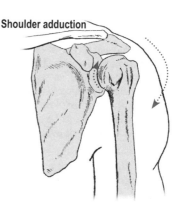

Concave on Convex rule: when a concave surface moves on a convex surface **roll and slide occur in the *same* direction**. Conversely, when a convex surface moves on a concave surface roll and slide occur in the *opposite* direction

Close-packed (tight) position (CPP): synovial joint position where the articular surfaces become maximally congruent; occurs when the joint capsule/ligaments becomes twisted causing the joint surfaces to become maximally approximated or compressed; usually occurs near end range of motion (eg. full extension knee or elbow - when standing joints are in close pack position - little or no muscle contraction is needed)

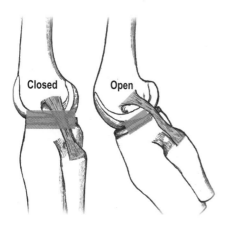

Open-packed (loose) position (OPP): synovial joint position where the joint surfaces become separated and the joint capsule/ligaments are relaxed or untwisted

Capsular pattern of restriction: predictable pattern of restriction that occurs when pathological conditions exist which affects the whole joint capsule. Patterns are named from the most restricted ROM to least restricted (eg. elbow when flexion > extension)

Accessory Motion/Joint Play - cannot be performed voluntarily but needs muscle relaxation and application of passive movement by an examiner (**essential for pain free joint function and used by clinicians for assessment & treatment**)

- **Distraction**
- **Lateral/Medial glide**
- **Anterior-Posterior (AP or PA) glide**
- **Rotation**

In order to control movements, the nervous system must receive continuous sensory information from muscles, fascia & joints. Joints have proprioceptors (Pacini & Ruffini) that provide us with movement & position information. Muscles contain spindles which have sensory nerve receptors & intrafusal muscle fibers. Muscle spindles are sensitive to muscle length (stretch) because they are parallel with the contractile fibers. Specifically, they measure the amount of muscle stretch, rate and speed of lengthening.

Muscle spindle fibers are walled off from the rest of the muscle by a collagen sheath. This sheath has a spindle or "fusiform" shape, hence the name "intrafusal." Intrafusal fibers are still able to contract & are wrapped with sensory receptors; extrafusal muscle fibers are far more numerous & are responsible for generating power.

As a muscle is lengthened, the spindle sends impulses to the CNS, letting the brain know the muscle is being stretched. To prevent overstretching or tearing of the muscle, there is a reflex stimulation that results in contraction of the muscle. This reflex is known as a 'myotatic reflex,' 'stretch reflex,' 'muscle spindle reflex' or 'deep tendon reflex.' - **Deep tendon reflexes assess neuroarticular and muscular function**

Golgi Tendon Organ (GTO)

The **propriocetive sensory** endings of the Golgi tendon organ are interwoven with collagen fibrils in the tendon. If the muscle contracts hard enough to be in danger of tearing, the GTO is triggered to make the muscle 'let go' - acting like a breaker or safety switch. - It is possible override this safety switch and tear muscles, ligaments and tendons.

Because changes in muscle tension will provide different degrees of pull on the tendon, the Golgi tendon organ provides information about muscle tension. Many think that a muscle stretch would also pull on the tendons & stimulate the Golgi tendon organ; however, most of the force of a stretch is absorbed by the muscle itself, so a muscle contraction is a much better stimulus for the Golgi tendon organ.

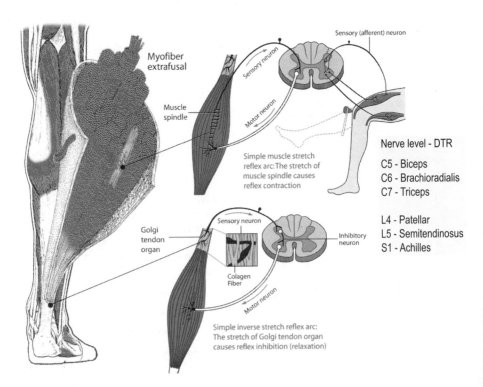

Myofiber extrafusal

Muscle spindle

Sensory (afferent) neuron

Sensory neuron

Motor neuron

Simple muscle stretch reflex arc: The stretch of muscle spindle causes reflex contraction

Golgi tendon organ

Sensory neuron

Colagen Fiber

Inhibitory neuron

Motor neuron

Simple inverse stretch reflex arc: The stretch of Golgi tendon organ causes reflex inhibition (relaxation)

Nerve level - DTR

C5 - Biceps
C6 - Brachioradialis
C7 - Triceps

L4 - Patellar
L5 - Semitendinosus
S1 - Achilles

There are four types of mechanoreceptors embedded in ligaments/joint organs. All are myelinated and rapidly transmit sensory information regarding joint positions to the central nervous system

Type	Function	Location	Behavior
1	Posture	**Superficial Capsule**	Slow adapting, postural kinetic awareness (tonic stabilizers) Stimulated by oscillations at end ROM (joint play or manip)
2	Dynamic	**Deep Capsule**	Fast adapting, movement sensation (phasic movers) Silent at rest, fire as movement begins - proprioceptive Stimulated by all motion, esp. oscillations at mid ROM
3	Inhibitive	**Ligaments**	Defensive receptor (provides reflex inhibition of muscle) - function similar to golgi tendon organ (in structure & function) Proprioceptive
4	Pain	**Most Tissues**	Nociceptive protection (help produce muscle guarding) Stimulated by excessive pressure or tissue damage

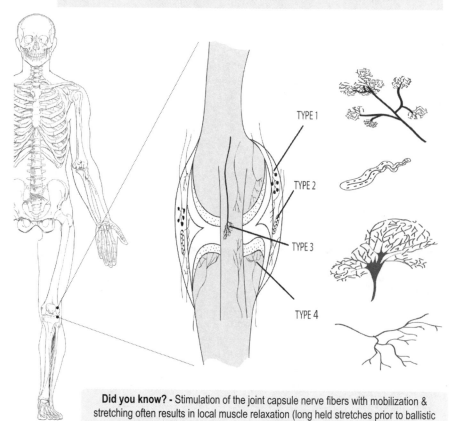

Did you know? - Stimulation of the joint capsule nerve fibers with mobilization & stretching often results in local muscle relaxation (long held stretches prior to ballistic activity may increase injury risk but stretching after activity improves flexibility)

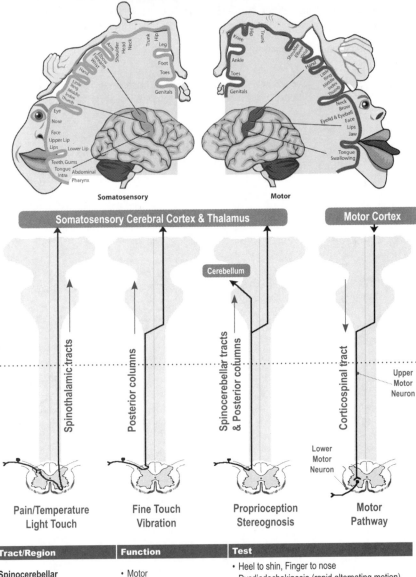

Tract/Region	Function	Test
Spinocerebellar (cerebellum)	• Motor • Gait	• Heel to shin, Finger to nose • Dysdiadochokinesia (rapid alternating motion) • Heel to toe (tandem walk)
Posterior Columns	• Sensory • 2 point discrimination • Vibration • Position sense	• Romberg, stand with eyes closed • 2 pins, paper clip • 128 Hz tuning fork • Passive toe movement
Corticospinal	• Motor	• Muscle strength tests • Deep tendon reflexes
Lateral Spinothalamic Anterior Spinothalamic	• Sensory, light touch • Pain & Temperature	• Sharp/dull • Hot & cold test tubes
Vestibulospinal	• Sensory • Auditory	• Balance reflexes • Weber, Rinne, hearing

The gate control theory of pain suggests that **non-painful input closes "gates" to painful input,** which prevents pain sensation from traveling to the central nervous system. **Stimulation by non-noxious input is able to suppress pain** (example we can often rub away the pain or mommy can kiss it better ☺)

Psychological factors play a role in pain perception and physical pain is not a direct result of activation of pain receptor neurons, but rather its perception is modulated by interaction between different neurons. **Neurons that fire together, wire together (this is how we groove pain and movement patterns)**

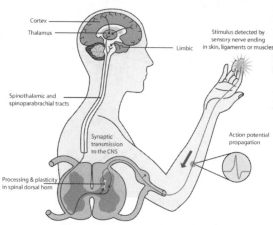

Cortex
Thalamus
Limbic
Spinothalamic and spinoparabrachial tracts
Synaptic transmission to the CNS
Processing & plasticity in spinal dorsal horn
Stimulus detected by sensory nerve ending in skin, ligaments or muscles
Action potential propagation

Most activities and treatments close pain gates

The three systems located in the spinal cord act to influence perception of pain...
1. Substantia gelatinosa in the dorsal horn
2. Dorsal column fibers
3. Central transmission cells

The **dorsal horn** is responsible for passing on information which can be interpreted as pain. This area is referred to as the '**gate**' as it prevents the brain from receiving too much information too quickly.

Neurons involved in pain conduction include
1. Primary: from 'nociceptors' to dorsal horn
2. Secondary: from dorsal horn to the thalamus
3. Tertiary: from thalamus to cortex & awareness

Nerve fibers Involved include
- Smaller, unmyelinated A (delta) and C nerve fibers sense pain such as sharp burning and aching feelings
- Larger, myelinated A (beta) skin nerves which carry senses of touch, heat, cold and pressure
- A (beta) nerves are faster, and also have priority which effectively blocks out the pain messages to the brain and closes the gate

The **dorsal horn** is responsible for passing on information which can be interpreted as pain. This area is referred to as the 'gate' as it prevents the brain from receiving too much information too quickly.

Stimulation of the large-diameter fibers (A-Fibers) inhibits the transmission of pain ('closing the gate').

Stimulation of the small-diameter fibers (C-Fibers) stimulates the transmission of pain (opening the gate). When the gate is closed, signals from small diameter pain fibers do not excite the dorsal horn transmission neurons. When the gate is open pain signals excite dorsal horn transmission cells. Gating mechanism is influenced by nerve impulses that descend from the brain (you can over-ride the pain)

Factors that influence opening/closing of the gate
- Amount of activity in the pain fibers
- Amount of activity in other peripheral fibers
- Messages that descend from the brain

Pain gates are CLOSED by...

- **Physical pain** - analgesic remedies
- **Emotional pain** - being in a 'good' mood
- **Mental factors** - not concentrating on the injury (work, family, TV, friends, books, sex)
- **Relaxation, contentment, meditation**
- **Activity** - movement, exercise, yoga & sleep
- **Counter-stimulation** - heat, cold, massage, acupuncture, stretching, IASTM, mobilizations

Pain gates are OPENED by...

- **Physical factors** - bodily injury or prior injury
- **Emotional factors** - anxiety & depression
- Mental factors - focusing on the pain and catastrophization (fear)
- **Lack of activity** from disuse or avoidance through ADLs or treatment

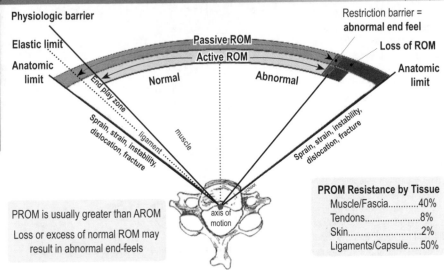

Physiologic barrier

Restriction barrier = abnormal end feel

Elastic limit

Passive ROM

Loss of ROM

Active ROM

Anatomic limit

Anatomic limit

End Play Zone

Normal

Abnormal

Sprain, strain, instability, dislocation, fracture

ligament

muscle

Sprain, strain, instability, dislocation, fracture

axis of motion

PROM is usually greater than AROM

Loss or excess of normal ROM may result in abnormal end-feels

PROM Resistance by Tissue
Muscle/Fascia............40%
Tendons....................8%
Skin...........................2%
Ligaments/Capsule.....50%

The purpose of ROM assessment is to establish a patient baseline of ability (outcome marker) & locate dysfunction generators (muscles activated, tissue stretched, motion restrictions)

Active ROM - patient moves body part themselves

- Amount of joint motion attained by a subject during unassisted voluntary joint motion

- Provides examiner with information regarding subjects willingness to move, coordination, muscle strength and overall ROM - **important to get a baseline of function and reassess throughout treatment**

- Can be pain limited due to contraction or stretching of 'contractile' tissues (muscles & fascia) or due to stretching or compression on 'non-contractile' tissues (i.e. ligaments, joint capsules, bursa, etc.)

- If a subject can easily & painlessly complete an active ROM, then further testing/investigation is probably not needed

- If active ROM is limited, painful, or awkward, then additional testing needs to be pursued to clarify the problem

Passive ROM - movement done by examiner without patient assistance - involuntary joint motion

- Normally passive is greater than active

- Testing provides examiner with information about articular surfaces, joint capsules, ligaments, fascia, nerve tension and muscles

Resisted ROM (RROM) - patient performs active ROM against examiner's resistance

- Helps determine strength of muscle contraction through full range

Physiologic barrier - end of active joint movement (as far as the patient can move)

Elastic limit - elastic resistance that is felt at end of passive range of movement; further motion towards anatomic barrier may be induced passively by examiner

Anatomic limit - limit of anatomical integrity; limit of motion imposed by anatomic structures; forcing movement beyond this barrier will produce tissue damage (sprain/strain/fracture)

Joint play - discrete, short-range movements of a joint independent of action of voluntary muscles, determined by springing each joint in neutral position

End Play (end feel) or Passive Over Pressure (POP) - discrete, short-range movements of a joint independent of action of voluntary muscles *at the end or start of PROM*

Paraphysiological space - area of increased movement beyond elastic barrier available after cavitation (popping sound) within joint's elastic range (grade 5 mob. osseous manipulation zone)

prohealthsys

Realize that any mobilization (grade 1-4) can be made into a manipulation (grade 5) with the addition of a high velocity thrust (HVT) & vice versa with the lack of a HVT

Grades of Oscillations

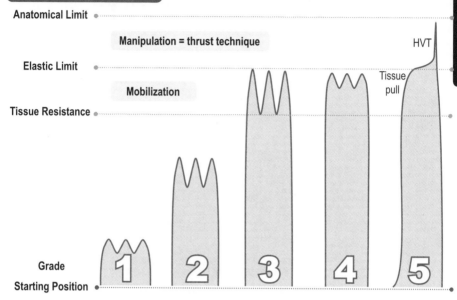

Grade	Definition	Use
1	Slow, small amplitude, rhythmic oscillations at the beginning of available joint play range (between initiation of movement and tissue resistance)	Used to establish initial contact, assessment, pain management & warm up
2	Slow, larger amplitude, rhythmic oscillations within the midrange of available joint play range (between initiation of movement and tissue resistance)	
3	Slow, large amplitude, rhythmic oscillations from the middle to the end of available joint play range (within tissue resistance & backing out again - below elastic limit)	Used to mobilize and stretch the joint capsule, fascia & ligaments and muscle tendon units
4	Slow, small amplitude, rhythmic oscillations to end of available joint play range (within tissue resistance, but below elastic limit)	
5	High velocity thrust (HVT) **at the elastic limit** (end of PROM) osseous manipulation or an adjustment; which **may** be accompanied by a 'popping' sound or *cavitation (tribonucleation)* as gas is released from synovial fluid in the joint cavity	Used to reduce joint motion restrictions or malpositions, induce local muscle relaxation, stretch shortened ligaments & joint capsules

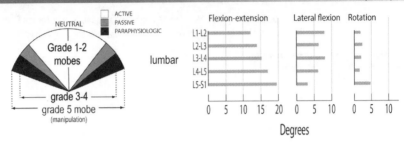

SIDE POSTURE: Neutral Position

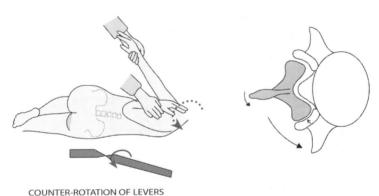

SIDE POSTURE: Limit of Active R.O.M

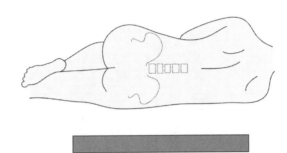

COUNTER-ROTATION OF LEVERS

Know the limit, play within it

Grade 1-4 mobilizations are generally in a safe ROM and have a very low chance of injury

Grade 5 mobilizations (manip) require the application of a High Velocity Low Amplitude (HVLA) thrust at the anatomical limit of a joint – movement beyond the anatomical limit results in strains/sprains and tissue tearing – even the best most controlled thrust stretch the joint capsules causing micro trauma as part of the healing process. Repetitive attempts at adjusting the same segment often results in smaller tears becoming larger and affecting surrounding tissues (muscles, nerves, blood vessels) in severe cases this may result in instability, 'whiplash' type injury or even neurovascular rupture

Clinicians should **limit high velocity thrusts (HVT) to 2-3 attempts maximum**
to limit the potential for negative side effects of over treatment

Patient position for adjustment (when possible have patient move under their own power)

- Prone
- Side lying
- Supine
- Seated
- Knee-chest
- Standing

Head piece up or pillow to save neck- spine should be relatively neutral

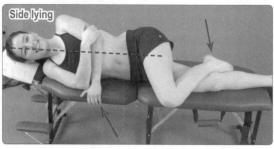

Side lying

Clinician's position

- Head of table, side of table; seated, squatting, fencer, kick-start
- Straddle flexed knee
- Thigh-to-thigh
- Double thigh to shin
- Split leg (need patient permission)
- Square stance (perpendicular to table)

proTip: foot position and clinicians center of gravity are FOUNDATIONAL for any mobilization setup - if the foundation is off the whole house will be off

Don't fight the table, make sure your stance leg foot is not under the table. If you are not balanced and relaxed the patient will autonomically sense this and respond with muscle guarding (~70% of communication is non-verbal)

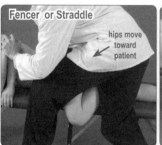

Fencer or Straddle

hips move toward patient

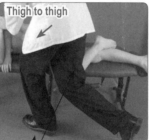

Thigh to thigh

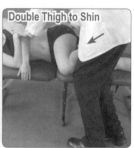

Double Thigh to Shin

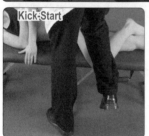

Kick-Start

Most of the weight is in the front foot (80%) and **rear thigh** (~20%)

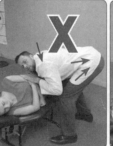

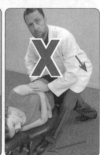

Do NOT over flex at hips - keep your head up

Foot should never be under the table (makes it impossible to get weight over patient)

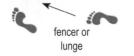

cervical

square

Foot direction dictates the direction of the joint mobilization forces you will generate

fencer or lunge

proTip: sternum over contact with chest up when ever possible; work in your 'Strike Zone'

1. Pisiform
2. Hypothenar
3. 5th metacarpal (knife edge)
4. Digital (finger pads/tips)
5. Distal interphalangeal*
6. Proximal interphalangeal*
7. Metacarpal phalangeal*
8. Web
9. Thumb (pad)
10. Thenar
11. Palmar
12. Base (calcaneal or heel)

*5, 6, 7 = **Index contact** - the specific point used will depend on clinician size vs. patient size

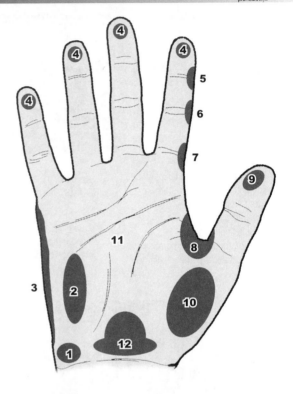

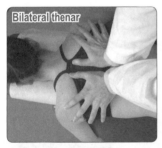

Bilateral thenar

Selected Patient Contacts

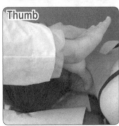

Thumb

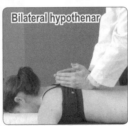

Bilateral hypothenar

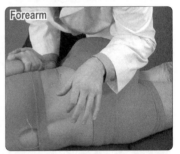

Forearm

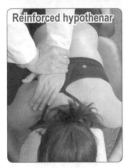

Reinforced hypothenar

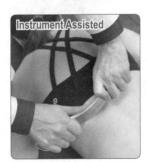

Instrument Assisted

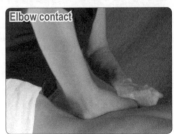

Elbow contact

Contact points (anatomical location)

- Clinician's anatomical structure in contact with patient (thenar, hypothenar, index, forearm) - will vary depending on patient and clinician size

- Hand placement & specific location of patient anatomy used as lever
  - eg. hypothenar PSIS P-A glide

- *Stabilization (s)* points used by "non mobilization" or "indifferent" hand

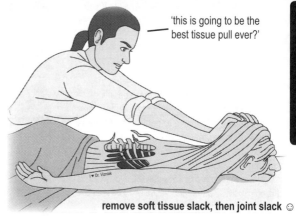

'this is going to be the best tissue pull ever?'

remove soft tissue slack, then joint slack ☺

Tissue pull: reduction of soft tissue slack by applying traction in the direction of the mobilization - **remove soft tissue slack, then joint slack**

- The set-up of **pre-tension is the most important factor in influencing the success of a given treatment**. The better the set-up the less force is required to successfully complete the maneuver, which ultimately results in increased effectiveness & patient satisfaction

Hypothenar Spinous Push

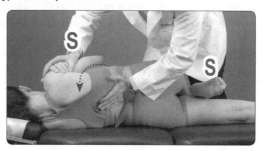

Vectors ('line of drive') - generally vectors or force follow the direction of the forearm

- Push, pull or combo (push-pull)
- I-S = inferior to superior;
- S-I = superior to inferior
- M-L = medial to lateral;
- L-M = lateral to medial
- P-A = posterior to anterior;
- A-P = anterior to posterior
- R = rotational; T = torque

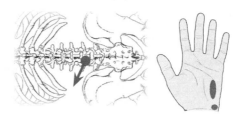

tissue pull I-S, P-A, develop tension by pre-setting the patient in an extended position; at tension mobilize by dropping body & pushing through lumbar contact hand

proTip: in order to be successful the clinician must land mark contacts accurately and have balance in their own body. As a basic rule try to get **sternum over contact** and be relaxed in your treatment position - it can take many hours of practice to accomplish this

S = stabilization (indifferent hand)
● = contact
⟶ = examiner force
····▶ = patient motion

There are many sounds made by joints, these vary depending on the actual cause, size and shape of the joint, region of the body and prior joint activity. Sounds or 'cracks' do not occur without motion and vary significantly with body regions and patients.

Joint popping may be due to cavitation (gas bubble formation); secondary to the production of a momentary partial vacuum produced by joint separation (see MRI image to right[2]). The contents of this vacuum are thought to contain water vapor, nitrogen, oxygen, and carbon dioxide under reduced pressure. According to Unsworth et al, synovial fluid in a joint is composed of 15% gas, 80% of which is carbon dioxide. Roston and Wheeler-Haines show joint spacing, stating that the pressure in a joint right before release is –3.5 atm (normal is 1 atm - atmospheric pressure).

Following cavitation there is an overall gain of 5-10% in PROM and often a reflex muscle relaxation.

Unsworth and Sandoz both report that patients who were unable to relax muscles near the affected joint could not produce an effective result that led to articular release with audible sound. They also found that "the joint did not open or, at best, opened erratically as the subject attempted to relax at intervals."

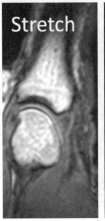
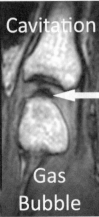

'Any patient readily learns, even without being told, that the crack is a necessary condition for a successful manipulation, and conversely that a failure to obtain the crack means an unsuccessful manipulation. And we must frankly admit that for the manipulator, the crack represents also an important, although not an absolute nor a sufficient, criterion for a good manipulation." - Sandoz

Cavitation is NOT required for success!

Below is a table to summarize many of the more common articular sounds:

Term	Definition
Cavitation (articular release)	**Audible "pop" or "crack" sound** (often accompanies mobilization). The volume of the joint increases suddenly as the joint ligaments are stretched and surfaces are gapped or spread apart, breaking the surface tension of synovial fluid results in a negative pressure that leads to a rapid gas bubble formation and popping sound. (**cannot be repeated for ~20 min** - can have a refractory period of several hours)
Clunk	**Repeatable 'thud' or 'shift'** as the joint clunks around due to ligament laxity, instability or muscle firing pattern issues - often observable through AROM with an awkward shift or palpable clunk - Example: GH instability or TMJ disc subluxation
Crepitus	**Repeatable clicking and grinding sensation** - patient may state 'it feel like sand paper in my joint' - reproducible with grinding and scour type orthopedic tests - indicates cartilage surface roughening (patellar grind test on a knee with OA would be a prime example where damaged surfaces are rubbed together)
Rupture (tendon, ligament or fascia)	**Non-repeatable, tearing or 'pop'** sound often accompanied by sudden onset of pain (achilles or biceps tendon rupture would be a prime example - patient may actually hear the snapping, popping or tearing at time of rupture)
Snap or Strum	**Repeatable 'snap'** secondary to tight ligaments, tendons or fascial structure rolling over a bone or solid prominence. Snapping hip is a prime example (internal snapping hip iliopsoas snaps over lesser trochanter or external snapping hip)

Force Displacement Curve for Joint Separation & Cavitation

(Adapted from Brodeur R. The audible release associated with joint manipulation. JMPT 18:155, 1995)
(Protapapas, M. Joint Cracking and Popping Understanding Noises with Articular Release. JAOA 102:5, 2002)

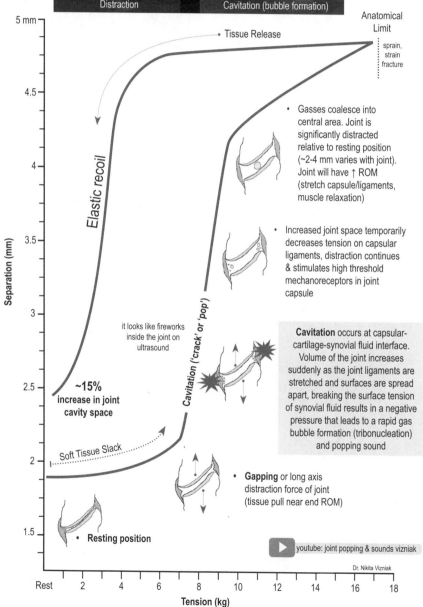

Distraction

Cavitation (bubble formation)

As the joint separates, rapid bubble formation distends the joint capsule stimulating local receptors

Anatomical Limit

sprain, strain fracture

Tissue Release

Elastic recoil

- Gasses coalesce into central area. Joint is significantly distracted relative to resting position (~2-4 mm varies with joint). Joint will have ↑ ROM (stretch capsule/ligaments, muscle relaxation)

- Increased joint space temporarily decreases tension on capsular ligaments, distraction continues & stimulates high threshold mechanoreceptors in joint capsule

it looks like fireworks inside the joint on ultrasound

Cavitation ('crack' or 'pop')

Cavitation occurs at capsular-cartilage-synovial fluid interface. Volume of the joint increases suddenly as the joint ligaments are stretched and surfaces are spread apart, breaking the surface tension of synovial fluid results in a negative pressure that leads to a rapid gas bubble formation (tribonucleation) and popping sound

~15% increase in joint cavity space

Soft Tissue Slack

- **Gapping** or long axis distraction force of joint (tissue pull near end ROM)

- **Resting position**

youtube: joint popping & sounds vizniak

Dr. Nikita Vizniak

Separation (mm) — 5 mm, 4.5, 4, 3.5, 3, 2.5, 2, 1.5

Tension (kg) — Rest, 2, 4, 6, 8, 10, 12, 14, 16, 18

Subluxation (world health organization): "A lesion or dysfunction in a joint or motion segment in which alignment, movement integrity and/or physiological function are altered, although contact between joint surfaces remains intact. It is essentially a functional entity, which may influence biomechanical and neural integrity."

Potential Subluxation Causes (joint restriction)

- Muscle hypertonicity or guarding
- Joint malposition (biomechanical)
- Lack of joint surface congruency (common in SI with rough surfaces & high force loads)
- Meniscoid (joint capsule) entrapment
- Nerve compression
- Antalgic posture (pain avoidance)
- Nucleus pulposus malposition
- Effusion/swelling
- Connective tissue/adhesions (scar tissue) or contracture

Osseous Manipulation/Adjustment - a therapeutic procedure utilizing controlled force, leverage, direction (vector), amplitude (depth) and velocity; most commonly applied as a high velocity low amplitude (HVLA) thrust to the spine utilizing parts of the vertebra and contiguous structures as levers to correct articular malposition (subluxation), restrictions of movement or other dysfunctions of the body

Indications - potential reasons for choosing a given technique or method are dependent largely on the examiner's physical assessment skill & anatomical understanding - realize that multiple findings may exist simultaneously (e.g. C2-C3 rotation restriction with associated suboccipital muscle tightness and muscle tension headache).

Indications for mobilization = P-STAR

P - Pain (local or referred)

S - Symptom reproduction

T - Tissue change (tone, temp)

A - Asymmetry, alignment

R - ROM (joint play, end feel)

Muscles **create** movement

Ligaments **resist** movement

Joints **guide** movement

Bones **support** movement

Nerves **control** movement

Do NOT get addicted to crack - while joint popping is common, it is not required for successful treatment ☺

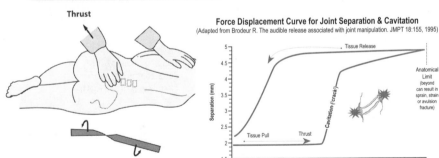

Thrust

Left rotation restriction mobilization L3-L4

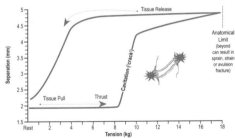

Force Displacement Curve for Joint Separation & Cavitation
(Adapted from Brodeur R. The audible release associated with joint manipulation. JMPT 18:155, 1995)

Mobilization Indications Detailed

- **Symptom reproduction** with a biomechanical mechanism or challenge
- **Pain** that changes with palpation or activity
  - Headaches, low back pain, local regional pain
- Local palpatory **muscle tightness** or spasm
- **Abnormal end feel** or joint play
- Specific segmental **lack of motion** (e.g. C2-C3 right rotation restriction)
- **Asymmetry**/bone out of place (e.g. Left ilium extension malposition - PI ilium)
- Patient states '**it feels stuck**' or 'it just needs to move or be popped'

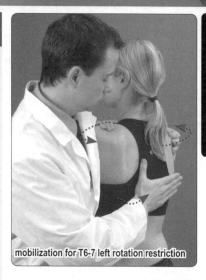

mobilization for T6-7 left rotation restriction

Mobilizations name = clinician contact + patient body part + direction of force

(eg. hypothenar transverse push or P-A glide)

5 rules for great spinal mobes

1. Foot & body position
2. Relaxed hands & body
3. Sternum over contact (work in your 'strike zone')
4. Correct contacts & tissue pull
5. Use breathing technique (force on exhale)

Therapeutic Considerations

Clinician considerations

- What are the goals of treatment?
- Confidence with particular technique based on skill level & prior experience
- Specialized knowledge
- Physical fitness, i.e. stamina, strength & flexibility
- Time available for treatment
- Physical limitations: extent of reach based on height, length of arms, girth, table height & width - size of hands & digits in relation to size of structure being treated

Patient considerations

- Overall health & age of the patient
- Presenting condition/pathology & stage of dysfunction(acute, subacute, chronic)

- Side effects of medication
- Personal goals of treatment & preference
- Prior treatment experience
- Pain threshold/ level of sensitivity
- Tissue: type, tone, texture, location (depth), shape, contour, resistance, size, pliability, reaction

Other considerations

- Physiological effects of technique - is it physically taxing on the patient or clinician?
- Length of treatment
- Type of instruments (drop table, activator, stone) or lubricant used (oil, lotion, powder, etc.)
- Gowning or clothed treatment
- Patient mobility or psychosocial issues

Introduction

Contraindications (CIs) exist when certain therapeutic techniques are *NOT* indicated for a given condition or situation. When a modality is contraindicated, a clinician must **modify or omit** the type of treatment given. The value of the treatment must be considered with respect to the risk to the patient & to the clinician. Contraindication guidelines exist to protect the patient from further exacerbation of a condition & to help avoid legal action being taken against the clinician.

If in doubt, it is best to omit the involved area or the treatment altogether until you are sure you can safely treat the patient. As clinicians gain experience & knowledge in clinical sciences & pathologies, some of the **absolute** contraindications **may** become **relative** contraindications.

Types of contraindications

- **Systemic (general) contraindication** exists when situation or condition affects the whole body

- **Local contraindication** is when the situation or condition affects a particular region or body part

- **Absolute contraindication:** pathological conditions or symptoms that cannot be treated under any circumstances. Absolute contraindications can be *systemic or local.*

- **Relative contraindication:** pathological conditions or symptoms that are generally less acute or in a state of remission may be **treated with caution or modification** of technique(s). Relative contraindications can be *systemic or local.*

Contraindications to Mobilization

CI	Absolute	Relative	** 5Ds And 3Ns
Misc.	☐ Lack of consent (PAR-Q) ☐ Intoxication or drug influence ☐ Recent surgery or malingering	☐ Recent spinal trauma ☐ Prior 'bad experience' with mobes. ☐ Undiagnosed lump, hypochondriasis	For c-spine mobilizations
Arthro	☐ Severe instability (spondylolis., Down's, Marfan's) ☐ Severe sprain strain ☐ Dislocation or fusion ☐ Disc prolapse	☐ Mild sprain/strain ☐ Acute inflam. arthritis (RA, AS) ☐ Ankylosing spondylitis ☐ Atlantcoccipital OA	**Dizziness**, vertigo, giddiness **D-LOC** (decreased level of conscious) **Diplopia** (or other visual disturbances)
Osteo	☐ Congenital malformation (posterior arch aplasia) ☐ Bone destruction (cancer, avascular necrosis, **osteomyelitis, fracture, severe osteoporosis**) ☐ Spinal fusion surgery	☐ Hypermobility (mild instability)* ☐ Benign bone tumor ☐ Demineralization (osteopenia, long-term steroid use) ☐ Mild spondylolisthesis ☐ Scheurmann's disease	**Dysarthria** **Dysphagia** **Ataxia**
Neuro	☐ Cauda equina syndrome ☐ Recent TIAs or Stroke	☐ Neurologic deficits (radiculopathy) ☐ Lack of peripheral sensation (diabetes, herniation)	**Nausea & vomiting** **Numbness**
Vascular	☐ Stroke or CVA ☐ Aneurysm ☐ VBI signs & symptoms**	☐ Calcified abdominal aneurysm ☐ Anti-coagulant therapy ☐ Atherosclerosis	**Nystagmus**

CVA = cerebral vascular accident - *Generally joint mobilizations should not be applied in the direction of hypermobility of a joint. However, it is possible for the same joint to be hyper mobile in one direction, but hypermobile in other directions, meaning that hypermobile joints can be mobilized into directions of hypomoblility with specific dedicated treatments

Potential 'Positive' Effects

1. **Pain reduction** & prevention - muscle, bone, ligament, fascia, cartilage, nerve & viscera

2. **Faster healing time** & prevention of chronic conditions - shortened time to recover from acute back pain

3. **Stretches contracted** (hypertonic) muscles to induce relaxation (decrease muscle spasm)

4. **Reduce soft tissue adhesions** (stretch of contracture and scar tissue)

5. **Increase in passive range of motion** (PROM)

6. **Restore myofascial**/joint optimal position & biomechanical function to prevent future injury & promote optimal performance

7. Increase local blood flow to promote healing (basic fact: **more blood flow = better healing!**)

8. **Relieve nerve compression,** irritated sympathetic chain ganglia & potentially modify organ function (correct abnormal somatovisceral reflexes, improve digestion, bowel function)

9. **Stress reduction,** decreased anxiety & improved mental attitude (therapeutic touch)

10. **Placebo effect** (very powerful) - the belief of future wellness is key to healing - do NOT underestimate the importance of placebo

11. **Neuromodulation** via pain processing networks, motor & sensory cortex, muscle/joint proprioception (golgi tendon etc.)

12. **Reduced medication** intake for pain

13. **Improved immune function**

14. **Muscle relaxation** (joint capsule nerve ending stimulation reflex - similar to GTO)

SIDE POSTURE: limit of Passive R.O.M

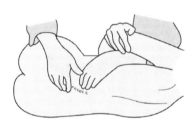 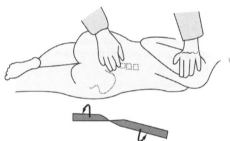

MOBILIZATION

Potential 'Negative' Side Effects

1. **Local soreness** or mild bruising (should disappear after ~24-48 hrs)

2. **Mild strain/sprain** of local tissue, hypermobility of ligaments (instability) - do NOT over mobilize as it may induce injury (2-3 attempts maximum to reduce risk of injury)

3. **Headache**, tiredness, lowered blood pressure (fainting - usually from orthostatic hypertension)

4. **Vertebral & rib fractures** (osteoporotic patients)

5. **Stroke** (patients are no more likely to suffer a stroke following osseous manipulation than they would after visiting their family doctor's office *(SPINE, Feb, 2008)* extremely low risk - estimated that only 1 of every 1-100 million mobilizations have serious side effects - controversial evidence, some suggest there may be under reporting of issues)

----------- **Evaluating Risk of Various Treatment Options** -----------

When evaluating the risk associated with given therapeutic procedures or different practitioners, an extremely valid method to use is evaluation of malpractice insurance premiums - insurance companies are in the business of assessing risk and charging premiums based upon these risks (more risk = higher premium). Joint mobilization providers pay the lowest premiums in the healthcare arena!

Introduction

Spinal mobilization is among several options for pain reduction secondary to back pain (exercise, massage). Spinal mobilization appears to work as well as conventional treatments such as applying heat, using a firm mattress, and taking pain-relieving medications - often with **fewer side effects**. In one study for neck pain in 2012, spinal mobilization had a **statistically significant advantage** over medication after 8, 12, 26, and 52 weeks, and home exercise therapy was superior to medication at 26 weeks.[1]

Gay, et. Al. (2014) have shown **brain activity between regions of the PPN (pain processing network) before and after MT** (manual therapy); specific and treatment-dependent changes measured using resting-state fMRI (functional MRI).[2]

Daligadu et. al (2013) has shown that neck mobilization may provide a modulatory effect on the motor cortex by reducing the amount of intracortical inhibition and influence cerebellar modulation of motor output.[3]

A theoretical framework exists from which hypotheses about the neurophysiological effects of spinal mobilization can be developed. An experimental body of evidence exists indicating that **spinal mobilization impacts primary afferent neurons** from paraspinal tissues, the motor control system and pain processing.[4]

The data suggest that the high-velocity, short-duration load delivered during the impulse of a spinal mobilization can stimulate muscle spindles and Golgi tendon organs more than the preload. The physiologically relevant portion of the mobilization may relate to its ability to **increase as well as decrease the discharge of muscle proprioceptors.** In addition, the preload, even in the absence of the impulse, can change the discharge of paraspinal muscle spindles. Loading of the vertebral column during a sham mobilization may affect the discharge of paraspinal proprioceptors.[5]

There appears to be a complex relationship between deep paraspinal muscle inhibition during dynamic activity and non-voluntary guarding behavior during static activity. The relationship between these findings and palpable tissue change is speculative, but increased activity, decreased activity, or both may be responsible for paraspinal tissues detected as abnormal with palpation.[6]

There is also evidence to support pain reduction and potential improved immune function following spinal mobilization; plasma levels of substance P (SP) before and after treatment in sham treated subjects did not differing significantly; however, **elevated plasma SP was observed in subjects after spinal mobilization.**[7, 8]

The Evidence, suggests spinal mobilization stimulate mechanoreceptors and nociceptors of the joints resulting in afferent discharges and subsequently causing CNS modulation - potentially leading to pain reduction, muscle relaxation and nociceptor desensitization.

1. Bronfort G. Evans R. et al. Spinal Mobilization, Medication, or Home Exercise With Advice for Acute and Subacute Neck Pain: A Randomized Trial. Annals of Internal Medicine. Jan 3, 2012.
2. Gay, CW., Robinson, ME., George, SZ., Perlstein, WM., & Bishop, MD. Immediate changes after manual therapy in resting-state functional connectivity as measured by functional magnetic resonance imaging in participants with induced low back pain. JMPT 2014, 37(9), 614-627.
3. Daligadu, J., Haavik, H., Yielder, P. C., Baarbe, J., & Murphy, B. . Alterations in cortical and cerebellar motor processing in subclinical neck pain patients following spinal mobilization. JMPT 2013, 36(8), 527-537.
4. Pickar, JG. Neurophysiological effects of spinal mobilization. Spine J. 2002 Sep-Oct;2(5):357-71 - NCBI accessed feb 4 2018
5. Pickar JG, Wheeler JD. Response of muscle proprioceptors to spinal manipulative-like loads in the anesthetized cat. J Manipulative Physiol Ther. 2001 Jan;24(1):2-11.
6. Fryer G, Morris T, Gibbons P. Paraspinal muscles and intervertebral dysfunction: part two. J Manipulative Physiol Ther. 2004 Jun;27(5):348-57.
7. Nansel D, Szlazak M. Enhanced phagocytic cell respiratory burst induced by spinal mobilization potential role of substance P (and) enhanced neutrophil respiratory burst as a biological marker for mobilization forces duration of the effect and association with substance P and tumor necrosis factor. J Manipulative Physiol Ther. 1993 Sep;16(7):505-7.
8. Amir Qaseem, MD, PhD, MHA; Timothy J. Wilt, MD, MPH; Robert M. McLean, MD; Mary Ann Forciea, MD. Noninvasive Treatments for Acute, Subacute, and Chronic Low Back Pain: A Clinical Practice Guideline From the American College of Physicians. Annals of Internal Med. 14 Feb 2017.

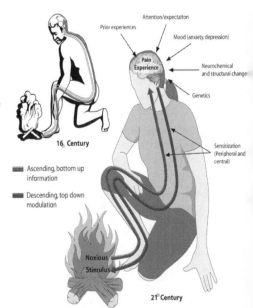

Attention/expectaiton
Prior experiences
Mood (anxiety, depression)
Pain Experience
Neurochemical and structural change
Genetics
16. Century
Sensitization (Peripheral and central)

■ Ascending, bottom up information

■ Descending, top down modulation

Noxious Stimulus

21ˢᵗ Century

Evidence of Manipulation Effectiveness

Spinal manipulation received the highest level of evidence awarded any intervention in the 1994 Agency for Health Care Policy and Research (AHCPR) Guidelines, recommending the use of manipulation in the care of acute low back pain.[1]

In 2010, the Agency for Healthcare Research and Quality (AHRQ) noted that spinal manipulation offers additional options to conventional treatments, which often have limited benefit in managing back and neck pain (**spinal manipulation was more effective than placebo and as effective as medication in reducing low-back pain intensity**).[8]

Other research listed below has shown that...

- spinal manipulation (2012) is as effective as other interventions for reducing pain and improving function.[21]

- there is strong evidence that spinal manipulation is effective for chronic low-back pain and moderate evidence of its effectiveness for acute low-back pain.[3]

- strong evidence that spinal manipulation/mobilization works as well as a combination of medical care and exercise instruction

- moderate evidence that spinal manipulation combined with strengthening exercises works as well as prescription nonsteroidal anti-inflammatory drugs combined with exercises

- limited-to-moderate evidence that spinal manipulation works better than physical therapy and home exercise.

- level 1b evidence spinal mobilization as one of the most preferable approaches for the management of LBP due to disk degeneration[26]

- "NCCIH examined long-term effects in more than 600 people with low-back pain, results suggested that care involving spinal manipulation was at least as effective as conventional medical care for up to 18 months. However, less than 20 percent of participants in this study were pain free at 18 months, regardless of the type of treatment used." [25]

1. Bigos S et al. Acute Low Back Problems in Adults. Edited by the Agency for Health Care Policy and Research, Public Health Service. , Rockville, Md: US Department of Health and Human Services, 1994.
2. Bialosky JE, Bishop MD, Robinson ME, et al. Spinal manipulative therapy has an immediate effect on thermal pain sensitivity in people with low back pain: a randomized controlled trial. Physical Therapy. 2009;89(12):1292–1303.
3. Bronfort G, Haas M, Evans R, et al. Effectiveness of manual therapies: the UK evidence report. Chiropractic & Osteopathy. 2010;18(3):1–33.
4. Bronfort G, Haas M, Evans R, et al. Evidence-informed management of chronic low back pain with spinal manipulation and mobilization. Spine Journal. 2008;8(1):213–225.
5. Bronfort G, Haas M, Evans RL, et al. Efficacy of spinal manipulation and mobilization for low back pain and neck pain: a systematic review and best evidence synthesis. Spine Journal. 2004;4(3):335–356.
6. Cagnie B, Vinck E, Beernaert A, et al. How common are side effects of spinal manipulation and can these side effects be predicted? Manual Therapy. 2004;9(3):151–156.
7. Cherkin DC, Sherman KJ, Deyo RA, et al. A review of the evidence for the effectiveness, safety, and cost of acupuncture, massage therapy, and spinal manipulation for back pain. Annals of Internal Medicine. 2003;138(11):898–906.
8. Chou R, Huffman LH. Nonpharmacologic therapies for acute and chronic low-back pain: a review of the evidence for an American Pain Society/American College of Physicians clinical practice guideline. Annals of Internal Medicine. 2007;147(7):492–504.
9. Chou R, Qaseem A, Snow V, et al. Diagnosis and treatment of low-back pain: a joint clinical practice guideline from the American College of Physicians and the American Pain Society. Annals of Internal Medicine. 2007;147(7):478–491.
10. Dagenais S, Tricco AC, Haldeman S. Synthesis of recommendations for the assessment and management of low back pain from recent clinical practice guidelines. Spine Journal. 2010;10(6):514–529.
11. Elder WG Jr, King M, Dassow P, et al. Managing lower back pain: you may be doing too much. Journal of Family Practice. 2009;58(4):180–186.
12. Ferreira ML, Ferreira PH, Latimer J, et al. Comparison of general exercise, motor control exercise and spinal manipulative therapy for chronic low back pain: a randomized trial. Pain. 2007;131(1-2):31–37.
13. Ferreira ML, Ferreira PH, Latimer J, et al. Efficacy of spinal manipulative therapy for low back pain of less than 3 months' duration. Journal of Manipulative and Physiological Therapeutics. 2003;26(9):593–601.
14. Furlan A, Yazdi F, Tsertsvadze A, et al. Complementary and Alternative Therapies for Back Pain II. Evidence Report/Technology Assessment, no. 194. Rockville, MD: Agency for Healthcare Research and Quality; 2010. AHRQ publication no. 10(11)–E007.

15. Hoiriis KT, Pfleger B, McDuffie FC, et al. A randomized clinical trial comparing chiropractic adjustments to muscle relaxants for subacute low back pain. Journal of Manipulative and Physiological Therapeutics. 2004;27(6):388–398.
16. Hurwitz EL, Morgenstern H, Kominski GF, et al. A randomized trial of chiropractic and medical care for patients with low back pain: eighteen-month follow-up outcomes from the UCLA low back pain study. Spine. 2006;31(6):611–621.
17. Kinkade S. Evaluation and treatment of acute low back pain. American Family Physician. 2007;75(8):1181–1188.
18. Machado LAC, Kamper SJ, Herbert RD, et al. Analgesic effects of treatments for non-specific low back pain: a meta-analysis of placebo-controlled randomized trials. Rheumatology. 2009;48(5):520–527.
19. National Institute of Arthritis and Musculoskeletal and Skin Disorders. Handout on Health: Back Pain. National Institute of Arthritis and Musculoskeletal and Skin Disorders Web site. Accessed at www.niams.nih.gov/health_info/back_pain/default.asp on April 11, 2012.
20. Oliphant D. Safety of spinal manipulation in the treatment of lumbar disk herniations: a systematic review and risk assessment. Journal of Manipulative and Physiological Therapeutics. 2004;27(3):197–210.
21. Rubinstein SM, van Middelkoop M, Assendelft WJ, et al. Spinal manipulative therapy for chronic low-back pain. Cochrane Database of Systematic Reviews. 2011;(2):CD008112. Accessed at www.thecochranelibrary.com on April 11, 2012.
22. Santaguida PL, Gross A, Busse J, et al. Complementary and Alternative Medicine in Back Pain Utilization Report. Evidence Report/Technology Assessment no. 177. Rockville, MD: Agency for Healthcare Research and Quality; 2009. AHRQ publication no. 09–E006.
23. van Tulder MW, Koes B, Malmivaara A. Outcome of non-invasive treatment modalities on back pain: an evidence-based review. European Spine Journal. 2006;15(suppl 1):S64–S81.
24. National Center for Complimentary and Integrative Health (NCCIH). Spinal manipulation for Low Back Pain. (2013) https://nccih.nih.gov/health/pain/spinemanipulation.htm - Accessed January 2, 2018
25. Beattie, et al. The Immediate Reduction in Low Back Pain Intensity Following Lumbar Joint Mobilization and Prone Press-ups is Associated With Increased Diffusion of Water in the L5-S1 Intervertebral Disc. Journal of Orthopaedic & Sports Physical Therapy, 2010 Volume:40 Issue:5 Pages:256–264 DOI: 10.2519/jospt.2010.3284 - - Accessed January 2, 2018
26. Krekoukias, et al. Spinal mobilization vs conventional physiotherapy in the management of chronic low back pain due to spinal disk degeneration: a randomized controlled trial. JMPT 2016 - http://dx.doi.org/10.1080/10669817.2016.1184435

----------- Explaining to Patients How Mobilization Works -----------

Most of us have changed body position and felt a knee or elbow that doesn't feel like it is moving quite right, this is a joint dysfunction (biomechanical fault); the natural response is to kick out the knee or flick the arm, a little click or shift is often heard and the problem is corrected - that was a self induced manipulation. Given the complexity of anatomy, freedom of movement and specific biomechanical issues, many joint dysfunctions are difficult if not impossible to correct by ourselves. This is where professionals trained in specific mobilization techniques are able to offer a world of benefit to their patients

prohealthsys

Wash your hands & clean your table between every patient, visit to the bathroom or meal. If you have a transmittable condition, such as a cold or flu, use a mask to prevent or reduce the chances of spreading this disease to your patients, classmates & instructors. If you have an open wound on your hand, protect yourself from infection & spreading possible infection to your patient. If your condition is a concern do NOT offer treatment.

Performing manual medicine procedures can & will cause you to perspire heavily on occasion. In order to avoid dripping perspiration on your patient keep a towel or tissue nearby to wipe your brow. Strong breath odours resulting from some herbs & seasonings (e.g. garlic/onions) or cigarettes can also be offensive to others in close proximity. Either brush your teeth (and tongue) or use natural fresheners.

As manual medicine providers we also need to pay particular attention to the cleanliness & smoothness of our hands & finger nails. Finger nails must be cleaned, trimmed & filed regularly; calluses need to be filed. Longer nails can carry bacteria & along with exposed nails, unfiled nails or rough skin, can be uncomfortable for the patient when performing many techniques.

Before treatment: always wash hands, remove all jewellery & watch, ensure that your equipment is clean & ready, have a towel available to wipe your hands or wipe off perspiration.

After treatment: wipe tables down, especially the face piece (replace face paper), with viral/bacterial cidal solution; wash hands, first with warm or hot water, then finish with cool or cold, leave room neat & tidy!

Washing Hands

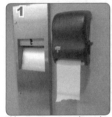

Have paper towel ready from dispenser

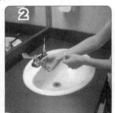

Remove jewelry & watches

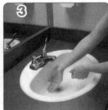

Turn on water, make sure it is warm

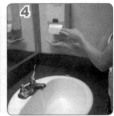

Wet hands & forearms & apply soap

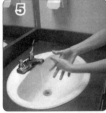

Rub hands together for **~20 seconds**; pay particular attention to your finger nails & webs of fingers

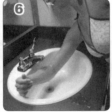

Rinse forearms down to fingertips

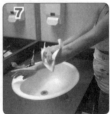

Dry forearms down to finger tips

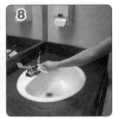

Use paper towel to turn off water & dry sink area

Coughing & Sneezing

Cough into your elbow to help keep you hands bug free!!!

Do NOT cough into your hand (arrows denote location of bacteria - see image)

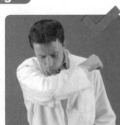

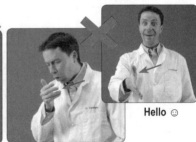

Hello ☺

Biomechanics

- **Manual medicine providers must always be aware of their biomechanics**, especially foot positioning, back, shoulders & hands
- Pick the correct table height (use an adjustable table in practice):
  - **Soft tissue mobilization** - STM (massage) - with arms relaxed at sides, fingers or knuckles should brush table top when standing
  - **Osseous mobilization** - base of patella should be level with table top when standing
  - With clinical skill, practitioners evolve specific styles based on body and table size that works best for them (always adapt & explore)
- Anticipate direction of movement & try not to finish in an awkward position
- Adjust posture & biomechanics according to the technique being applied & the body part being treated, to facilitate smooth transition from one body part to another, & from one technique to another
- **Keep shoulders relaxed**; there is a tendency to raise shoulders when trying too hard or when the therapist is fatigued Elbows are flexed & wrists are relaxed for all light & moderate techniques; be careful not to "whip" or "snap" wrists during rapid applications (hyper-radial/ulnar deviation)
- **Stand with feet shoulder width apart**, point feet in the **direction of movement**; knees & hips should be slightly flexed, back is straight, shoulders relaxed
- **Lift heavy patient limbs close to your body**; use other parts of your body (legs, arms), bolsters, pillows or the table to support whenever possible
- **Use your body weight whenever possible**

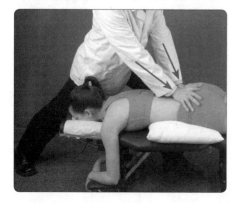

Passive Patient Movement

- Physical contact creates non-verbal communication that can be sensed by the patient; if you are nervous or not confident, patients can sense it & often react in a counter productive manner to the treatment
- Clinicians must overcome the patient's tendency to muscle guard or 'help' move the limb
- Support joints with your hands, another part of your body (arms, leg, etc.) or the table; this mainly refers to proximal joints (elbows or knees), which can become very unstable if not supported
- Distal joints (ankle & wrists) may not have to be supported at all times through the whole range, provided that there is no threat of compromising the joint

Other patient movement tips:

- **Practice:** continually refine your skills to be more proficient ("perfect practice makes perfect")
- Teach the patient to have **awareness of when they are guarding** or moving limbs for you; the majority of the time patients do not even realize they're guarding or moving the limb for you
- **Firm & solid hand contacts:** this will communicate to the patient that the limb is secure & that you have complete, safe control
- **Voice commands** to the patient are helpful. "Let me take the weight of your arm," "Let your body sink into the table," "Take a nice deep breath," "Close your eyes," "Rest your tongue on the roof of your mouth," - these phrases are all helpful cues that do **not** include the word **RELAX,** which may make it even more difficult for the patient to prevent guarding
- **Smooth movements:** jerky movement will stimulate joint proprioceptors which results in the muscles contracting around that joint to stabilize it; this prevents smooth mobilization of the limb
- **Always support injured joints:** prevents further injury & helps relax the patient
- Slight **axial distraction (traction)** of the limb may help inhibit stimulation of joint receptors, which will in turn prevent muscle guarding

Consider using grounding intention exercises or visualization. Feel your feet on the floor, balance in your body, deep breath in & out, be present with the anatomy, your patient and visualize goal.

prohealthsys

Confidence in ability & skill

- Patients sense & respond both positively & negatively to the perceived ability of their clinician
- Physical medicine skills are best learned through repetition and experience
- Mental visualization of the structures contacted and forces to be applied is an excellent technique to use

Relaxation/mood

- Both the patient & clinician must be relaxed to ensure maximum therapeutic effect from their treatment
- Patients easily sense irritation, anger and other emotions & respond to them accordingly

Appropriate set-up

- **Mobilization is 90% setup & 10% movement.** Proper set-up result in more gentle actions, better "patient experience" & higher success rate
- Select the appropriate & specific contacts for the selected adjustment
- Whenever possible clinician's center of gravity should be as close to contact points as possible
- Minor adjustments in position or tension should be made prior to adjusting
- Do NOT 'let-up' or 'back-off' of pre-adjustive tension just before thrusting - consider practicing with an analogue bathroom scale to show even momentum & force generated with weight transfer (see image)

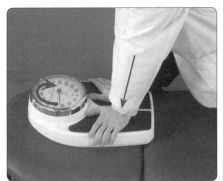

Analog scale used to measure force loading rate and generation - excellent method to give instant visual feedback

Thrust technique

- The thrust must be delivered as a **high velocity low amplitude** movement (learning skills usually start with the more painful and uncomfortable *low* velocity *high* amplitude thrust - otherwise known as 'Hammer Hands' ☺)
- Stability of the upper extremity must be maintained, but avoid biomechanically compromising positions (many physical medicine providers have suffered career ending injuries when applying their therapy)
- When appropriate, there should be a weight transfer to help generate momentum during a body drop for thoracic, lumbar and sacroiliac procedures

Breathing technique

- Breathing technique should always be used (whether vocalized or not)
- **Method 1:** Instruct patient, "Take a deep breath in & let it all the way out." As the patient nears the completion of exhalation, then mobilize

  Common errors
  1. Mobilize/thrust too early – uncomfortable, patient may guard
  2. Thrust too late – patient gets 'winded'. It is a poor practice management strategy to consistently knock the wind out of patients ☺

- **Method 2:** timing mobilize with patient's natural breathing cycle, rather than instructing breathing. Involves more skill & may surprise patient (mobilization is still with patient expiration)

Anti-Guarding Technique

- Many patients have a tendency to guard or fail to relax musculature enough to ensure effective adjusting. Distraction techniques should be used with caution as they may surprise or alarm patients

  - **Method 1:** Instruct patient to relax, "make your head heavy in my hand" or "try to let go of the tension in your muscles"
  - **Method 2:** Distraction – ask patient to wiggle toes, make a fist & unclench it, tickle patient ear/neck. During or slightly after distraction, then mobilize

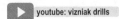 youtube: vizniak drills

Synergistic Myofascial Assisted Release Techniques (SMART ☺)

- This technique is useful for patients who find it consistently difficult to relax their muscles completely (works particularly well in the cervical spine, can be used in any region).

- **The key:** rather than attempting to fight through muscle resistance – *have the muscles work for you* (not against you), to assist in the action you are attempting to accomplish. Instruct patient to move (only slightly) their spine in the direction you (the clinician) are attempting to restore normal motion.

Eg: C4/5 left rotation, right lat. flexion restriction

1. Set-up & contact as usual normally

2. Demonstrate with your hands on the patient's head/ neck the direction you want them to move (turn patients head to left & laterally flex to right). Tell them '*you are going to help you with this motion by using their muscles*' (patients love to help their clinicians & it allows them to become more involved in their treatment)

3. Ask patient to demonstrate once or twice "Give me a demonstration of what I have just shown you" – positive affirmation is always good, "Not quite, do it again, good… that's perfect"

4. **IMPORTANT:** patient assisted motion should be < 5% of total motion at that joint – just enough to facilitate muscles at that motion segment in the direction you are attempting to move

5. Have patient perform the motion, with *your mobilization occurring immediately after the patient starts moving*

6. Result – same mobilization performed with much less resistance by the patient & much less force by the clinician

Note: by using this technique, clinicians can improve patient comfort, reduce the chance of injury & become known (through patient referrals) as a much more gentle & competent practitioner (try it out & make up your own mind... it works for me ☺)

Positive affirmation

- Whenever possible & appropriate tell patients they are "…doing well" or "That worked wonderfully" or "You are doing better than I had expected from our initial consultation."

- People like to know that things are above average, going well & that you are able to help get them there (the healing power of a positive attitude can not be overstated!).

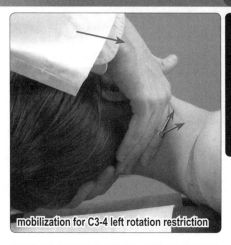
mobilization for C3-4 left rotation restriction

Soft or gentle end-range

Use a **soft or gentle end range to reduce guarding and discomfort**. When learning do NOT hold people in a hard end-ROM - relax your hands and body for more effective application.

Other considerations

- Realize that the cavitation is often used as a required sign of a successful mobilization, but is NOT an absolute necessity

- Repeating the mobilizations shortly after the joint has cavitated without an audible release, aiming to "get an audible," may cause damage as the joint is potentially stretched beyond its anatomical range of movement (sprain or strain)

- The audible joint cavitation may have a powerful placebo effect on both the patient and practitioner. It is not unreasonable to assume that the patient expects to hear a cracking sound during the treatment and interprets this sound as a sign of a successful adjustment (correction can be made without cavitation - explain this to the patient)

--- Informed Consent ---

PAR-Q (procedures, alternatives, risks, Qs)

Legally required for every new procedure

- **Procedures** (what you would like to do)
- **Alternatives** (other treatment options)
- **Risks** (common & catastrophic/serious)
- **QUESTIONS** (from patient)

Obtain <u>written</u> informed consent to proceed with treatment - verbiage/terms used in communication must be at a level the patient understands

Basic Body Drop

Clinicians must realize that the strength and power of their adjustment is developed from the body drop and is ultimately generated from the lower body and weight transfer **(force = mass x acceleration)**

Adjusting Hand at Center of Gravity: whenever possible the clinician's adjusting hand contact should be located below the base of the clinicians sternum to ensure good body biomechanics and optimum thrust delivery (the further away from this position the clinician gets the less force can be delivered and greater the chance for injury)

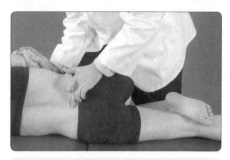

F = ma (force = mass x acceleration) - either get heavier or faster to develope force
Force vectors have to be correct

Load, Load, Drop - slowly load by transferring body weight to forward leg (loading is performed to eliminate force robbing soft tissue slack); the thrust is then delivered by allowing forward knee to flex & dropping body (the drop simulates a HVLA thrust) - the drop must be a **controlled and tight**, high velocity, low amplitude impulse (most students start with the variation of LVHA (low velocity high amplitude ☺)

Scale Thrust

Position: clinician in fencer stance, bilateral hand placement on scale

Force: slowly load scale by transferring body weight to forward leg, thrust is then delivered by allowing forward knee to flex & dropping body (load, load, drop) - load simulates removal of soft tissue slack - the drop can simulate a HVLA thrust or mobilization

Clinical notes: this method is probably the best single drill for side posture, prone & supine manipulations, as it offers instant visual feed back to the clinician

It is crucial that the needle on the scale ALWAYS continues in an increasing direction until the thrust is done for most techniques

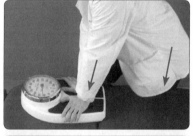

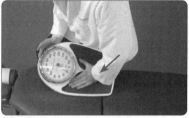

Common errors:

1. Hyperextension of the wrists - during thrust delivery proper technique requires good biomechanics to prevent practitioner injury - repetitive wrist hyperextension can result in wrist sprains, strains & instability

2. Load, load, LIFT, thrust - clinician loads, then releases pressure just prior to thrust - this is very uncomfortable for the patient and defeats the purpose of the initial loading tissue pull to remove soft tissue slack

S = stabilization (indifferent hand),　　● = contact,　　——▶ = examiner force,　　·········▶ = patient motion

Pillow Thrust

Position: clinician in fencer stance, bilateral hand placement on pillow

Force: slowly load pillow by transferring body weight to forward leg, thrust is then delivered by allowing forward knee to flex & dropping body (load, load, load, drop)

Common errors: same as scale thrust

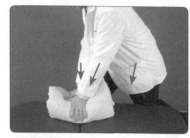

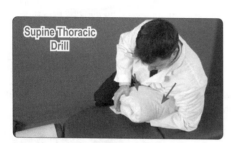

Supine Thoracic Drill

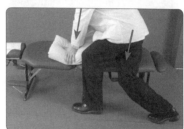

Cervical Thigh & Wrist Thrust

Thigh-Cervical simulation: clinician seated, wraps hands around own thigh (to simulate cervical spine) and practices tissue pull & controlled HVLA thrusts or mobilizes into thigh

Wrist-Cervical simulation: clinician seated - partner has hands interlocked with wrists together, clinician wraps hands around partners wrists (to simulate cervical spine) and practices tissue pull & controlled mobilization or HVLA thrusts into wrists depending on your scope of practice

Cervical manipulation requires a huge amount of speed and control to prevent injury; as such, regular practice is absolutely critical!

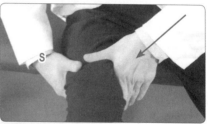

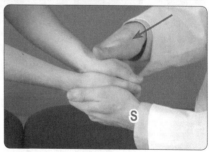

Simulated Patient Thrust

Position: patient side posture, clinician in fencer stance, clinician's inferior hand over patients upper lateral thigh or gluteal region; stabilization over the patients shoulder or elbow

Force: slowly load patient by transferring body weight to forward leg, thrust is then delivered by allowing forward knee to flex & dropping body (load, load, load, drop)

Common errors: same as scale thrust

 youtube: vizniak drills

Exercises to build clinician strength/skill should include push-ups, lunges & Brazilian jujitsu.

S = stabilization (indifferent hand), ● = contact, ⟶ = examiner force, ┈┈┈▷ = patient motion

prohealthsys

Realize that joint mobilization is an extremely difficult skill to even begin to perform effectively, much less master. While many professionals may make it look effortless and easy, realize that you are looking at thousands of hours of practice and clinical experience.

When you first start, the forms and postures are going to seem very awkward and even mildly uncomfortable - this is normal! When setting-up if it doesn't feel correct - step back, reassess and ask - what is wrong here? If you are not comfortable there is no way your patient will be comfortable & relaxed. Stay focused & relaxed and you will have more success, and remember "practice does NOT make perfect"... "*Perfect* practice makes perfect."

Below are some errors that are funny in the classroom but should be avoided in real practice.

"Dropsie Daisy"

Patient is not positioned correctly - clinician is so focused on their own position they fail to realize the patient is slowly falling off the table. Usually the legs will slide off the table or, in worst case scenario, the upper body starts to roll off the table

Correction: ensure proper patient position during initial set-up and as the soft tissue slack is being removed

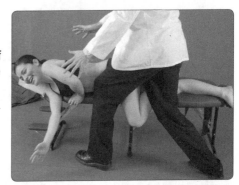

"The Straddler"

Student attempts yoga warrior pose over patient - feet too far apart results in no room for weight transfer to develop body drop force - student comment "I feel like I have no-where to drop"

Correction: stand with feet closer together & knees bent have space between body & patient

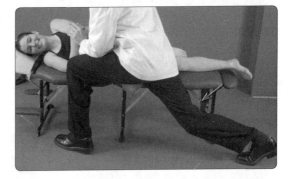

"Incidental Contact"

While it may occur accidentally on occasion, genital or breast contact with patient is never recommended (either when the patient's thigh is straddled or at end of thrust) see arrow in picture

Correction: position patient correctly and be conscious of your body position, consider the use of a protective device (pillow or towel) - **instructor tip** - carry a whistle & yellow card during the class and hand tem out (fun ☺)

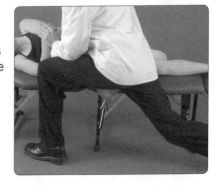

Introduction

"The Grip of Death"

Clinician is quivering in place & maintaining a huge amount of muscle tension to hold their own body & patient position; often a painfully tight grip on the patient (see arrow)

Correction: relax (take a deep breath), if you are working that hard reassess your set-up position - both the patient & clinician must be relaxed

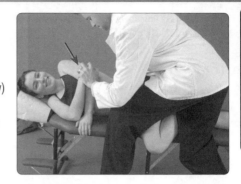

"The Shoulder Ripper"

Clinician moves away from center of gravity - increases chance of clinician injury (many physical medicine providers have sustained career ending injuries secondary to poor biomechanical set-ups - rotator cuff tears, wrist injuries, carpal tunnel syndrome)

Correction: ensure adjusting contact hand is near the center of gravity (below sternum)

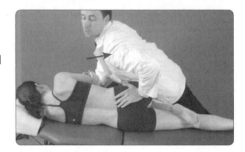

"The Bilateral Thruster"

Clinician applies force with both adjusting contact hand and stabilization hand (common in weight lifters and cross fitters)

Correction: only deliver thrusting force through contact hand (not stabilization hand); be conscious of patient experience

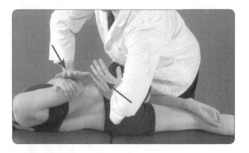

Other Common Error's

'Macho man muscler' - often male practitioners, with more upper body strength, will use this technique with success on smaller patients; however once larger patients or more difficult issues are addressed this biomechanical disadvantage will result in a significant treatment handicap

Lack of lower body weight transfer results in a loss of 50%-75% of potential force generation - common practitioner compensation is attempted through upper body muscle force

Correction: flex your knees & drop body - use your body weight to your advantage

'Sky butt' - clinician's gluteal muscles are higher than their head, placing center of gravity too high (clinician gets 'beached on patient'). Clinician correction is to stand up straighter, bend knees and bring pelvis closer to patient ('tail bone tuck')

'Hammer Hands' - Load, load, **LIFT**, mobe - Clinician looses tension and slides off of adjustment contact point or thrust too deep

Mobilizations are 90% set-up, and 10% movement/thrust

Introduction

Typical forces & time for given regional manipulations (grade 5 mobes)

Manipulation	Peak Force (lbs-force)	Time (ms)
Supine Cervical	100 N (22 lbs)	80-100 ms
Prone Thoracic	~400-960 N (90-215 lbs)	96-150 ms
Side-lying Sacroiliac	220-550 N (50-125 lbs)	100-185 ms

- In general SI side posture manipulations develop force that is ~30%-75% of the treating clinician's body weight
- Realize that peak force and pre-tension vary greatly between clinicians, given body size and specific technique used

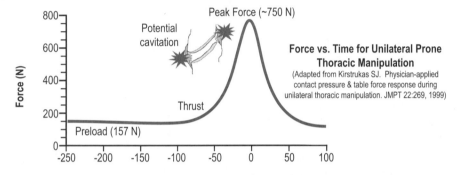

Peak Force (~750 N)

Potential cavitation

Thrust

Preload (157 N)

Force (N)

Force vs. Time for Unilateral Prone Thoracic Manipulation
(Adapted from Kirstrukas SJ. Physician-applied contact pressure & table force response during unilateral thoracic manipulation. JMPT 22:269, 1999)

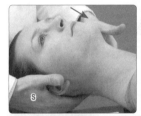
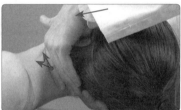

Supine Cervical
(index pillar push for C3-4 right rotation restriction)

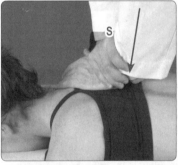
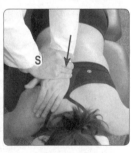

Prone Thoracic
(reinforced hypothenar transverse push for T4-5 left rotation restriction)

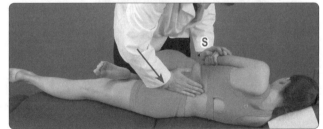

Side-lying Sacroiliac
(heel sacral push for sacral counter nutation restriction - nutated sacrum)

Thrust: application of a controlled directional force generated by a combination of the clinician's weight transfer, muscular force and line of drive (HVT = high velocity thrust; HVLA = high velocity low amplitude)

- **Non-pause thrust** - HVT is delivered as the soft tissue slack is removed; this method may also be applied with breathing with the thrust delivered at the end of expiration, and is particularly useful to help maintain adjustive momentum & reduce patient muscle guarding

- **Pause thrust** - tissue slack is removed, clinician pauses then applies HVT

- **Double thrust** - tissue slack is removed, apply mild oscillations at end range, then apply HVT thrust (good technique to help avoid patient guarding)

- **Recoil thrust** - HVT thrust with passive tissue recoil accomplished by rapid removal of the contact hand immediately following the adjustment

- **Impulse thrust** - HVT thrust followed by the maintenance of mild pressure with contact hand for a short duration following adjustment

- **Mechanical assist techniques** - mechanical devices used to help accomplish given treatment

  - Drop table - section of table drops away when force is applied

  - Instrument Assisted - impact tools or instruments to assist in force delivery (activator, thumper, proSTM2, etc.)

  - Motorized tables - provide rhythmic distraction to help set up pre-adjustive tension

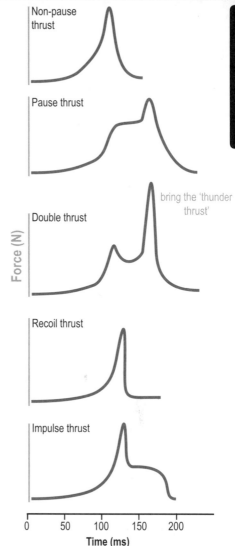

Why grade 5 manipulation vs. grade 3 or 4 mobilizations? - There is application for both...

When addressing hypomobility secondary to contracture of soft tissues or hypertonicity of muscle; mobilizations work up to the elastic limit and do NOT reach the anatomic limit that manipulation does (given the difference in apical impulse force and energy). This increased force allows for **greater soft tissue stretching potential, local segmental neurologic stimulation** and muscle relaxation reflex to counteract hypertonicity, that cannot be accomplished as quickly with grade 1-4 mobilization.

If you only address the joints with manipulation you are missing the larger soft tissue component - conversely soft tissue methods that fail to rectify the specific underlying joint biomechanics result in transient short term effects. **Joints are the moving foundations of motion** - massage, stretch & strengthen all you like, if there foundational issues causing functional compensations, unless addressed you are just putting band-aids over a deep issue - **proximal stability is needed for distal mobility**

Quiz & References

prohealthsys

1. Vizniak, NA. Human Cadaver Dissections. 1999-2018
2. GN Kawchuk, J Fryer, JL Jaremko, H Zeng, L Rowe. Real-time visualization of joint cavitation. Published: April 15, 2015 https://doi.org/10.1371/journal.pone.0119470
3. Gregory D Cramer, et. al. Accelerometer Assessment of Spinal Joint Crepitus Before and After Spinal Manipulation. April 2017. The FASEB Journal vol. 31 no. 1 Supplement 902.16
4. Brodeur R. The audible release associated with joint manipulation [review]. J Manipulative Physiol Ther. 1995;18(3):155-164.
5. Hembrow CH. Symposium. Manipulative treatment. Med J Aust. 1967; 1(25):1274-1280. Cited by: Heilig D. The thrust technique. J Am Osteopath Assoc. 1981;81:247.
6. Kelso AF. Physiology. In: Northup GW, ed. Osteopathic Research: Growth and Development. Chicago, Ill: American Osteopathic Assoc; 1987:66-67.
7. Meal GM, Scott RA. Analysis of the joint crack by simultaneous recording of sound and tension. J Manipulative Physiol Ther. 1986;9(3):189-195.
8. Nordheim Y. Eine neue Methode, den Gelenkknorpel, besonders die Kniegelenkmenisken, röntgenologisch darzustellen (ohne Zuhilfnahme eingespritzten Kontrastmittels). Fortschr. Röntgenstr. 1938;57:479-495. Cited in: Sandoz R. The significance of the manipulative crack and of other articular noises. Ann Swiss Chiro Assoc. 1969;4:47-68.
9. Sandoz R. The significance of the manipulative crack and of other articular noises. Ann Swiss Chiro Assoc. 1969;4:47-68.
10. Unsworth A, Dowson D, Wright V. Cracking joints. A bioengineering study of cavitation in the metacarpophalangeal joint. Ann Rheum Dis. 1971;30(4):348- 358.
11. Brodeur R. The audible release associated with joint manipulation [review]. J Manipulative Physiol Ther. 1995;18(3):155-164.
12. Garry JP, McShane JM. Postcompetition elevation of muscle enzyme levels in professional football players. MedGenMed. Mar 3 2000;[sic]:E4.
13. Hembrow CH. Symposium. Manipulative treatment. Med J Aust. 1967; 1(25):1274-1280. Cited by: Heilig D. The thrust technique. J Am Osteopath Assoc. 1981;81:247.
14. Kelso AF. Physiology. In: Northup GW, ed. Osteopathic Research: Growth and Development. Chicago, Ill: American Osteopathic Assoc; 1987:66-67.
15. Maigne R. Les manipulations vertébrales. Expansion scientifique française. 1960. Cited in: Sandoz R. The significance of the manipulative crack and of other articular noises. Ann Swiss Chiro Assoc. 1969;4:47-68.
16. Meal GM, Scott RA. Analysis of the joint crack by simultaneous recording of sound and tension. J Manipulative Physiol Ther. 1986;9(3):189-195.
17. Mennell JM. Joint pain: Diagnosis and treatment using manipulative techniques. Boston, Mass: Little Brown & Co; 1964:136-137.
18. Nordheim Y. Eine neue Methode, den Gelenkknorpel, besonders die Kniegelenkmenisken, röntgenologisch darzustellen (ohne Zuhilfnahme eingespritzten Kontrastmittels). Fortschr. Röntgenstr. 1938;57:479-495. Cited in: Sandoz R. The significance of the manipulative crack and of other articular noises. Ann Swiss Chiro Assoc. 1969;4:47-68.
19. Sandoz R. The significance of the manipulative crack and of other articular noises. Ann Swiss Chiro Assoc. 1969;4:47-68.
20. Swezey RL, Swezey SE. The consequences of habitual knuckle cracking. West J Medicine. 1975;122:377-379. 21. Castellanos J, Axelrod D. Effect of habitual knuckle cracking on hand function. Ann Rheum Dis. 1990;49:308-309
21. Unsworth A, Dowson D, Wright V. Cracking joints. A bioengineering study of cavitation in the metacarpophalangeal joint. Ann Rheum Dis. 1971;30(4):348- 358.
22. Boal RW, Gillette RG. Central Neuronal Plasticity, Low Back Pain and Spinal Manipulative Therapy. JMPT 27(5):314-326, 2004.
23. Bodgduk N, Tynan W, Wilson AS. The nerve supply to the human intervertebral discs. J Anat 1981;132:39-56.
24. Bogduk N, Jull G. The theoretical pathology of acute locked back: a basis for manipulative therapy. Man Med 1985;1:78-82.
25. Boline PD, Haas M, Meyer JJ, Kassak K, Nelson C, Keating JC., Jr Interexaminer reliability of eight evaluative dimensions of lumbar segmental abnormality: Part II. JMPT. 1993 Jul–Aug;16(6):363–374.
26. Boline PD, Haas M, Meyer JJ, Kassak K, Nelson C, Keating JC., Jr Interexaminer reliability of eight evaluative dimensions of lumbar segmental abnormality: Part II. JMPT. 1993 Jul–Aug;16(6):363–374.
27. Bolton PS. Reflex Effects of Vertebral Subluxations: The Peripheral Nervous system. An Update. JMPT 23(2):101-103, 2000.
28. Bolton PS. The Somatosensory System of the Neck and Its Effects on the Central Nervous System. JMPT 21(8): 553-563, 1998.
29. Brennan PC, Cramer GD, Kirstukas SJ, Cullum ME. Basic science research in chiropractic: state-of-the-art and recommendations for a research agenda. JMPT 1997;20(3).
30. Brennan PC, Triano JJ, McGregor M, Kokjohn K, Hondras MA, Brennan DT. Enhanced neutrophil respiratory burst as a biological marker for manipulation forces: duration of the effect and association with substance P and tumor necrosis factor. JMPT 1992;15:83-9.
31. Brodeur R. The audible release associated with joint manipulation. JMPT 1995;18:155-64.
32. Budgell B, Igarashi Y. Response of Arrhythmia to Spinal Manipulation: Monitoring by ECG With Analysis of Heart-Rate Variability. JNMS 9(3):97-102, 2001.
33. Budgell B, Polus B. The Effects of Thoracic Manipulation on Heart Rate Variability: A Controlled Crossover Trial. JMPT 29(8):603-610, 2006.
34. Budgell BS, Sato A. The Cervical Subluxation and Regional Cerebral Blood Flow. JMPT 20(2):103-107, 1997
35. Budgell BS. Reflex Effects of Subluxation: The Autonomic Nervous System.
36. Buerger AA. Experimental neuromuscular models of spinal manual techniques. Man Med 1983;1:10-17.
37. Bugdell BS, et al. Reflex Responses of Bladder Motility After Stimulation of Interspinous Tissues in the Anesthetized Rat. JMPT 21(9):593-599, 1998.
38. Carrick FR. Changes in Brain Function Afrter Manipulation of the Cervical Spine.
39. Cassidy JD, Lopes AA, Yong-Hing K. The immediate effect of manipulation versus mobilization on pain and range of motion in the cervical spine: a randomized controlled trial. JMPT. 1992 Nov–Dec;15(9):570–575.
40. Cavalcanti FS, de Freitas GG. Alternative medicine in a patient with juvenile chronic arthritis. J Rheumatol. 1992 Nov;19(11):1827–1828.
41. Cherkin DC, MacCornack FA. Patient evaluations of low back pain care from family physicians and chiropractors. West J Med. 1989 Mar;150(3):351–355.
42. Christensen HW, Vach W, et al. Palpation of the Upper Thoracic Spine: An Observer Reliability Study. JMPT 25(5):285-292, 2002.
43. Christian GH, Stanton GJ, Sissons D, How HY, Jamison J, Alder B, Fullerton M, Funder JW. Immunoreactive ACTH, beta-endorphin and cortisol levels in plasma following spinal manipulative therapy. Spine 1988:13:1411-7.
44. Clarke, Judy MA ; van Tulder, Maurits PhD; Blomberg, Stefan MD, PhD, et al. Traction for Low Back Pain With or Without Sciatica: An Updated Systematic Review Within the Framework of the Cochrane Collaboration. Spine. 31(14):1591-1599, June 15, 2006.
45. Coderre TJ, Katz J, Vaccarino AL, Melzack R. Contribution of central neuroplasticity to pathological pain: review of clinical and experimental studies. Pain 1993;52:259-85.
46. Collaca JC, et al. Neurophysiological Responses to Intraoperative Lumbosacral Spinal Manipulation. JMPT 23(7):447-457, 2000.
47. Conway PJW, Herzog W, Zhang Y, et al. Forces required to cause cavitation during spinal manipulation in the thoracic spine. Clin Biomech 1993;8:210-4.
48. Cornwall MW, et al. The Effect of Physical Activity on Ligamentous Strength. J Orth Sports Phys Ther 5(5):275-277, 1984.
49. Cox JM, Fromelt KA, Shreiner S. Chiropractic statistical survey of 100 consecutive low back pain patients. JMPT. 1983 Sep;6(3):117–128.
50. Cox JM, Shreiner S. Chiropractic manipulation in low back pain and sciatica: statistical data on the diagnosis, treatment and response of 576 consecutive cases. JMPT. 1984 Mar;7(1):1–11.
51. Cox JM. Patient benefits of attending a chiropractic low back wellness clinic. JMPT. 1994 Jan;17(1):25–28.
52. Deboer KF, Harmon R, Jr, Tuttle CD, Wallace H. Reliability study of detection of somatic dysfunctions in the cervical spine. JMPT. 1985 Mar;8(1):9–16.
53. DeVocht JW, Pikar JG, Wilder DG. Spinal Manipulation Alters Electromyographic Activity of Paraspinal Muscles: A Descriptive Study. JMPT 28(7):465-471, 2005.
54. Deyo, Richard A. MD, MPH; Mirza, Sohail K. MD, MPH; Martin, Brook I. MPH. Back Pain Prevalence and Visit Rates: Estimates From U.S. National Surveys, 2002. Spine. 31(23):2724-2727, 2006.
55. Dishman JD, Ball KA, Burke J. Central Motor Excitability Changes After Spinal Manipulation: A Transcranial Magnetic Stimulation Study. JMPT 25(1):1-9, 2002.
56. Dishman JD, Cunningham BM, Burke J. Comparison of Tibial Nerve H-Reflex Excitability After Cervical and Lumbar Manipulation. JMPT 25(5):318-325, 2002.
57. Donatelli R, Owens-Burkhart H. Effects of Immobilization on the Extensibility of Periarticular Connective Tissue.J Ortho Sports Phys Ther 3(2):67-72, 1981.
58. Downey BJ, Taylor NF, Niere KR. Manipulative physiotherapists can reliably palpate nominated lumbar spinal levels. Man Ther. 1999 Aug;4(3):151–156.
59. Driscoll MD, Hall MJ. Effects of Spinal Manipulative Therapy on Autonomic Activity and the Cardiovascular System: A Case Study Using the Electrocardiogram and Arterial Tonometry. JMPT 23(8):545-550, 2000.
60. Ernst E, Canter PH. "A systematic review of systematic reviews of spinal manipulation". J R Soc Med 99 (4): 192–6. 2006.
61. Eskelund Hansen B, Simonsen T, Leboeuf-Yde C. Motion Palpation of the Lumbar Spine – A Problem With The Test or the Tester? JMPT 29(3):208-212, 2006.
62. Fjellner A, Bexander C, Faleij R, Strender LE. Interexaminer reliability in physical examination of the cervical spine. JMPT. 1999 Oct;22(8):511–516.
63. Frach JP, Osterbauer PJ, Fuhr AW. Treatment of Bell's palsy by mechanical force, manually assisted chiropractic adjusting and high-voltage electrotherapy. JMPT. 1992 Nov–Dec;15(9):596–598.
64. French SD, Green S, Forbes A. Reliability of chiropractic methods commonly used to detect manipulable lesions in patients with chronic low-back pain. JMPT. 2000 May;23(4):231–238.
65. Fryer G, Morris T, Gibbons P, Briggs A. The Electromyographic Activity of the Thoracic Paraspinal Muscles Identified as Abnormal With Palpation. JMPT 29(6):437-447, 2006.
66. Frymann VM, Carney RE, Springall P. Effect of osteopathic medical management on neurologic development in children. J Am Osteopath Assoc. 1992 Jun;92(6):729–744.
67. Gagnier, Joel J. ND, MSc, PhD(cand.); van Tulder, Maurits W. PhD; Berman, Brian MD]; Bombardier, Claire MD Herbal Medicine for Low Back Pain: A Cochrane Review. Spine. 32(1):82-92, January 1, 2007.
68. Gal JM, Herzog W, Kawchuk GN, Conway PJ, Zhang Y-T. Forces and relative vertebral movements during SMT to unembalmed post-rigor human cadavers: peculiarities associated with joint cavitation. JMPT 1995;18:4-9.
69. Giesen JM, Center DB, Leach RA. An evaluation of chiropractic manipulation as a treatment of hyperactivity in children. JMPT. 1989 Oct;12(5):353–363.
70. Giles LGF, Harvey AR. Immunohistochemical demonstration of nociceptors in the capsule and synovial folds of human zygapophyseal joint capsule and synovial fold innervation. Br J Rheumatol 1987;26:993-8.
71. Giles LGF. Mechnisms of Neurovascular Compression Within the Spinal and Intervertebral Canals. JMPT 23(2):107-111, 2000.
72. Gillette RG, Kramis RC, Roberts WJ. Spinal Neurons Likely to Mediate Low Back and Referred Leg Pain. Society for Neuroscience Abstracts Vol 16, 294-7.
73. Gillette RG. Spinal cord mechanisms of referred pain and neuroplasticity. In Gatterman MI (ed). Foundations of Chiropractic: Subluxation. St. Louis, MO: Mosby, 1995.
74. Gonnella C, Paris SV, Kutner M. Reliability in evaluating passive intervertebral motion. Phys Ther. 1982 Apr;62(4):436–444.
75. Gonnella C, Paris SV, Kutner M. Reliability in evaluating passive intervertebral motion. Phys Ther. 1982 Apr;62(4):436–444.
76. Good CJ, Mikkelsen GB. Intersegmental sagittal motion in the lower cervical spine and discogenic spondylosis: a preliminary study. JMPT. 1992 Nov–Dec;15(9):556–564.
77. Gotlib, A & Rupert R. Chiropractic manipulation in pediatric health conditions – an updated systematic review. Chiropractic & Osteopathy 2008, 16:11
78. Grice AS. Muscle tonus changes following manipulation. J Can Chiropr Assoc 1974;18:29-31.
79. Haas M. How to evaluate intraexaminer reliability using an interexaminer reliability study design. JMPT. 1995 Jan;18(1):10–15.
80. Haas M. Statistical methodology for reliability studies. JMPT. 1991 Feb;14(2):119–132.
81. Haas M. The reliability of reliability. JMPT. 1991 Mar–Apr;14(3):199–208.
82. Haldeman S. Neurologic Effects of the Adjustment. JMPT 23(2):112-114, 2000.
83. Hammer WI, Pfefer MT. Treatment of Subacute Lumbar Compartment Syndrome Using the Graston Technique. JMPT 28(3):199-204, 2005.
84. Hartvigsen, Jan DC, PhD; Christensen, Kaare MD, PhD Active Lifestyle Protects Against Incident Low Back Pain in Seniors: A Population-Based 2-Year Prospective Study of 1387 Danish Twins Aged 70-100 Years. Spine. 32(1):76-81, January 1, 2007.
85. Hawk C, Phongphua C, Bleecker J, Swank L, Lopez D, Rubley T. Preliminary study of the reliability of assessment procedures for indications for chiropractic adjustments of the lumbar spine. JMPT. 1999 Jul–Aug;22(6):382–389.
86. Hawk C, Phongphua C, Bleecker J, Swank L, Lopez D, Rubley T. Preliminary study of the reliability of assessment procedures for indications for chiropractic adjustments of the lumbar spine. JMPT. 1999 Jul–Aug;22(6):382–389.
87. HEILIG D. Principles of vertebral manipulation in the cervical area. J Am Osteopath Assoc. 1952 Oct;52(2):109–114.
88. Herzog W, Conway P, Kawchuk G, et al. Forces exerted during spinal manipulative therapy. Spine 1993a;18:1206-12.
89. Herzog W, Conway PJ, Zhang YT, et al. Reflex responses associated with manipulative treatments on the thoracic spine. JMPT 1995;18:233-6.
90. Herzog W, Scheele D, Conway PJ. Electromyographic Responses of Back and Limb Muscles Associated With Spinal Manipulative Therapy. Spine 24(2):146-153, 1999.
91. Herzog W, Zhang YT, Conway PJ, et al. Cavitation sounds during spinal manipulative treatments. JMPT 1993b;16:523-26.
92. **Full list of 210 available on request**

Quiz (actual answer page)

1. How many hours per day is the average North American sitting/laying)? (2) _____
2. What is the first known written record of joint mobilization? (3) ________________
3. According academic calendars, what profession has the most training in joint mobilization and manips? (5) ___________
4. Define the Term 'Subluxation' according to the World Health Organization (7) ________
5. As levers get longer what happens to their speed and power? (9) _____________
6. What are the names of forces that can act on joints and bones? (12) ____________
7. Proteoglycans are hydrophilic? T/F (13)
8. What are the Osteokinematic motions? Arthrokinematic motions? (14) ___________
9. What is the Concave on Convex Rule? (15) ________________________
10. Define Closed packed? Open packed? (15)
11. List the sensory pathways? (18) __________
12. List the types and functions of receptors in joints, and muscles? (17) __________
13. Define the grades of mobilization? (21) ____
14. Give examples of patient positions, tissue contacts and force vectors ________ (23-27)
15. Give a list of potential causes for joint sounds? (26) ________________
16. What are the indications for joint mobilizations? (28) ________________
17. What are the contraindications for joint mobilizations? (30) ______________
18. What are the potential positive & negative effects for joint mobilizations? (31) _______
19. During informed consent, what is does acronym PAR-Q stand for? (37)
20. List common technique errors? (40) ______
21. Mobilizations are ____ % set-up and ____ % movement/thrust (41) ______________
22. Perform some basic joint mobilization drills? (38) - and have fun - youtube: vizniak drills

Learning Objectives

After completing this chapter, students will be able to:

1. Develop effective assessment flow based around the o-HIP-MNRS DDx protocol

2. Identify and create a differential diagnosis (DDx) list and rule in/rule out fractures in office

3. Perform a detailed chief **concern** history and recognize red flags for serious pathology

4. Discuss application of outcome markers and pain assessment scales and differentiate tissue specific injuries and visceral pain referral patterns

5. Perform a detailed postural assessment (standing, seated & sleeping) and gait analysis and discuss the biomechanical changes in bare-foot vs shoed running

6. Create detailed palpation protocols for static, bony, muscle, ligament and motion palpation integrated with joint-play end-feels

7. Discuss joint ROM, goniometry application, lever systems, open and closed kinetic chains, and tight and loose packed joint positions

8. Recognize spinal joint listing systems and the spectrum of joint dysfunction

9. Choose appropriate assessment and treatment options based on hyper or hypo mobility of tissue

10. Accurately chart/record findings and treatments

Joint Assessment

Determining Joint Mobility

- Can be difficult to assess
- Quantity - graded in millimeters
- Quality - graded by "end feel"
- Poor intra/inter-examiner reliability
- Compare bilaterally (unaffected side)

Direct Method (most common)

- Hands on evaluation of accessory motions (joint play or PROM with over pressure) in all directions

Indirect Method

- Observational application of convex/ concave rules to determine the direction of limited mobility while observing AROM, motion, posture & gait

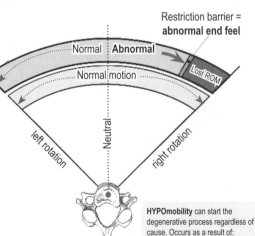

Restriction barrier = abnormal end feel

Normal : Abnormal

Normal motion

Lost ROM

left rotation — Neutral — right rotation

HYPOmobility can start the degenerative process regardless of cause. Occurs as a result of:
- Injury, inactivity, contracture
- Loss of coordination/proprioception
- Muscular atrophy
- Thickened joint capsules/ligaments

Below is a sample clinical exam flow that can be used as a framework for individuals to use as a foundation to develop their own specific exam style (detailed exams are covered in the Physical Assessment Texts)

Observation, history & inspection should be performed first; following steps may be done depending on patient's clinical presentation. With more acute & potentially serious injuries, vascular & neurological screens should be done earlier during the physical exam.

O - observe

H - history

I - inspection

P - palpation

M - motion

N - neurovascular

R - referred pain

S - special tests

DDx = differential diagnosis

Tx = treatment

1. Observe

- Patient's general appearance, posture & mobility (how do they walk into office?)
- Emotional status (happy, sad, anxious) - are they comfortable?

2. History (basic considerations)

- Where is the problem? - point to it exactly, When did start?
- What makes it better or worse? (self care) - Prior treatment or injuries?
- Quality of issue? (numbness, tingling, weakness, sharp, dull)
- Severity (scale from 0-10)? - Gradual or sudden onset?
- What are the patients goals for treatment?

3. Inspection

- **Posture (standing & seated), gait**, bony deformity, trouble with ADLs

- Obvious discomfort (painful expression, unable to sit comfortably, limp)
- Bony & soft tissues (deformity, bruising, swelling, color, sweat/dry, scars, calluses, bunions, atrophy, ulcers)
- Foot wear (supportive, wear patterns on shoes, assisting devices such as orthotics or braces)

4. Palpation

- Ask permission before performing a hands on assessment
- Temperature, Texture, Tone, Tenderness (4 Ts)
- **Anatomy review** (bone, tendons, muscle, ligaments, fascia, blood vessels, nerves, lymph, viscera)
- Swelling, pain, inflammation, myospasm, scar tissue

5. Motion

- Functional screen (ADLs & functional movements)
- **Active ROM** (provides baseline outcome marker)
- **Passive ROM** with over pressure (joint play)
- **RROM** = resisted ROM = isometric testing (break test)

Movement	Muscle	Ligament	Nerve
AROM	Pain	Pain	Weak
PROM	-	Pain	-
RROM	Pain	-	Weak

Tissue specific DDx on following pages

Joint Assessment

6. Neurovascular screen

- ☐ Dermatomes, reflexes (DTRs), cranial nerves, pathologic reflexes

- ☐ Muscle strength (myotomes), proprioception, coordination

- ☐ Pulses, nail bed or skin blanching, temperature

7. Referred pain (screen adjacent areas & spine)

- ☐ MFTPs referral, nerve root impingement, visceral origin, infection, psychogenic origin/overlay

8. Special tests

- ☐ Orthopedic tests or injection of local anesthesia in specific tissue (pain reduction shows damaged tissue)

- ☐ Diagnostic imaging: X-rays, U/S, CT, MRI, thermography

- ☐ Lab tests: blood, urinalysis, biopsy etc.

Assessment is Therapeutic!

Many assessment methods may be used as treatment techniques. Example - patient presents with pain between the shoulders and limited mid thoracic extension - the AROM you do in office may be the only time the patient goes through FULL ROM, passive ROM to assess extension restriction also stretches the tight soft tissues fibers & is a mobilization

Specific assessment, treatment and a rapid DDx review are shown in each chapter

 youtube: Vizniak fracture screen

Fracture Screen

Fractures must be ruled out prior to joint play, mobes & manip. (there are documented malpractice cases of clinicians mobilizing & manipulating fractures - you can be tricked...). Below is a list of commonly performed fracture screen tests based around the Canadian C-spine rules and general practice experience, more positive criteria increase the likelihood of fracture - remember **x-rays are NOT 100% diagnostic!** - For example, in scaphoid fractures there will be fractures present that do NOT show up on xray ~20% of the time (which are later confirmed in MRI) - **Treat the patient NOT their pictures.**

- *Four step* test (4 steps without pain or altered gait?) - **this test is still valid for upper extremity and spinal injuries** (observe for abnormal arm swing, rigid spine and very soft foot strike with each step)

- **History of significant *trauma*?** (FOOSH, fall from height, ballistic impact with force)

- **Older than 55?** (with age bones become less flexible & soft tissues are more fibrous)

- **Dark black bruising?** (darker, rapid onset bruising indicates more severe vascular rupture)

- *Resisted* isometric contraction (activated muscles pull on periosteum and bone attachments - with fracture patient is unable to develop muscle tension due to pain - excellent way to assess without displacing fragments)

- *Percussion*, light palpation, **Pain with squeeze** of bone (yes you can gently squeeze fractured bones, or even flex bone as in a sternal compression test)

- 128 Hz tuning fork, ultrasound (many false negatives - higher reliability in very acute fractures)

- **Limited or inability to move damaged area?**

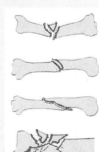

Red Flags* for More Serious Pathology

History of...
- Violent trauma
- Carcinoma
- Systemic steroid use
- Drug abuse, HIV, Hepatitis
- Recent unexplained weight loss
- Constant, progressive non-mechanical pain
- Bowel and/or bladder dysfunction

Signs & symptoms
- Temperature > 100° F / 37.8° C
- Blood pressure > 160/95 mm Hg
- Resting pulse > 100 bpm
- Resting respiration > 25 bpm
- Auscultation of bruits - carotid, abdominal
- Widespread neurological deficits
- Saddle anesthesia

*Red flag = pathognomonic sign or symptom that is very suggestive & almost always associated with a given condition (e.g. shooting or electrical pain radiating down the back of the leg into the heel is a "red flag" for lumbar radiculopathy)

The parameters below are to be used only as guidelines for the development of a management plan. These are estimates of treatment and/or healing time for commonly encountered categories of neuromusculoskeletal conditions. Individual patients will vary in the amount of time required for their healing & rehabilitation depending upon their specific clinical presentation & dedication to treatment.

0-6 weeks of treatment
- Mild-moderate strain, mild sprain
- Mechanical/joint dysfunction (uncomplicated)
- Acute facet syndrome, contusion
- Mild-mod. tendinitis, capsulitis, bursitis, synovitis
- Mild sacroiliac syndrome
- Acute myofascial pain syndrome
- Mild symptomatic degenerative joint disease
- Headaches: vertebrogenic, muscle contraction, migraine, vascular
- Torticollis (acquired)

~2-12 weeks of treatment
- Moderate-marked strain, moderate sprain
- Post traumatic mild-moderate myofibrosis
- Post traumatic periarticular fibrosis & joint dysfunction with marked tendinitis, bursitis, capsulitis
- Chronic tendinitis, bursitis, capsulitis
- Chronic facet syndrome
- Moderate sacroiliac syndrome
- Chronic SI syndrome with marked myofascial pain syndrome
- Chronic myofascial pain syndrome
- Mechanical/joint dysfunction (complicated)
- Mild inter-vertebral disc syndrome without myelopathy
- Chronic headaches: vertebrogenic, muscle contraction, migraine, vascular
- Mild temporomandibular joint dysfunction
- Symptomatic spondylolisthesis
- Mild clinical joint instability

1-6 months of treatment
- Chronic facet syndrome associated with clinical vertebral instability
- Marked strain associated with post traumatic myofibrosis and/or joint dysfunction
- Marked sprain w/ associated instability/dysfunction
- Thoracic outlet syndromes
- Moderate inter-vertebral disc syndrome w/o myelopathy
- Peripheral neurovascular entrapment syndromes
- Moderate to marked temporomandibular joint dysfunction
- Adhesive capsulitis (frozen joint)
- Partial or complete dislocation

2-12 months of treatment
- Marked inter-vertebral disc syndrome w/o myelopathy, with or without radiculopathy
- Lateral recess syndrome
- Intermittent neurogenic claudication
- Acceleration/deceleration injuries of the spine with myofascial complications (whiplash)
- Cervicobrachial sympathetic syndromes
- Sympathetic dystrophies
- Severe strain/sprain of cervical spine with myoligamentous complications

Joint Assessment

LOC-Q-SMAT

Review intake questionnaire

- Prior to beginning the patient history, review intake questionnaire to help better point out specific areas of interest or coexisting conditions
- CC = 'chief concern' is better than 'complaint' as the word 'complaint' has negative connotations -
- Who wants to go to work and listen to complaints all day? ☺

Why are they seeking care
How can I help you today?

1. Location

- **Where? Point to it**, indicate L or R
- Write as accurate a location as possible ("low back" is too general, "lumbosacral" is better, "shoulder" is too general, "anterior & lateral right shoulder" is better)
- •Does it radiate? Where? How far? (elbow, wrist, hand, fingertips?)
- What aspect/surface? (lateral/medial/posterior)

2. Onset (what happened & when?)

- When did it happen? Gradual or sudden? What caused it?
- What is the **mechanism of injury?** - Look for specific actions, changes in activities, posture, work (worker's compensation)

3. Chronology/Timing (symptom patterns)

- Constant or intermittent (episodic)
- If constant, is it truly 24 hours a day? Does it prevent sleep?
- If intermittent: is it **associated with specific circumstances?** (e.g. eating certain foods? certain activities? Time of day?)
- Frequency & duration of the episodes
- Diurnal patterns (worse in morning? end of day?)
- Is there night pain (wake or prevent sleep?)
- Getting worse (progressive)? Getting better? Staying the same?
- Prior history: **has this ever happened before?** When? How long? What did you do about it?

4. Quality

- Ask patient to **describe symptoms in their own words**, use patient's words in quotations
- Describe pain or symptoms (sharp, dull, etc.)

5. Severity/effect on ADL

- Pain mild, moderate or severe?, **Pain scale (0-10)**

ADLs: can you go to work? Affect performance? Affect hobbies? Sexual activity? Simple activities such as putting on a shirt? **Get specific activities & how the patient is affected (excellent source of functional outcome markers)**

6. Modifying factors

- What increases the symptoms or pain? Be specific
- **What makes it better? What makes it worse?** Avoiding what? Changing posture? Rest? Medications, supplements (dose & frequency?)

7. Associated symptoms

- Do you have any **other symptoms or problems that you feel are related to this issue?**
- Additional specific questions are asked based on what the patient presents with & what the examiner thinks it could be; for example:
  - Neck or back complaint: is there numbness, tingling, or weakness in an extremity?
  - Low back: does your back ever catch or get locked? Change in bowel habits? Change in bladder habits? Change in sexual function? Change in menses?
  - Knees: any popping, clicking, snapping? Knee ever lock? Swell? Give way?

8. Treatment previous

- Who did they see? When? What tests done?
- What diagnosis? **What treatment? Did it help?**

9. Relevant injuries/x-rays

- When? What happened? Eventual outcome/ residual effects?
- Where x-rays taken? What were the results?

10. Review of Systems (if indicated)

11. Goals

- What is patient's treatment goals?
- If long standing problem, why did they come in now?

Is there **anything else you can tell me about your condition that I have not asked?**

Create a differential diagnosis list to help direct physical exam, select special tests or referral for co-management

Outcome markers are used to monitor patient treatment progression. Any parameter that has the ability to be proven valid & reliable & can be objectively measured has the potential to become a clinical outcome marker. Listed below are some commonly accepted outcome markers:

Pain (subjective) - see below
- **Visual analogue scale (VAS)**
- Verbal pain scale (0-10) - printable scale on website - prohealthsys.com/central/clinic-forms/
- **Medication or botanical use & dosage (decreased intake is a good thing)**
- Centralization of symptoms, duration, frequency

Activities of Daily Living (ADLs)
- The **best functional outcome measure**
- Walking, sitting, chewing food, range of motion
- Ability to perform specific tasks
- Playing sports, hobbies, intercourse
- Days of missed work in a set time frame

Orthopedic tests / Range of Motion
- Active & passive motion before symptoms, utilizing a goniometer, inclinometer
- Change in response to provocative testing

Strength
- Muscle grading (0-5)
- Dynamometer, grip strength
- Ability to lift weight (kg/ lbs & number of reps)

Endurance
- Walk/run set distance (meters, km)
- Back extension repetition, sit-ups
- Ability to maintain position

Flexibility (ROM)
- Global range of motion (AROM, PROM)
- Touch toes (measure finger distance from floor)
- Reach behind back (measure distance to C7)
- Inclinometer, goniometer

Neurological
- Normalization of DTR's, loss of pathologic reflexes
- Centralization of symptoms - decreased sensory deficits, muscle strength (dynamometer)
- Improvement on nerve conduction studies

Quality of Life
- Patients that report a lower quality of life may be predisposed to poor treatment outcomes
- Ask the patient "Think of the last week, how would you rate your quality of life?" - excellent, very good, moderate, bad, very bad

Outcome Assessment Questionnaires
- While Questionnaires show good reliability many patients find it time consuming & somewhat inconvenient to repeatedly fill out multipage forms prior to each treatment
- Oswestry Low Back Pain Disability Questionnaire
- Roland/Morris Disability Questionnaire
- Pain Disability Index, McGill Pain Questionnaire

Pain Parameters

- **Dermal Pain:** from superficial soft tissues, usually well localized (eg. cut in skin)
- **Sclerotomic Pain:** from deep somatic tissues typically deep, aching & somewhat localized (eg. muscle strain)
- **Visceral pain:** from internal organ capsule distension or ischemia, deep achy, cramping pain that may be sharp at times, often poorly localized and may be immobilizing in more severe cases (eg. intestinal cramps, heart attack, appendicitis)
- **Radicular Pain:** from nerve roots, often described as shooting, electrical and/or burning & in a dermatomal pattern (nerve root compression) - Nerve compression distal to the nerve roots may result in a peripheral nerve distribution pattern of pain
- **Phantom pain:** arises from direct changes in neural pathways & perception of the brain, felt by amputees in the area of the missing limb

 30+ Questionnaires on website

- **Referred pain:** pain felt at a site other than where the cause is situated; pain in internal organs or myofascial trigger points (MFTP) is often referred to other locations (mechanisms of referred pain are complex - theories include convergent projection, convergent facilitation, axon reflex & hyper excitability)

Pain Duration
- **Acute Pain:** generally refers to pain associated with the acute stage of inflammation, however can be described as pain that is unbearable, usually first 48-72 hours.
- **Sub Acute:** pain after the acute stage but not yet chronic (> 72 hrs)
- **Chronic Pain:** refers to pain associated with the stages healing after the resolution of the inflammatory response. - is commonly used in reference to pain of long duration (> 3 months)

Joint Assessment

Definition of pain: **an unpleasant sensory and emotional experience associated with actual or potential tissue damage, or described in terms of such damage**[15]

Pain is one of the best determinants of disability[9] and low back pain (LBP) is predictive of work resumption within the year following related short-term absence.[10]

Three main meth ☺ ods are used to measure pain intensity: visual analogue scale (VAS), verbal rating scale (VRS), and numerical rating scale (NRS).[23,25,26] Pain scales have been demonstrated to be both a reliable & valid instrument for measuring the patient's sense of pain.[21, 29, 33, 34] The faces pain scale is recommended for use with younger children & elderly in parallel with numerical self-rating scales (0-10).

Application: ask the patient to "**rate current pain on a scale from 0-10, 0 being no pain, 10 being totally incapacitated.**" Patient states a number or points to corresponding pain level. Separate body regions should be rated individually; for example, in a patient with LBP & leg pain (which may or may not be related) there should be a pain rating for the LBP and a second rating for leg pain.

Other Considerations

1. **Ask separate questions**
   - What is your current pain? What is the usual pain level?
   - What is the pain at its worst?
   - What is the pain at its least?

2. Tissue sensitivity to pain

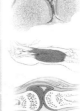

Least sensitive
- Fibrocartilage
- Articular cartilage
- Synovium

- Cortical bone
- Muscle
- Fascia

- Tendons
- Ligaments
- Subchondral bone

Most sensitive
- Fibrous capsule
- Periosteum
- Skin

3. **Chronic pain cases**
   - Consider recording the "least pain" the patient has been experiencing (research suggests patients recall "least pain" more accurately than "usual or worst")

4. **Measuring symptoms other than pain**
   - 0-10 scale can be applied to different symptoms (discomfort, nausea, fatigue, stress, etc.)
   - Simply substitute the word "pain" with the given symptom you wish to measure

> **'Pain should be respected, but challenged'**
> For most rehab., a low amount of pain is OK
> **up to a 3/10 is usually a safe place to work**
>
> **If pain is sharp or stops your breath then it is too much - look for the joyful discomfort ☺**

Numeric Rating Scale (NRS)

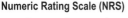

0	1	2	3	4	5	6	7	8	9	10
No Pain					Moderate Pain					Worst Possible Pain

Visual Analog Scale (VAS)

No Pain	Mild Pain	Moderate Pain	Severe Pain	Very Severe Pain	Worst Possible Pain

Faces Pain Scale (as used on ProHealth Goniometer & Posture wall chart)

Alert smiling	Serious face CAN BE IGNORED	Furrowed brow INTERFERES WITH TASKS	Raised upper lip INTERFERES WITH CONCENTRATION	Slow blink INTERFERES WITH BASIC NEEDS	Moaning - crying BEDREST - REQUIRED

NO PAIN →→→ Totally Incapacitated

prohealthsys

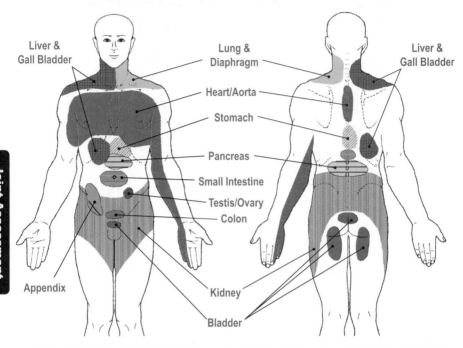

Liver & Gall Bladder

Lung & Diaphragm

Liver & Gall Bladder

Heart/Aorta

Stomach

Pancreas

Small Intestine

Testis/Ovary

Colon

Appendix

Kidney

Bladder

Visceral/organ pathology usually has musculoskeletal manifestation (myospasm, loss of ROM, local tenderness) - visceral cofactors must be ruled out if treatment is offering poor results after 2-3 sessions - '**Address the symptoms but treat the cause**' - Dr Vizniak

Differential Diagnosis by Location of Pain

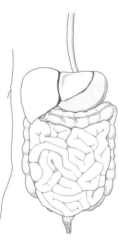

Right Upper Quadrant
1. Pleurisy
2. Hepatitis
3. Cholecystitis
4. Perforated duodenal ulcer
5. Appendicitis
6. Perforated colon
7. Fallopian tube (rupture)

Left Upper Quadrant
1. Pleurisy
2. Splenic rupture or infarct
3. Perforated gastric ulcer
4. Pancreatitis
5. Diverticulitis
6. Perforated colon (cancer)
7. Fallopian tube (pregnancy, abscess)

Right Lower Quadrant
1. Appendicitis
2. Acute Crohn's disease
3. Pelvic inflammatory disease
4. Perforated duodenal ulcer
5. Acute cholecystitis
6. Inguinal hernia
7. Leaking aortic aneurysm

Left Lower Quadrant
1. Sigmoid diverticulitis
2. Pelvic inflammatory disease
3. Sigmoid carcinoma
4. Gastric ulcer
5. Inguinal hernia
6. Leaking aortic aneurysm
7. Constipation

Joint Assessment

Condition	AROM	PROM	RROM	Comments
Muscle Injury (strain or tendinopathy)	↓ AROM (painful)	WNL (pain at end ROM)	Pain	• Dull ache - sharp pain when challenged • **Pain with palpation, stretching or contraction of damaged muscle** (possible weakness) • *Unidirectional* pain with motion in muscle fiber direction
Fascial Strain (adhesion or scaring)	↓ AROM (painful)	↓ PROM (painful)	WNL (painless)	• May have palpatory subcutaneous adhesions, limited ROM or non-dermatomal pain & posture changes
Ligament Injury (sprain)	↓ AROM (painful)	↓ PROM (painful)	WNL (painless)	• Injured at full end ROM with tearing • **Pain with palpation or stretching** of ligament (passive over pressure) • **Instability** due to full ligament rupture may show an empty end feel, ↑ PROM or repeatable 'clunk' with motion
Capsulitis	↓ AROM (painful)	↓ PROM (painful)	WNL (painless)	• Pain with direct capsule palpation or *multidirectional* pain with motion - pain in a single direction indicates muscle or tendon damage
Joint Injury (arthropathy)	↓ AROM (painful)	↓ PROM (painful)	WNL (painless)	• Mild loss of ROM or pain • **Crepitus with scour test** • AROM may show repeatable 'snapping' & 'popping' • Pain may change with weather
Joint Dysfunction (subluxation)	WNL or limited segmental ROM	Limited in specific ROM	WNL or weak	• Pain or point tenderness • Asymmetry/misalignment • **PROM abnormality or restriction** - joint "feels stuck"
Bone Injury (fracture)	↓ AROM (painful)	↓ PROM (painful)	↓ RROM (painful)	• Hx of trauma - **perform fracture screen** • Pin point tenderness, dull ache but very sharp when challenged
Nerve Injury	↓ or WNL	WNL	Weak	• **Numbness, tingling or muscle weakness** & shooting electrical pain with stretch or compression of nerve
Visceral Injury				• Writhing or **cramping pain** secondary to internal organ capsule distension or vascular compromise, deep achy, often **poorly localized** & may be immobilizing in more severe cases (eg. intestinal cramps, PMS, appendicitis) - pain is often **NOT relieved by change in body position**

↑ = increase, ↓ = decrease, WNL = within normal limits, Hx = history, **World Health Organization 'Subluxation' definition** - "A lesion or dysfunction in a joint or motion segment in which alignment, movement integrity and/or physiological function are altered, although contact between joint surfaces remains intact. It is essentially a functional entity, which may influence biomechanical and neural integrity." Vascular injuries often present with bruising, throbbing pain, changes in local body temperature and altered capillary refill times (> ~2 sec). Cutaneous (skin) injuries are easy to locate and visualize. The table above is for common general presentations, patients often have ranges of presentation depending on the specific scope of their injury or condition.

Posture Definition: evaluation of a person's body position and/or structure in standing; **assessed in 4 positions.** It is used for overall observation, gathering assessment information, monitor patient progress, and noting positional changes. It is useful to **observe a patient in a seated or work positions** (especially office workers) or in the stance they spend most of their day (cashiers, machinist) - in addition smart practitioners also **evaluate sleeping positions**

Postures are used to perform activities with the least amount of energy and we can hold a variety of postures for a long period of time. Postural relationships of body parts can be altered/controlled voluntarily, but such control is short-lived because it requires concentration; long-term changes are more difficult

When discomfort sets in from joint compression, ligamentous tension, continuous muscle contraction (fatigue) or circulatory occlusion (hypoxia) we typically move and stretch our joints and muscles as we settle into a new posture - **the body is designed to move - 'move it or lose it' makes clinical sense!**

Changing posture habits long term requires:
- Increases in ROM (mobilization)
- Stability (if unstable or weak)
- Muscle strength/endurance
- Training (neuronal programming in both proprioception and motor activity)

Long term postures without position change can lead to decreased ROM (atrophy/contracture), deformity (slow strains/creep), tissue damage and hypoxia (ulcers/amputation in sever cases)

Procedure: patient is examined in their habitual, relaxed standing position

- Explain procedure to the patient - but **do NOT use the word posture!** - "I would like to observe how you normally stand" - "try and stand as relaxed as possible." - have them "shake it out" or 'take a few steps'

- Observe body in 4 different positions (anterior, right lateral, left lateral, & posterior view)

- **Performed from the feet up to the head** - plumb line is suspended from the ceiling or use a posture poster (can use a laser)

- Patient is best **observed in shorts, underwear, swim suit or unitard** ☺

- Patients using orthotics should first be viewed with corrective devices in place, and then without (be sure to record type of device)

Postural Sway

The standing human body has a high Centre of Gravity (COG) (~S2 level - slightly higher in men, lower in women) and a small base of support – this leads to an unstable equilibrium; the constant displacement and correction of the position of the COG within the base of support is called **Postural Sway**. Postural sway is controlled by motor, visual, vestibular systems and proprioceptive organs

Postural sway is most stable between ages of 20-60, when vision accounts for 30% of stability; over 60, stability decreases by 50% with eye closure. Regular **participation in movement therapies can slow the decline** (yoga, Tai Chi)

Factors Affecting Posture

Structural	Functional (neuromyofascial)	
• Anatomical variation	• **Pain** (pain avoidance)	• Work position (seated, standing)
• Leg length discrepancy	• Muscle spasm or imbalance	• Poor habits (work, sport, rest)
• Scoliosis	• Ligament laxity or contracture	• Excess weight (pregnancy, fat)
• Age (osteoporosis & DJD)	• Fascial adhesion & scar tissue	• Shoes (heels, abnormal wear)
• Respiratory conditions	• Neurologic inhibition or over activation (movement patterns)	• Peer pressure (younger tall girls, large breasts)
• Orthotics/prosthetics	• Joint dysfunction (subluxation)	• Fatigue or depression

Realize that **structural changes can cause functional compensation**; myospasm (muscle stabilizing unstable or damaged area), hypomobility (long term contracture/adhesions & loss of ROM; hypermoblilty (ligament laxity or muscle firing pattern errors) -

Functional changes can lead to structural problems; atrophy (disuse muscle weakness abnormal neural pathways), instability & degeneration (wearing of cartilage & tenosynovial sheaths)

Start at the feet (foundation) and work up - done standing, seated & sleeping

Anterior View

Vertical Landmarks:
- ☐ Pubic symphysis
- ☐ Umbilicus
- ☐ Xiphoid
- ☐ Suprasternal notch
- ☐ Nasal bones

Horizontal Landmarks
- ☐ Foot angle, arches, malleoli
- ☐ Fibular heads level
- ☐ Knees straight (varum/valgum)
- ☐ Patellae point straight ahead
- ☐ Level at symphysis pubis
- ☐ ASIS level
- ☐ Iliac crest level
- ☐ Palms (hands) face body in relaxed position
- ☐ Elbows carrying angle (5°-15°)
- ☐ Waist angles (equal, arms equal distance to waist, IR/ER)
- ☐ Ribs/sternum, clavicles/ AC Joint (level & symmetrical)
- ☐ Shoulders (level, dominant arm is usually lower)
- ☐ Trapezius neck (slope on dominant may be greater)
- ☐ Nose (midline)
- ☐ Jaw (in resting position)
- ☐ Head (straight, tilting, rotation)

Lateral View x 2

Vertical Landmarks:
- ☐ Anterior to lateral malleolus
- ☐ Fibular head
- ☐ Greater trochanter
- ☐ Acromion
- ☐ Bodies of cervical vertebrae
- ☐ External auditory canal

Horizontal Landmarks
- ☐ Knees (slightly flexed 0-5°)
- ☐ Pelvic angle (normal male 0-10°, female 15-30°)
- ☐ Chest (pectus excavatum/ pectus carinatum)
- ☐ Muscles of abdomen
- ☐ Chest and back
- ☐ Shoulders (anterior rotation or military stance)
- ☐ Spine (normal spinal curvatures)
- ☐ Ear lobe - align with acromion and iliac crest other vertical landmarks

Posterior View

Vertical Landmarks:
- ☐ S2
- ☐ L5-C7 SPs
- ☐ Inion (EOP)

Horizontal Landmarks
- ☐ Heels (straight, angled in/out)
- ☐ Achilles tendon (straight, angled in/out)
- ☐ Popliteal fossa levels
- ☐ Gluteal folds (level, symmetry)
- ☐ PSIS level
- ☐ Arms (equal distance from body)
- ☐ Waist angles (equal/level, equal distance from body)
- ☐ Ribs (protruding)
- ☐ Spine (straight, curved laterally)
- ☐ Scapulae (inferior angles level, winging out posteriorly)
- ☐ Shoulders level
- ☐ Head (midline)

Joint Assessment

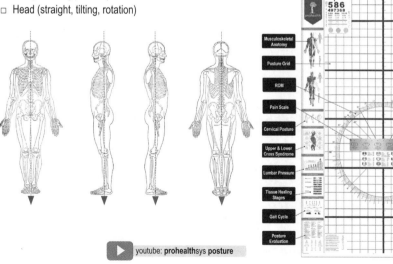

youtube: prohealthsys **posture**

Typical ADLs for North Americans

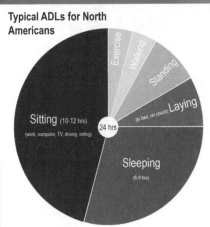

24 hrs

Sitting (10-12 hrs)
(work, computer, TV, driving, eating)

Exercise

Walking

Standing

(in bed, on couch) Laying

Sleeping
(6-8 hrs)

The human body is designed to move.

For 1,000's of years, that's exactly what we did. With urbanization & technological advances (cars, TV, computers, tractors) physical activity levels have been steadily dropping. As technology does more of the heavy lifting, people become increasingly sedentary.

Sitting disease - *metabolic syndrome & ill-effects of an overly sedentary lifestyle*

Did you know? Physical Inactivity is the 4th leading cause of mortality...

1. Smith L, Hamer M, Ucci M, et al. Weekday and weekend patterns of objectively measured sitting, standing, and stepping in a sample of office-based workers: the active buildings study. BMC Public Health. 2015;15:9.
2. Aggio D, Wallace K, Boreham N, Shankar A, Steptoe A, Hamer M. Objectively Measured Daily Physical Activity and Postural Changes as Related to Positive and Negative Affect Using Ambulatory Monitoring Assessments. Psychosomatic Medicine. 2017;79(7):792-797. doi:10.1097/PSY.0000000000000485.
3. The pandemic of physical inactivity: global action for public health.
4. Kohl HW 3rd, Craig CL, Lambert EV, Inoue S, Alkandari JR, Leetongin G, Kahlmeier S, Lancet Physical Activity Series Working Group. Lancet. 2012 Jul 21; 380(9838):294-305.

Limit all types of screen time and have **consistent changes of body position** through the entire day - **(sitting < 3 hrs/day day increase life expectancy by ~2 years).** Prolonged sedentary time is independently associated with negative health outcomes regardless of physical activity! **Sitting disease = prolonged sitting is the new smoking.** Average North American: 13 hrs/day sitting (computer, driving, phone, eating) + 8 hrs/day lying (sleep, lounging) = ~21 hrs/day of inactivity

(Aviroop, B. et. al. Sedentary Time and Its Association With Risk for Disease Incidence, Mortality, and Hospitalization in Adults: A Systematic Review and Meta-analysis. Annals of Internal Medicine. Jan, 2015.)

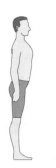 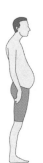 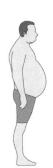 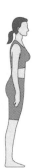 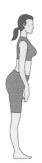 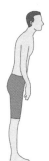 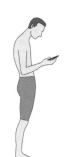

Attention! **Military spine**	**Sway** **Back**	**Base Drum** **Pregnancy**	**'Normal'** **Posture**	**The** **Duck**	**Head** **Start**	**Kyphotic** **Lordotic**

'Text Neck'

Also known as computer spine from excessive computer use

Neutral - 0°	**15°**	**30°**	**60°**	**45°**
~10 lbs (4.5kg)	**~27 lbs** (12kg)	**~40 lbs** (18kg)	**~60 lbs** (27kg)	**~49 lbs** (22kg)

Smart phone connect you to those far away, but disconnect you from the people close to you

Clinical Tip: have a section of clinic wall painted with a grid for more accurate postural and AROM assessment - posture exam form and Evidence Based Posture Assessment Chart on website

prohealthsys

Seated postures - ask patient to have co-workers/fellow student to **take a few pictures of them throughout the day so they can get a true evaluation of their habits** and allow their clinician a more accurate assessment.
Realize most texts on posture do not evaluate seated or sleeping postures...

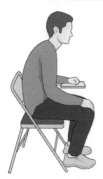 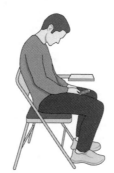 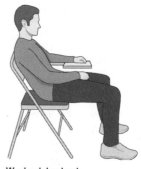

Student Standard / 'Office Express'
- Upper cross syndrome (chin poked, scapulae protracted, thorax in flexion, arms int. rot.)
- Shallow breath cycle

Crotcher (cell phone)
- Head bent (forehead parallel to ground), chin tucked
- Shoulders collapsed
- Shallow breath cycle

Wayback Layback
- Spine is a giant C
- Stretch of posterior elements
- Shallow breath cycle
- Does take pressure off spine

Sleeping Postures

Most common: short upper trap, lev. scap. pecs, abdominals, psoas, hip flexors & hamstrings

Stretched or inhibited posterior spine, rhomboids & mid trap (reinforces upper cross syndrome)

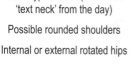
FETUS   YEARNER

too thin   too thick

Neck hyperflexion (reinforces 'text neck' from the day)

Possible rounded shoulders

Internal or external rotated hips

SOLDIER   VAMPIRE

Neck rotation bias

Possible neck hyperextension or hyperflexion

Shoulder & thoracic outlet issues

FREEFALLER   CACTUS

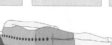
matress too firm ❌

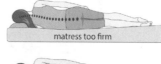
matress too soft ❌

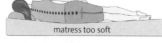
'spine in line, feeling fine' ✓
also consider a pillow between the knees

~30% of our life is spent sleeping it is crucial to evaluate sleep systems, habits & positions

"...when sleeping a busy mind makes for a lumpy pillow."
Good sleep requires a clear and relaxed mind and body, develope a relaxing sleep routine

- Many conditions of desk-bound workers, students & vehicle operators are associated with poor posture habits (headaches, muscle aches, stress, rotator cuff syndromes, carpal tunnel syndrome, thoracic outlet, respiratory issues, functional scoliosis, etc.)

- **Upper back rounded forward, shoulders become shrugged**

- **Head pushes forward & chin pokes (extension of cervical spine)**

- **Chest breathing predominates over belly breathing**

- **These postural faults result in standard muscle patterns of tightness & weakness referred to as upper & lower cross syndromes**

The supporting ligaments and joint capsules will also be shortened with prolonged postures (tissue contracture)

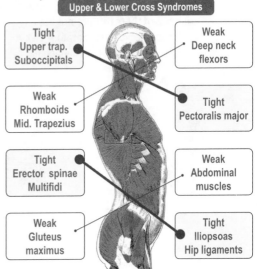

Upper & Lower Cross Syndromes

Tight Upper trap. Suboccipitals

Weak Deep neck flexors

Weak Rhomboids Mid. Trapezius

Tight Pectoralis major

Tight Erector spinae Multifidi

Weak Abdominal muscles

Weak Gluteus maximus

Tight Iliopsoas Hip ligaments

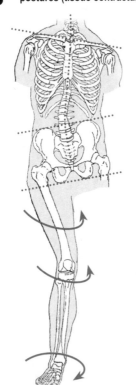

Over pronation causes medial rotation of the lower extremity and greater stresses across the ankle & knee

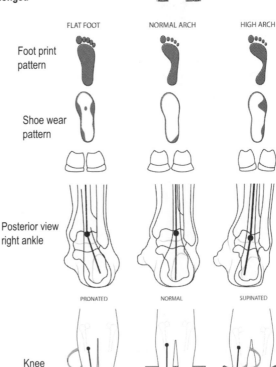

FLAT FOOT   NORMAL ARCH   HIGH ARCH

Foot print pattern

Shoe wear pattern

Posterior view right ankle

PRONATED   NORMAL   SUPINATED

Knee changes

Gait analysis is simply the observation of moving posture

video of gaits at prohealthsys.com

Type	Description	Potential causes
Antalgic Limp	Stance phase shortened More gentle heel-strike in painful limb	Secondary to lower extremity injury/ pain avoidance
Cerebellar or Ataxic	Unsteady, reeling to one side, slow start, unexpected/erratic (looks intoxicated)	Stroke, tumor, mid-cerebellar tumor
Back Knee Gait	Knee locked in hyperextension during stance phase May place hand on thigh to assist Difficulty with stairs	Quadriceps &/or gluteus maximus weakness
Drunken/Staggering	Inability to tandem walk (straight line heel to toe)	Alcohol, multiple sclerosis, brain tumor, drugs, paresis
Hemiplegic	Swinging/circumduction of affected leg	Stroke; hip or knee disease, immobility, sacroiliac fusion
Hysterical	Varies - usually grotesque movements, bizarre & inconsistent	Hysteria, possible malingering Diagnosis by exclusion
Mincing/Short Step	Little tiny steps that are slow from obvious pain	Lumbar disc syndrome Diffuse cerebellar disease
Propulsion/ Festination	Slow to fast; falling forward, arms held at sides; steps are short & shuffling	Parkinson's disease
Scissors	Spastic paraplegia - knees are pulling together & body swings laterally from the stepping limb	Cerebral palsy, some myodystrophies
Short Leg Limp	Limp may be disguised by pelvic tilt (scanogram, leg length check, Allis)	Congenital, post traumatic bone healing (especially femur)
Steppage or Foot Drop	Toe drop (slap): has to raise thigh of affected side excessively high to compensate (usually will not recover)	Unilateral peroneal neuritis, L5 disc herniation, compartment syndrome, muscle atrophy - Bilateral - polio
Tabetic or Ataxic	Wide stance, heel slapping Spinal ataxia - feet apart, looking at ground; Romberg positive	Syphilis, posterior column disease which causes proprioception loss
Trendelenberg Gait	Lurching gait with the pelvis tilting dramatically down on the affected side during swing phase	Gluteus medius &/or minimus weakness or paralysis
Waddling/Clumsy	Patient waddles side to side, Gower's/ Minor's sign - patient climbs up front of their thighs upon rising from a chair	Myo-Dystrophy, weak hip

Joint Assessment

prohealthsys

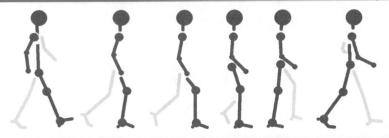

Stance Phase (60%)

Heel strike (~27%)	Midstance (~40%)	Take-off (~33%)

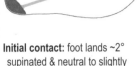 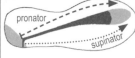 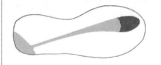

pronator / supinator

Initial contact: foot lands ~2° supinated & neutral to slightly dorsiflexed. Rapid ankle plantar flexion is controlled by leg muscles, especially tib. anterior

Foot adapts to ground by pronating & collapsing of arches to absorb shock

Forefoot strike: followed by rapid ankle dorsiflexion & pronation. Tibialis anterior eccentrically controls pronation, gastrosoleus controls dorsiflexion & absorbs shock

Loading response: knee flexes 15° while ankle plantar flexes ~15° (energy-conserving)

Hamstrings & ankle dorsiflexors remain active; quads & glutes act during loading & midstance to maintain hip & knee stability

Lower limb rotates internally, same hip adducts slightly & pelvis drops to opposite side. Controlled by gluteus med/min

Begins with contralateral toe off & ends when the center of gravity is directly over the reference foot

Momentum carries body over fixed foot. COG over a single stance limb

Foot starts fully pronated. It supinates through neutral & ends slightly supinated

Mid-foot: with mid-foot pronation the ankle dorsiflexes

Supination: foot inverts, adducts & ankle dorsiflexes at mid tarsal & subtalar joints

Concentric contractions of gluteus maximus & quadriceps only with resistance (ie. hills/wind)

Terminal stance: begins when the center of gravity is over the supporting foot & ends when the contralateral foot contacts the ground

Begins at contralateral initial contact & ends at toe off

COG anterior to stance limb

Preswing, knee flexes ~35° & ankle plantar flexes ~20°

Gastrosoleus lift (plantar flexes) heel

Tibialis posterior rapidly inverts heel at start

Supination of foot is complete (rigid foot) - subtalar locks mid tarsals

Toes passively extend (foot rolls like a wheel)

Increase weight on larger 1st toe. Metatarsal break helps distribute weight to other toes

Toe flexors eccentrically control toe extension aided by tension of the plantar fascia (Windlass effect)

Fibularis longus & big toe flexors stabilizes 1st ray & transverse arch & plantar flex 1st metatarsal

Thigh & leg extend & externally rotate

Step - advancement of a single foot

Stride - advancement of both feet (one step by each side of your body)

Double support - both feet on ground

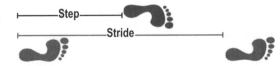

prohealthsys

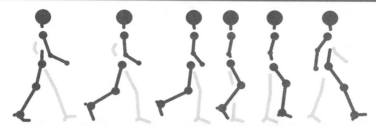

Swing Phase (40%)

Initial swing	Mid swing	Terminal swing
Starts with toe off & continues until maximum knee flexion (~60°) occurs **Knee flexes**, hip extends Completion of leg & thigh external rotation **Anterior thigh** (hip flexors) decelerate/ stop (eccentric contraction) Very little initial swing in walking, increases with increased speed	Change in direction, from maximum knee flexion until the tibia is vertical or perpendicular to the ground **Early:** hip flexors & quads 'whip' limb forward ('bowling ball effect') - concentric contraction **Late** (after swing limb crosses stance limb): hip extensors & knee flexors (glut max. & hamstrings) decelerate/ stop forward motion (eccentric contraction) **Dorsiflexors/ toe extensors:** hold foot dorsiflexed/ toes extended; otherwise accentuated hip/ knee flexion or toes drag on ground: 'foot drop' may also occur during foot strike **Internal hip rotators** (adductors) & hip capsule internally rotate hip	Change in direction, begins where the tibia is vertical & ends at initial contact **Hip & knee** extensors rapidly concentrically pull limb back to ground speed Amount of rotation affects foot orientation (toe-in or toe-out) during foot strike of next stance phase **Foot strike** = heel strike = end of swing phase

Velocity - stride length/cycle time (m/s); **Cadence** - steps /minute;
Float phase - neither foot is on the ground; **COG** - centre of gravity

Running Gait - during running stance phase decreases (~40%) & swing phase increases (~60%); the two periods of double support are replaced by periods of double float, and stance time is less than swing time. As speed increases the foot contact time with the ground decreases & float time increases

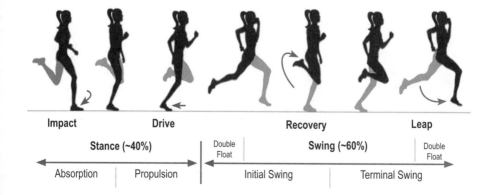

Impact	Drive		Recovery	Leap	
Stance (~40%)		Double Float	Swing (~60%)		Double Float
Absorption	Propulsion		Initial Swing	Terminal Swing	

Walking Speed

Every individual has a 'free' or comfortable walking speed on a smooth, level surface **that is most energy efficient** for them; changes to speed will affect all aspects of gait including time & distance measures, energy expenditures & muscle activity. The mean velocity for adults at a 'free' pace is: 5 km/h (3 mph), average stride length is 1.4 meters, mean cadence is ~112 steps per minute - on average, men tend to walk faster than women with a longer stride and slower cadence

- Men's average 100-120 steps/min
- Women's average 105-125 steps/min

Increasing walking speed results in decreased duration of stance and double support phase - in Olympic walking there must always be 1 foot on the ground or you are running (float phase)

Effects of age on Walking

Infants start walking at 11-15 months

- They contact the floor with a flat foot
- Use a wide base of support, prolonged stance phase
- Show marked external rotation of the hips with toes out at the feet
- Exhibit high guarding position of the arms
- Crash frequently!

By 2 years old:

- Heel strike & first knee flexion in stance appear
- Arms are lower, reciprocal arm swing appears
- External hip rotation occurs, base of support narrows

By age 4-5 years: children start to show adult type patterns

Note during rapid growth years and puberty there are often periods of incoordination and proprioceptive retraining that occur as the nervous system learns to use the change in limb length and muscle size

By age 60-65 years

- Slight changes to gait start to appear
- Tendency to walk slower
- Joint range of motion & stride length decrease, period of double support may increase, making a more stable gait

Energy Expenditure Walking

Walking speeds can vary greatly depending on many factors such as height, weight, age, terrain, surface, load, culture, effort, and fitness - average human walking speed is ~5.0 km/h (~3.1 mph). Walking uses about 3-4 times as much energy as resting (BMR)

Gait abnormalities increase energy expenditure due to:

- Excessive displacements of body's COG
- Muscles may have to work at high intensities or for prolonged periods
- Additional muscles may have to be recruited

Heal Stike Forces with Shoe

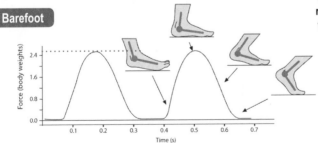

Net force is the same but how you get there is very different

The mid-foot strike of barefoot running drastically reduces the repetitive impact micro-trauma on the foot and body

Barefoot

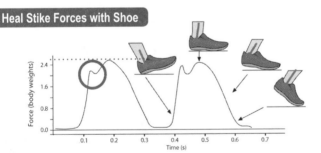

prohealthsys

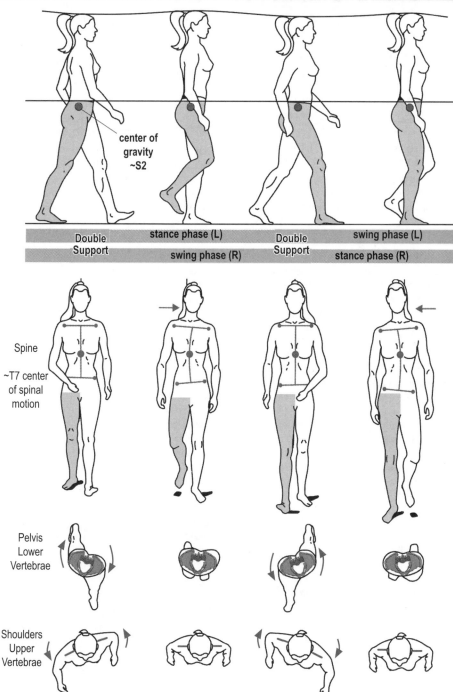

center of
gravity
~S2

| Double Support | stance phase (L) | Double Support | swing phase (L) |
| | swing phase (R) | | stance phase (R) |

Spine

~T7 center
of spinal
motion

Pelvis
Lower
Vertebrae

Shoulders
Upper
Vertebrae

Rotational movements occur in the vertebrae & hips. Clockwise & counter-clockwise rotation with
the point of minimal rotation at ~T7 - One arm & the opposite leg swing forward during gait.
At the Hip the pelvis rotates forward around the stance leg (called Pelvic Step)

Palpation Tips - For student & Instructors

- **Know anatomy terminology** - say the name out loud "with a smile"
- **Visualize** structure, **verbalize** the name, then **palpate on yourself** (confirm with instructor)
- **Visualize, verbalize, then palpate on classmate** (classmate should give feedback)
- **Palpate on other people and different body types & ages** (other classmates, friends, family)
- **Set up rotation stations** in class or during study time to move from body to body ("clinicians up, patients down on table... please locate the___, now ___, now __ ... and rotate")

- **Take a deep, grounding breath before you start.** Excellent palpation & physical skills demand relaxed hands, good anatomical understanding & hours of practice with direct mental concentration
- **Confident Hands.** people can quickly tell if their clinician is nervous or not comfortable, be patient with yourself, realize repeated practice is what develops confidence & skill
- **Stay in touch** (pun intended ☺) with your patient's comfort level - continually ask how they are doing & observe their mental & emotional affect (be present in the moment, ask for feedback & self analyze)
- Work in your **'strike zone'** to lower back fatigue

General Palpation

- Application of manual pressure to determine abnormalities (tenderness, pain, shape, size, pulsations, masses, position, tissue mobility & turgor) - **you should be able to give a list of all the structures below your hand**
- Excellent physical palpation skills demand hours of practice & **direct mental concentration** (do not palpate casually)
- **Use the least amount of pressure possible** (touch receptors respond best to light touch)
- Use a **broad or flat contact** whenever possible
- Closing eyes may increase palpatory sense
- **Develop a palpation routine** that is standard for you & apply it to all patients
- **Compare results bilaterally**
- Numerous studies show excellent inter-examiner reliability for the palpation of bony & soft tissue tenderness (palpation is one of the best tools a clinician can use)

Soft Tissue Palpation

- Dermal layer (skin): palpation & assessment of temperature, texture, mobility, tissue sensitivity (temperature assessment use back of hand - more sensitive to heat)
- Subcutaneous & deeper layers (fascia & muscle): palpation & assessment of texture, motility, tissue sensitivity, flexibility, muscle tenderness, myospasm, guarding or splinting, edema, asymmetry & muscle imbalance from side to side
- Consider using instruments to increase palpatory and treatment abilities (IASTM - proSTM1 or proSTM2)

Bony Palpation

- Purpose: location of landmarks, assess contours for tenderness or anomalies and to use as leverage for joint play & mobilization
- Procedure: generally palmar surface of fingers (most sensitive to touch)
- Bony tenderness may result from: joint dysfunction, direct trauma, fractures, bone infection, neoplasms, or osteoporosis

Motion Palpation

- Use of hands to assess and treat joint motion (may be active or passive)
- **Requires detailed understanding of functional anatomy, biomechanics, pathomechanics**
- Each joint has unique patterns & ROM
- Purpose: assessment of motion quality, quantity, end feel, joint play & symptoms that may occur
- Motion should be performed slowly & smoothly
- Compare results bilaterally
- Be sure to palpate both bones on either side of the joint & joint space if possible

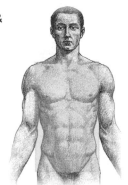

Strike zone

Work in this range for safer back biomechanics

It is important to **always use a well understood pain scale** during any physical assessment or treatment (palpation, massage, stretching, MET, IASTM, mobes, etc.). Establish pain reference at the beginning of each treatment (even if you have treated the patient, they may not always remember).

Keep in mind that telling the patient the pain scale doesn't mean that they will use it. Sometimes people feel like they should be able to deal with the pain, or they are too modest to tell you that they are in pain. Therefore, it is imperative that you not only use the pain scale and always check in with them but also watch their body language and facial expressions.

Subjective Pain Scale (verbal pain scale rating from 0-10 - ask patient to state where they are)

Descriptive Pain Intensity Scale

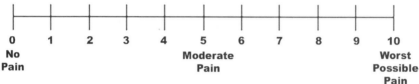

0	1	2	3	4	5	6	7	8	9	10
No Pain					Moderate Pain					Worst Possible Pain

Subjective Tenderness/Pain Scale - Palpation/Massage

Grade	Description
1	"Feel the pressure of my hand"
2	"A little pressure, but feels comfortable"
3	"Pressure, but is good" - 'joyful discomfort'
4	"Painful but you can breathe through it"
5	"STOP" - no longer tolerable

Objective Soft Tissue Tenderness/Pain Scale

Grade	Description
0	No tenderness
1	Tenderness with no physical response
2	Tenderness with grimace and/or flinch
3	Tenderness with withdrawal (= jump sign)
4	Withdrawal from non-noxious stimuli

Consistent pressure needs to be applied by the clinician pressure should be just enough to blanch fingernail capillary bed chart as a rating out of 4; e.g.; 0/4, 3/4, 2/4, 1/4, 0/4

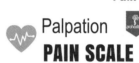
Palpation
PAIN SCALE

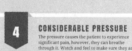

1 LIGHT PRESSURE
Therapist hands applying a light pressure, introducing their touch to the patient, used to stimulate superficial receptors on the skin.

2 SOLID PRESSURE
The pressure is felt as a slight weight applied to the body. This pressure is used for general massage techniques, usually for relaxation treatments.

3 THERAPEUTIC PRESSURE
The pressure is increased and there may be slight introduction of pain in tender areas. At this level, deeper tissues are targeted and is expected in a therapeutic treatment.

4 CONSIDERABLE PRESSURE
The pressure causes the patient to experience significant pain, however, they can breathe through it. Watch and feel to make sure they are consistantly breathing. Therapist can ask the patient to take in a deep breath and exhale.

5 STOP
Patient cannot breathe through the pain and needs to stop the treatment. Therapist may also notice that the patient is holding their breath.

! REMEMBER
When talking about the pain scale, also remind the patient that at any point throughout the treatment, they have the ability to request to stop for any reason.

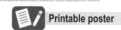 Printable poster

Realize that normal anatomical variation in bone size & shape may alter exact spinal levels being palpated

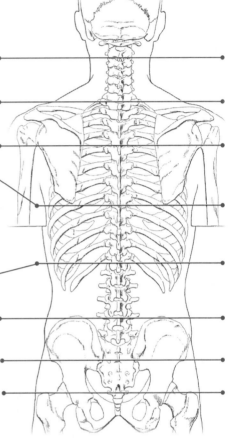

- **C2** - first palpable SP below the occipital bone

- **C7 or T1** - most prominent SP at base of neck (C7 will usually move from a palpating finger with cervical flexion/extension or rotation)

- **T4** - level with the root of the spine of scapula or apex of axillary fold

- **T7-T8** - level with the inferior angle of scapula

  Thoracic TP palpation Rule of 3s
  - **T1-T3 TPs:** at level of corresponding SP
  - **T4-T6 TPs:** ~½ segment *above* SP
  - **T7-T9 TPs:** ~1 segment *above* SP
    T10-T12 have TP's that project from a position similar to T9 & rapidly regress until T12 is like T1

- **T12** - level with the head of the 12th rib

- **L4** - level with the superior border of the iliac crest

- **PSIS & S2** - level with the most inferior portion of the PSIS

- **Sacral Apex** - level with upper greater trochanter (rotate patient's hip to locate trochanter)

Spinous process palpation using the scapular tip as a landmark vs a radiographic criterion standard . Journal of Chiropractic Medicine, Vol 6 , Issue 3 , PP 87-93. 2003. R. Cooperstein , M. Haneline

- *Method:* experienced palpator located inferior angle of scapular on 34 asymptomatic standing patients & positioned a 2-mm lead marker about 5 cm lateral to the nearest SP; markers were also placed at segments 3 above & below the 'T7' SP. The locations of the scapular tip and the spinal targets were determined by comparison with a radiological criterion standard.

- *Results:* the standing inferior scapular angle corresponded to the T8 SP on average (SD = 0.9)

- *Conclusion:* ~ 70% of patients have their inferior scapular angle at T7, T8, or T9; an experienced palpator can quite accurately locate vertebral levels 3 above or below a given landmark. Health professionals using the typical rule of thumb linking the inferior scapular tip to the standing T7 have likely been applying clinical interventions at spinal locations different from those intended (*this does not mean the treatment is ineffective, it is just not delivered at the exact level perceived by the practitioner*)

Factors Affecting ROM

Age

- **Infants:** typically have higher ROM for hip flexion / abduction / lateral rotation, dorsiflexion, and elbow motion (restricted ROM for hip extension, knee extension, and plantar flexion)

- **Older adults:** (60+ yrs) ROM decreases with age due to soft tissue contracture & atrophy; for limbs, losses in older adults typically are less than 15% however with **vertebral column ROM of older adults will decrease between 25% to 50% from their maximal ROM (regular stretching/yoga and mobilizations slows this process)**

Gender

- There are small to medium differences in ROM between women and men

- To determine if a ROM for an individual is impaired, compare the ROM values to the uninjured side (if possible) and ROM norms from a similarly age/gender sample *(see Prohealth Goniometer or Posture Chart)*

- During pregnancy women demonstrate increases in ROM due to increased ligament laxity (hormone Relaxin). This may last for up to 6 months post-partum

Injury

- Current or past injuries can limit ROM due to pain, scar tissue, atrophy, contracture or neurologic changes

Anatomical Variation

- Congenital (genetic) and developmental differences in joint shape, bone size, muscle, ligament and fascia or nerve supply can drastically affect ROM

- Genetic connective tissue disorders (Marfan, Loeys-Dietz, Ehlers-Danlos Syndrome)

Life-style

- Active lifestyle with regular stretching and motion (yoga) of soft tissues increases ROM and slows the aging process

Basic ROM Findings

- Full ROM without pain → normal finding
- Full ROM with pain → minor sprain/strain
- Hypomobility without pain → tissue contracture, adhesions or joint dysfunction
- Hypomobility with pain → acute sprain with possible muscle guarding or joint dysfunction
- Hypermobility without pain → complete ligament rupture
- Hypermobility with pain → partial ligament tear or sprain (intact fibers are being stressed)

Movement	Muscle	Ligament	Nerve
AROM	Pain	Pain	weak
PROM	-	Pain	-
RROM	Pain	-	weak

pain in multiple directions suggests joint/capsule damage, pain in a single direction indicates muscle, tendon or ligament damage

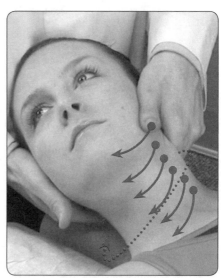

Index pillar mobilization into right rotation/left lateral flexion - note the angle of vectors changes as you move down the spine - it will also vary depending on specific patient anatomical variation (flexibility, bone shape, muscle tightness or discomfort)

Joint Assessment

Abnormal End Feel

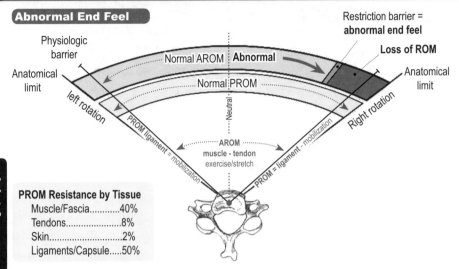

Restriction barrier = **abnormal end feel**

Physiologic barrier

Anatomical limit

Normal AROM **Abnormal**

Loss of ROM

Normal PROM

Anatomical limit

left rotation

Right rotation

PROM = ligament - mobilization

PROM = ligament - mobilization

Neutral

AROM
muscle - tendon
exercise/stretch

PROM Resistance by Tissue
Muscle/Fascia...........40%
Tendons.....................8%
Skin............................2%
Ligaments/Capsule.....50%

Schematic showing direction a joint or surrounding muscles & soft tissue can move towards a restriction barrier (abnormal end-feel) or towards a position of relative ease (normal). Osseous and/or soft tissue mobilization techniques may be applied to correct this fault.

Normal End Play (end feel)

	End Play	Definition (example)
Normal	**Tissue stretch**	Near end ROM hard/firm type of movement limited by tension in muscles & fascia (e.g. cervical lateral flexion)
	Soft tissue approximation	Squeezing quality, near end ROM where soft tissue compression prevents further motion (e.g. elbow flexion)
	Ligamentous	Hard, firm, painless end ROM, limited by tension in ligaments (e.g. normal knee extension)
	Bone to bone	Hard, non-giving, painless end ROM (e.g. elbow extension)

Normal end feels can be pathologic, if they happen at abnormal locations
eg. bony end feel in knee flexion, soft end feel in elbow extension

During ROM & end-feels clinicians need to identify the **DIRECTION of CORRECTION** to help restore function

Joint Assessment

Pathologic end feels occur either at a different place in the ROM than expected, or have an end feel that is not characteristic of the joint

End Play	Definition (example)
Bone to bone	Painful, hard end feel (osteophyte formation, ankylosis - fusion)
Muscle spasm	Guarded or splinting feel caused by movement reduction secondary to reactive myospasm to protect the injured tissue (apprehension, instability or trauma)
Capsular	Firm, decreased ROM accompanied with pain, but not myospasm (adhesions, adhesive capsulitis - scar tissue)
'Boggy'	Spongy end-feel secondary to diffuse swelling edema (eg. patellar ballottement)
Springy block	Bouncing or springy, seen in joints with menisci (knee mainly), associated rebound effect (internal derangement, meniscal tears)
Empty* / Absent	Lack of normal end ROM resistance, usually associated with an increase ROM (hypermobility, ligament rupture - normal end-feel is not there)
DNC	DNC - 'Did Not Complete' - patient stops movement of joint before resistance is felt (usually associated with fear of injury, pain or apprehension)

*Some authors erroneously call an incomplete exam an empty end-feel (David Magee-Orthopedic Physical Assessment, etc.). Case in point, if you were attempting to take blood pressure and the patient stopped the procedure you would NOT chart "empty blood pressure" - it is a DNC.

Abnormal (Pathologic)

Joint Assessment

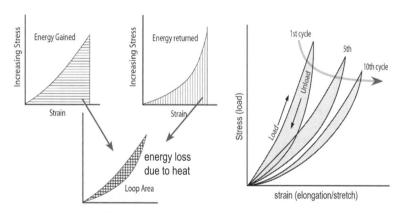

Hysteresis - energy loss from impulse loading & unloading heat generation

Creep - deformation from constant load

With repeated load-unload cycles there is a point of diminishing returns for tissue elongation (trend line - arrow)

Be aware that specific end-feels change with repeated loading as the tissue literally warms up, there is usually an increase in ROM (this is know as a *hysteresis loop* as the tissue stretches with serial loading and energy is lost in the gradual lengthening of tissue). Typically after 10 load/unload cycles the curves tend to flatten out with the largest change occurring in the first few cycles, and diminishing returns with each additional cycle. This is also why it is important to warm up prior to stretching and why joint mobilizations are so effective at increasing ROM. Be aware that older or damaged tissue will have lower functional capacity with the effects of immobilization or extreme activity being detrimental to healing.

Woo, SL. Anatomy, biomechanics of tendon, ligament and meniscus. Woo SL, Chan SS, Yamaji T: J Biomechics 30(5):431-439, 1997.

ABCs of Manual Muscle Testing

- **Active Range of Motion (AROM)** - region tested is taken through its full range of motion (establish a baseline of function, warms up muscle capillary beds & neuronal activation)

- **Break test** is a muscle strength test to determine effort exerted by a subject who is performing an **isometric contraction** (examiner applies a **gradual** buildup of pressure to the patient) - apply force along the fiber direction of the muscle (origin to insertion)

- **Concentric Contraction** - patient is asked to perform **concentric AROM** against resistance provided by the examiner (resist enough to **let the patient win**)

- **Stretch** muscle to determine flexibility & length (**PROM** origin away from insertion)

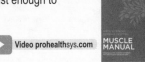

Video prohealthsys.com

MUSCLE MANUAL

Muscle Testing Rules

- Patient is positioned in optimum posture - if possible have the patient supine or prone to eliminate postural muscle action
    - Isolate specific muscle (as much as possible)
    - Stabilize region & have a confident flow
- Clinician states *"Don't let me move you"* or *"resist my force"* & demonstrates motion to be resisted
- Ask patient to hold position & relax when test is done ("hold, hold, hold, & relax")
    - **Typically patient holds position for 5 secs and may repeat 3x**
    - **If there is a high index of suspicion of muscle damage or neurologic compromise then...**
        - Hold for 5-10 seconds or,
        - Repeat for up to 10 repetitions (e.g. chart as 3/5 at 8x) or,
        - Test at multiple angles through ROM, and through eccentric, concentric, isometric contractions - remember muscles tend to have their maximum strength through the mid ROM of length

Functional Muscle Testing

Grade	Definition
Functional	5 sec hold, 5-6 reps
Fair	3-4 sec hold, 2-4 reps
Poor	1-2 sec hold, 1-2 reps
Non Functional	0 sec, 0 reps

- For a break test joint motion should be minimal (joint motion with muscle testing also challenges supporting ligaments and cartilage surfaces and can make interpretation more difficult)
    - Common error is to move joint too much, thereby testing many different muscles & joint capsule/cartilage
    - **Compare results bilaterally** & keep in mind dominant vs. non-dominant extremity
    - Palpate muscle tissue during test as biomechanics allow
- Examiner must remember to use good ergonomics & biomechanics
- For muscles that are typically stronger than examiner can resist, assess in a functional position. Example Gastrocnemius, start with standing bilateral plantar flexion, then unilateral dominant or good side then affected side

Stretch Muscle (Length Testing)

- Performed to determine if range of muscle length is normal, limited, or excessive
    - **Excessive length** usually indicates weak and allow adaptive shortening of opposing muscles and/or ligament laxity at the joint
    - **Short length** usually indicates strong and maintain opposing muscles in a lengthened position
- Muscle length testing consists of movements that increase the distance between origin and insertion (opposite of the concentric actions); use passive and/or active-assisted movements to determine muscle flexibility

An accurate & objective measurement of muscle strength is useful for many reasons:

- **Neurologic screen** - assessment of muscle strength also assesses motor nerve function

- **Diagnostic aid** - helps clinician identify specific muscles that are weak or damaged

- **Therapeutic aid** - creates an objective measure of progress through a treatment plan & allows the patient to witness the effect & necessity of treatment - also builds neuromuscular strength

Grading Muscle Strength

Grade		%	Definition
5	Normal	100%	Patient can maintain position against *full* examiner-applied resistance (4+ if shaking with resistance may indicate stabilizer weakness or proprioceptive issue)
4	Good*	~75%	Patient can maintain position against gravity & against *moderate* examiner-applied resistance (3+ resist *minimal* force)
3	Fair*	~50%	Movement against gravity but *not* against examiner's resistance
2	Poor*	~25%	Movement possible, not against gravity
1	Trace	~5%	Evidence of slight contractility; *little* or *no joint motion (twitch)*
0	Zero	0%	No palpable or perceivable evidence of contractility (*flaccid*)

% = % normal strength, ROM = range of motion, *Pain, muscle spasm or contracture may limit strength or ROM
Chart as a rating out of 5; e.g.; 5/5, 4/5, 3/5, 2/5, 1/5, 0/5

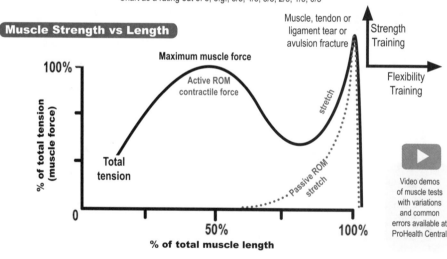

Muscle Strength vs Length

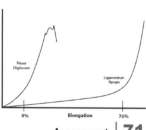

Video demos of muscle tests with variations and common errors available at ProHealth Central

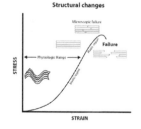

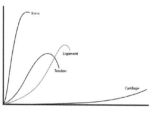

There are ~456 articulations in the adult skeleton.

It is difficult to count the number of joints in the body (depends on definition, age and anatomical variation)

Spine (177)

- **Cervical Spine (21)**
  - Atlanto-occipital joints (2)
  - Atlanto-dental joint
  - C1-C2 joints (2)
  - C2-C3 joints (2)
  - Zygapophyseal joints (10)
  - Intervertebral discs (6)
    1. C2-C3
    2. C3-C4
    3. C4-C5
    4. C5-C6
    5. C6-C7
    6. C7-T1

- **Thoracic Spine (98)**
  - Zygopophyseal (24)
  - Intervertebral discs (12)
    1. T1-T2
    2. T2-T3
    3. T3-T4
    4. T4-T5
    5. T5-T6
    6. T6-T7
    7. T7-T8
    8. T8-T9
    9. T9-T10
    10. T10-T11
    11. T11-T12
    12. T12-L1
  - Costovertebral (40)
    *lumbar/cervical ribs are possible
    1. T1 (4)
    2. T2 (4)
    3. T3 (4)
    4. T4 (4)
    5. T5 (4)
    6. T6 (4)
    7. T7 (4)
    8. T8 (4)
    9. T9 (2)
    10. T10 (2)
    11. T11 (2)
    12. T12 (2)
  - Costotransverse (20) (not at T11 or 12)

  **Scapulocostal (2 not a true joint)

- **Sternum (38)**
  1. Sternocostal (14)
  2. Costochondral (20)
  3. Manubriosternal (1)
  4. Xiphisternal (1)
  5. Sternoclavicular (2)

- **Lumbar, Pelvis & Coccyx (20)**
  1. Zygapophyseal (10)
  2. Intervertebral discs (5)
     - L1-L2
     - L2-L3
     - L3-L4
     - L4-L5
     - L5-S1
  3. Rarely can have L6 vertibra
  4. Sacroiliac (2)

5. S5-Co1
6. Co1-Co2
   *Co2-4 are usually fused
7. Pubic symphysis (1)

Upper Limb (88 joints)
1. Acromioclavicular
2. Glenohumeral
3. Humeralulnar
4. Humeroradial
5. Proximal Radioulnar
6. Distal Radioulnar

- **Hand & Wrist (76 joints)**
  1. Radioscaphoid
  2. Radiolunate
  3. Ulnatriquetrum (TFCC)
  4. Scaphotrapezium
  5. Scaphotrapazoid
  6. Scaphocapitate
  7. Scapholunate
  8. Lunatecapitate
  9. Lunotriquetrum
  10. Lunatehamate
  11. Triquetriumpisiform
  12. Triquetriumhamate
  13. Hamatecapitate
  14. Capitatetrapezoid
  15. Trapeziotrapezium
  16. Hamate MC5
  17. Hamate MC4
  18. Capitate MC3
  19. Capitate MC2
  20. Trapezoid MC2
  21. Trapezium MC1
  22. Trapezium MC2
  23. Metacarpal phalangal (5)
  24. Interphalangeal (thumb only)
  25. Proximal interphalangeal joints (4)
  26. Distal interphalangeal joints (4)
  27. Medial sesamoid-1st metacarpal
  28. Lateral sesamoid-1st metacarpal

Lower Limb (88 joints)
1. Acetabulofemoral
2. Tibiofemoral
3. Patellofemoral
4. Proximal Tibiofibular
5. Distal Tibiofibular

- **Foot & Ankle (78 joints)**
  1. Tibio-talus
  2. Fibulo-talus
  3. Calcaneo-talus
  4. Calcaneo-cuboid
  5. Talo-navicular
  6. Talo-cuboid
  7. Naviculo-cuboid
  8. Naviculo-medial cuneiform
  9. Naviculo-intermediate cuneiform
  10. Naviculo-lateral cuneiform
  11. Medial-intermediate cuneiform
  12. Intermediate-lateral cuneiform
  13. Cubo-lateral cuneiform
  14. Cubo-4th metatarsal
  15. Cubo-5th metatarsal

16. Lateral cuneiform-3rd metatarsal
17. Intermediate cuneiform-2nd metatarsal
18. Lateral cuneiform-2nd metatarsal
19. Medial cuneiform-1st metatarsal
20. 1st-2nd metatarsal
21. 2nd-3rd metatarsal
22. 3rd-4th metatarsal
23. 4th-5th metatarsal
24. Metatarsal phalangeal (5)
25. Interphalangeal (1) big toe
26. Proximal interphalangeal joints (4)
27. Distal interphalangeal joints (4)
28. Medial sesamoid-1st metatarsal
29. Lateral sesamoid-1st metatarsal

Skull (103 joints)
- **Temporomandibular (2)**
- **Teeth (32 gomphosis)**
- **Sutures in the skull (69)** - extra sutural
  bones are common
  - Left/right (2 sided): (62)
    1. parietal - sphenoid
    2. parietal - frontal
    3. parietal - temporal
    4. parietal - occipital
    5. frontal - nasal
    6. frontal - lacrimal
    7. frontal - maxilla
    8. frontal - sphenoid
    9. frontal - ethmoid
    10. frontal zygomatic
    11. occipital - sphenoid
    12. occipital - temporal
    13. temporal - sphenoid
    14. temporal - zygomatic
    15. nasal - ethmoid
    16. nasal - maxilla
    17. zygomatic - maxilla
    18. zygomatic - sphenoid
    19. lacrimal - maxilla
    20. lacrimal - ethmoid
    21. lacrimal - inferior nasal conchae
    22. inferior nasal concha - maxilla
    23. ethmoid - maxilla
    24. ethmoid - palatine
    25. ethmoid - inferior nasal conchae
    26. sphenoid - maxilla
    27. sphenoid - palatine
    28. vomer - palatine
    29. vomer - maxilla
    30. palatine - inferior nasal conchae
    31. palatine - palatine
  - One sided: (7)
    1. parietal - parietal
    2. nasal - nasal
    3. vomer - sphenoid
    4. vomer - ethmoid
    5. vomer - occipital
    6. ethmoid - sphenoid
    7. palatine - maxilla

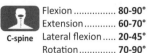

C-spine
Flexion .... **80-90°**
Extension .... **60-70°**
Lateral flexion ..... **20-45°**
Rotation .... **70-90°**

T-spine
Flexion .... **20-45°**
Extension .... **25-45°**
Lateral flexion ..... **20-40°**
Rotation .... **35-50°**

L-spine
Flexion .... **40-60°**
Extension .... **20-35°**
Lateral flexion . **15-20°**
Rotation .... **3-18°**

Shoulder
Flexion .... **160-180°**
Extension .... **50-60°**
Abd/add .... **180/35°**
Med/lat rotation. **90/80°**
Horizontal ab/ad. **45/130°**

Elbow
Flexion .... **~150°**
Extension .... **0 to -5°**
Supination* .... **~90°**
Pronation* .... **~90°**
*From neutral - 'thumbs up'

Wrist
Flexion .... **80-90°**
Extension .... **70-90°**
Ulnar flexion .. **30-45°**
Radial flexion . **~15°**
Sup/pro .... **85-90°**

Hip
Flexion (SLR) .... **~90°**
Flexion (knee bent) **~120°**
Extension .... **10-15°**
Abd/add .... **~40/30°**
Med/lat rotation. **~40/50°**

Knee
Flexion .... **130-150°**
Extension .... **0-15°**
Medial rot* .... **20-30°**
Lateral rot* .... **30-40°**
*knee must be flexed 90°

Ankle
Plantar flex ... **50°**
Dorsiflexion .. **20°**
Supination .... **45-60°**
Pronation...... **15-30°**
Big Toe
Flex MTP/IP **45/90°**
Ext MTP/IP . **70/0°**

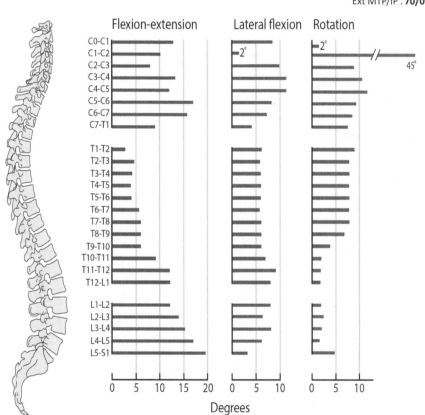

Flexion-extension | Lateral flexion | Rotation

C0-C1, C1-C2, C2-C3, C3-C4, C4-C5, C5-C6, C6-C7, C7-T1

T1-T2, T2-T3, T3-T4, T4-T5, T5-T6, T6-T7, T7-T8, T8-T9, T9-T10, T10-T11, T11-T12, T12-L1

L1-L2, L2-L3, L3-L4, L4-L5, L5-S1

0 5 10 15 20 | 0 5 10 | 0 5 10

Degrees

Depending numerous factors, functional AROM can vary greatly
(anatomical variation, bone/joint shape, flexibility, muscle mass, training adaptation, scar tissue, injury, pain, contracture, ligament laxity, posture, ADLs, genetics)

Adapted from: White, A & Panjabi, M. Clinical Biomechanics of the Spine. Lippincott, 1978. Hoppenfeld, S. Physical Examination of the Spine & Extremities. New York: Appleton-Century Crofts, 1976. Kapandji, LA. Physiology of the Joints. Vols. 1& 2, second edition. Demeter et al. Disability Evaluation. American Medical Association, Mosby 2003. American Academy of Orthopedic Surgeons 2018.

Gonia (G): angle, metron (G): measure

- Goniometry is the **measurement of angles at joints** by the bones of the body through ROM and requires 4 key concepts
  - Patient Position
  - Patient Stabilization
  - Goniometer Positioning
  - Recording Data
- Starting position for measuring all ROM, except for rotations in the transverse plane, is the anatomical position
- 0° - 180° notation is most commonly used
  - 0° starting at the anatomical, or 'start', position, and the body angle increasing towards 180°

Patient Position

- Place the joint in a consistent zero starting position
  - This affects the amount of tension present in soft tissue structures surrounding the joint
  - If any structures are tight, ROM will be affected
- **Stabilize the proximal joint segment**
- Must be the same for successive measurements of ROM in order to have a reliable basis for comparison - it should be the same examiner & goniometer each time
- Occasionally creativity is required to obtain ROM when normal testing positions are not possible (eg. patient injuries, specific conditions, etc.); in this case, record precisely the position used in the subject's records.

Patient Stabilization

- **Isolate motion to one joint** to ensure that a true measurement is obtained
- If both distal and proximal joint segments are able to move, it is difficult to determine ROM
- Examiner may provide additional stabilization manually using hand or body weight

Goniometer or inclinometer Position

- Align arms of goniometer with both proximal and distal segments of the joint - centre of goniometer should be over the axis of rotation
- Use bony landmarks & palpation to accurately visualize the joint segments (increases reliability and accuracy)
- *Goniometer*
  - **Stationary arm:** parallel to proximal segment of joint.
  - **Moving arm:** parallel to distal segment of joint. (In some situations, this may be reversed).
  - **Fulcrum of goniometer:** over joint axis
  - Read the goniometer at eye level
  - Understand the scale that you are using and read it correctly (know the intervals)
- *Inclinometer*
  - Requires the use of 2 instruments but is useful for rotatory movement of the spine and eliminating the effects of a lack of patient stabilization
  - Place one inclinometer on the above segment the other on the lower segment, zero out each instrument have the patient move can calculate the difference between the two

Recording Data

- Standard date - name, age, and gender along with examiners name
- Date, time and type of goniometer (eg. pain scale goniometer - 'PSG')
- Side of body, joint, and motion (eg. left knee flexion - compare bilaterally)
- Type of motion (active or passive)
- ROM – usually do 2 measures; if both are close, take the average
- Subjective (i.e. pain) and objective (i.e. spasm, crepitus) information with description of deviations from 'normal' testing positions
- Consider using star diagrams (below) to record data

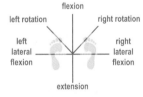

Spinal Joint

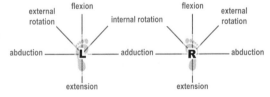

Peripheral Joint

Joint Assessment

Joint measurement reliability of goniometric instruments can be questionable – especially between different examiners

To **maximize reliability** always use the same:
- **Positioning, Procedure**
- **Goniometer, Examiner**

Protocols are shown by body region in individual chapters

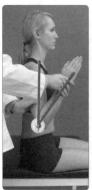
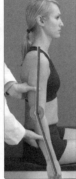

Goniometery Elbow Flexion
(normal 150°-160°)
- Patient prone or seated
- Fulcrum aligned with lateral epicondyle
- Stationary arm along the midline of the humerus, the moving arm is aligned with the radial styloid process
- Ask patient to flex elbow

Inclinometer Thoracic Flexion
(normal 50°-70°)
- Patient standing
- Zero inclinometers over T1 & T12
- Ask patient to flex trunk, subtract T1 inclination from T12 inclination = ROM
- 2 smart phones can also be used

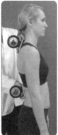
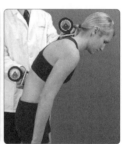

Pain Scale Goniometer (PSG)

Uses reference ranges from the American Academy of Orthopaedic Surgeons, is easy to use, portable durable and low cost - use of this instrument allows the creation of quantifiable clinical outcomes that can be tracked over time to gage patient response to treatment or collect data for research.

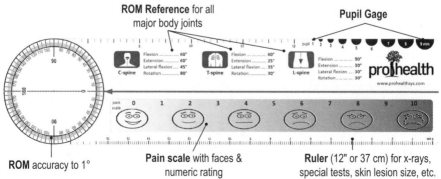

ROM Reference for all major body joints

Pupil Gage

	Flexion .... 60°
C-spine	Extension .... 60°
	Lateral flexion .... 45°
	Rotation .... 80°

	Flexion .... 60°
T-spine	Extension .... 25°
	Lateral flexion .... 35°
	Rotation .... 30°

	Flexion .... 90°
L-spine	Extension .... 30°
	Lateral flexion .... 30°
	Rotation .... 30°

prohealth
www.prohealthsys.com

ROM accuracy to 1°

Pain scale with faces & numeric rating

Ruler (12" or 37 cm) for x-rays, special tests, skin lesion size, etc.

Joint Assessment

Grade of Mobility		Treatment options
0	Fused	No motion (fusion/ankylosis) - do not mobilize
1	Severe hypomobility	Mobilization (will take time to see results), IASTM
2	Mild hypomobility	Mobilization-Manipulation, massage, stretching
3	Normal	No dysfunction = no treatment required
4	Mild hypermobility	Look for hypomobility/compensation in adjacent joints Exercise, taping, bracing, etc
5	Severe hypermobility	Look for hypomobility in other regions, biomechanical issues Exercise, taping, bracing, etc
6	Unstable	Look for hypomobility in adjacent joints Consider surgical consultation, bracing, casting

Grades 0-2 are labelled "Hypo"; grades 4-6 are labelled "Hyper"

*Pain, muscle spasm or contracture may limit ROM - remember joints can also be unstable through any part of their ROM
Chart as a rating out of 6; e.g.; 6/6, 5/6, 4/6, 3/6, 2/6, 1/6, 0/6

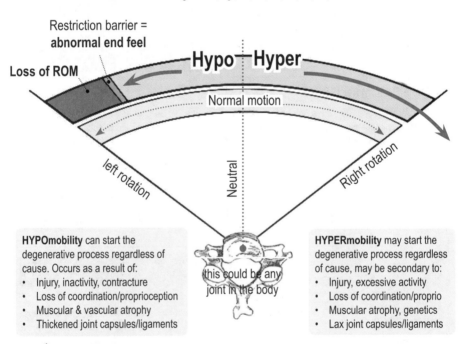

Restriction barrier =
abnormal end feel

Loss of ROM

Hypo — Hyper

Normal motion

left rotation

Neutral

Right rotation

HYPOmobility can start the degenerative process regardless of cause. Occurs as a result of:
- Injury, inactivity, contracture
- Loss of coordination/proprioception
- Muscular & vascular atrophy
- Thickened joint capsules/ligaments

this could be any joint in the body

HYPERmobility may start the degenerative process regardless of cause, may be secondary to:
- Injury, excessive activity
- Loss of coordination/proprio
- Muscular atrophy, genetics
- Lax joint capsules/ligaments

World Health Organization 'Subluxation' (joint dysfunction) Definition

"A lesion or dysfunction in a joint or motion segment in which alignment, movement integrity and/or physiological function are altered, although contact between joint surfaces remains intact. It is essentially a functional entity, which may influence biomechanical and neural integrity."

	Type & Description	Management Suggestions
Subluxation	**Incidental cavitation** or 'click'	Body corrects by itself (normal ADLs, ROM, stretch, yoga) - can be joint capsule, lig, muscle or fibrocartilage issue
	Intentional self correction	Person self corrects (non-specific twist of spine or lateral flexion of neck, flick of wrist or knee, etc.) - this non-specific technique can create segmental hypermobility
	'Superficial' subluxation	Often cavitates or shifts with mobilization or on set-up, is usually a hypermobile segment that moves first - may give a junior practitioner a false sense of confidence or ability
	Mild subluxation - very obvious end ROM, minimal muscle spasm or pain	Easy to mobilize by entry level practitioner - often requires minimal soft tissue work
	Moderate subluxation - more difficult to find end ROM, stronger level of muscle spasm and pain	Requires moderate skill and experience, clinician may choose to try and mobilize from the opposite side to reduce pain - requires some soft tissue treatment pre & post treatment - **~1 week follow up is usually OK**
	Severe subluxation - severe pain and muscle spasm - often too acute to adjust or mobilize directly	Requires significant soft tissue treatment pre & post mobilization - clinician must be very skilled to treat correctly - **1-2 day follow-up is required**
Luxation	**Mild dislocation**	Reducible through osseous mobilization - closed reduction (carpals, shoulder, finger, patella etc.) - **fracture must be ruled out**
	Severe dislocation	Requires surgical intervention - open reduction. Often associated with co-existing fracture - **ER referral**

Realize that joints usually have a **restriction of motion** in a specific direction with normal static position **(motion restriction)** or more rarely static malpositions may occur (bone out of place model)

Listings given refer to the position of the **superior vertebrae in relation to the inferior vertebrae**

Eg. C4-5 right rotation restriction

Dotted arrows show **direction motion restriction** and **direction of correction** with mobilization to restore normal ROM (vertebral bodies show malposition)

Neutral

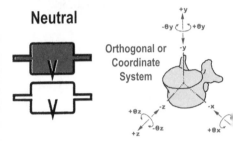

Orthogonal or Coordinate System

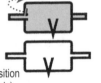

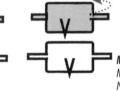

Motion: **Right Rot. Rest.**
Medicare: Left Rot. Malposition
National: LP (Left post. Body)
Gonstead: PR (Post. Right SP)
Orthogonal: +θy malposition
Osteopathic: L rotation lesion

Motion: **Left Rot. Rest.**
Medicare: Right Rot. Malpositic
National: RP (Right post. Body)
Gonstead: PL (Post. Left SP)
Orthogonal: -θy malposition
Osteopathic: R rotation lesion

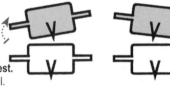

Motion: **Right Lat. Flex. Rest.**
Medicare: Left Lat. Flex. Mal.
National: LI (Left inf. Body)
Gonstead: none
Orthogonal: -θz malposition
Osteo: L side-bending lesion

Motion: **Left Lat. Flex. Rest.**
Medicare: Right Lat. Flex. Mal.
National: RI (Right inf. Body)
Gonstead: none
Orthogonal: +θz malposition
Osteo.: R side-bending lesion

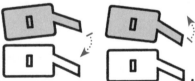

Motion: **Extension Restriction**
Medicare: Flexion Malposition
National: AI (Ant. Inf. Body)
Gonstead: none
Orthogonal: +θx malposition

*extension restrictions are very common in the thoracic spine

Motion: **Flexion Restriction**
Medicare: Extension Malpositic
National: PI (post. inf. body)
Gonstead: P (post. SP)
Orthogonal: -θx malposition

Rot. = rotation, Mal. = Malposition, SP = spinous process, inf. = inferior, sup. = Superior, post. = posterior, Ant. = anterior, Lat. = lateral, L = Left, R = Right, Rest. = Restriction, Flex
Flexion, Ext. = Extension, R_R = rotation right, R_L = rotation left, S_R = side-bending right, S_L = side-bending left, N = neutral (also be noted as F), NN = non-neutral (also be noted as E
= left, R = right, Csp = cervical spine, Tsp = thoracic spine, Lsp = lumbar spine

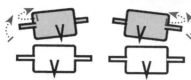

Motion: R Rot. R Lat Flex. Rest.
Medicare: L Rot. L Lat. Flex. Mal.
National: LPI (L post. inf. Body)
Gonstead: PRS (Post. R sup. SP)
Orthogonal: +θy, -θz mal.
Osteo: Csp: NNS_LR_L or NR_LS_L; Tsp/Lsp: NNR_LS_L

Motion: L Rot. L Lat. Flex. Rest.
Medicare: R Rot. R Lat. Flex. Mal.
National: RPI (R post. inf. Body)
Gonstead: PLS (Post. L sup. SP)
Orthogonal: -θy, +θz mal.
Osteo: Csp: NNS_RR_R or NR_RS_R; Tsp/Lsp: NNR_RS_R

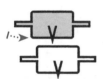

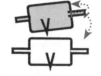

Motion: R Rot. L Lat. Flex. Rest.
Medicare: L Rot. R Lat. Flex. Mal.
National: LPS (L post. sup. body)
Gonstead: PRI (Post. R inf. SP)
Orthogonal: +θy, +θz mal.
Osteo: Tsp/Lsp: NS_RR_L (no Csp equivalent)

Motion: L Rot. R Lat. Flex. Rest.
Medicare: R Rot. L Lat. Flex Mal.
National: RPS (R post. sup. body)
Gonstead: PLI (post. L inf. SP)
Orthogonal: -θy, -θz mal.
Osteo: Tsp/Lsp: NS_LR_R (no Csp)

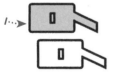

Motion: Right lateral restriction
Medicare: Left Lateral Listhesis
National: LL (Left Lat. body)
Gonstead: none
Orthogonal: +x malposition

Motion: Left lateral restriction
Medicare: Right Lateral Listhesis
National: RL (Right Lateral Body)
Gonstead: none
Orthogonal: -x malposition

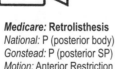

Medicare: Anterolisthesis
National: A (anterior body)
Gonstead: none
Motion: Posterior Restriction
Orthogonal: +z malposition

Medicare: Retrolisthesis
National: P (posterior body)
Gonstead: P (posterior SP)
Motion: Anterior Restriction
Orthogonal: -Z malposition

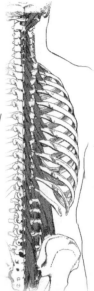

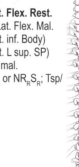

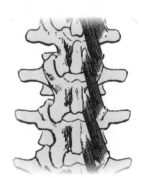

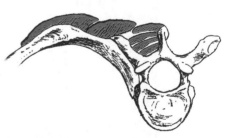

Do NOT only use static palpation and SP position to diagnose vertebral subluxation.
After 100s of cadaver dissections and 1000s of patients, it is this authors opinion, there is too much
anatomical variation in the size and shape of SPs, and bones in general for this practice to be accurate
- combined with AROM, PROM & end feel assessment for accurate evaluation -
remember bones shape, muscles, fascia and ligaments can alter vertebral motion

Joint Assessment

prohealthsys

Cause or ↓ ROM	Identification & treatment options
Soft Tissue Restriction	Palpable findings - pin and stretch, massage, IASTM
Shortened Extra-articular Muscle Groups	ROM affected by proximal or distal joint positioning - stretch, massage IASTM, PNF, MET
Muscle Weakness	Decreased muscle strength - Strengthen, neuromuscular retraining
Pain	Empty end-feel - Grade 1-2 mobilization
Nerve Root Adhesion	(+) nerve tension signs (SLR, brachial stretch) - neural mobilization
Intra-articular Adhesions or Pericaspsular Stiffness	ROM unaffected by proximal or distal joint positioning, capsular end feel - Joint Mobilization or Manipulation

Joint Assessment (sidebar)

Types of Hypermobility (instability)				
Generalized	Segmental	Functional	Structural	Surgical
Multiple joints	"Dysfunction"	Programming	Ligamentous damage	
May be genetic	Compensatory	Unstable mid-range	Unstable end-range	Very unstable
Significance? May be normal variation	*Reversible* Hypomobile segments around hypermobile	*Chronic/recurrent,* muscle imbalance (neuromuscular training)	*Difficult to reverse* (long term therapy & rehab.)	*Surgery* (grade 3-5 spon- dylolithesis)

No major structural damage → mild damage → moderate damage → serious damage

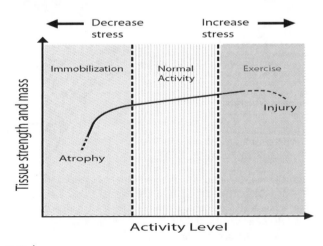

Decrease stress ←   Increase stress →

Tissue strength and mass (vertical axis)

Immobilization | Normal Activity | Exercise

Injury

Atrophy

Activity Level

Treatments and lifestyle choice must reach a balance in activities for optimal function

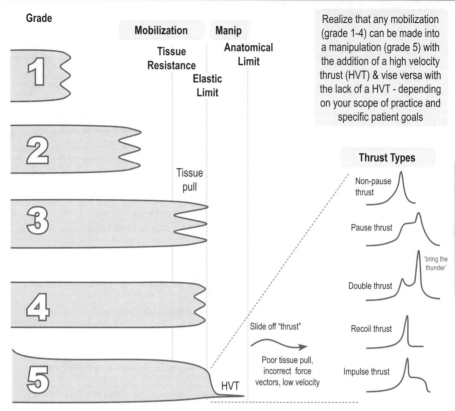

Grade

Mobilization **Manip**

Tissue Resistance **Anatomical Limit**

Elastic Limit

Realize that any mobilization (grade 1-4) can be made into a manipulation (grade 5) with the addition of a high velocity thrust (HVT) & vise versa with the lack of a HVT - depending on your scope of practice and specific patient goals

Thrust Types

Tissue pull

Non-pause thrust

Pause thrust

'bring the thunder'

Double thrust

Slide off "thrust"

Recoil thrust

Poor tissue pull, incorrect force vectors, low velocity

Impulse thrust

HVT

Joint Assessment

Grades 1-2

- Neurophysiological effect to reduce pain by neuromodulation on the sensory innervation of joint mechanoreceptors and pain receptors

- Gates pain achieved by the inhibition of transmission of nociceptive stimuli at the spinal cord and brain stem level

- Neutralizes joint pressure & reduces crepitus (grinding of rough surfaces with load)

Grades 3-5

- Increase ROM through promotion of capsular mobility and plastic deformation

- Mechanical distention and/or stretching of shortened tissues

- Grade 5 offers the deepest tissue stimulation

- Neurophysiological effects same as grade 1-2

Oscillations vs. Prolonged Hold

- Both stimulate type 1 & 2 mechanoreceptors
- Oscillations (60-120/min, 1-5 sets of 5-60 sec – generally used to treat pain)
- Prolonged Hold (5-30 sec. 1-5 reps, typically used at end range to treat stiffness) - stimulate type 3 mechano receptors & inhibit muscle guarding
- Variations include
  - Static Stretching
  - Post Isometric Relaxation (PIR),
  - Proprioceptive Neuromusc. Facilitation (PNF)
  - Post Facilitation,
  - Contract-Relax with Agonist Contract (CRAC),
  - Pin & Stretch (active release)

Use a **soft or gentle end range pressure to reduce guarding and discomfort**. When learning do NOT hold people in a hard end-ROM - relax your hands/body for more effective application.

S

Chief concern:
#1 – Mid-Back pain
#2 - Right mild subacute gastrosoleus strain (ddx from prior visit) "getting better"

O: Yesterday
Prog: "blow-drying my hair", all of a sudden it hurt to breath, experienced a sharp pain in left upper back
Pa: Moving slowly
Prov: Deep breathing, coughing, sneezing
Q: Dull achy sitting, sharp motion
R: None
S: 4/10, and 7/10 with deep breathing
T: No timing noted

Practice Building

Call new patients on the evening of their 1st visit to check in and follow-up - most clinician's forget this basic step as a way to go the extra distance to better engagement of their patients and evaluate the effectiveness of care - in most cases the patient will already be feeling better and associate you with those positive outcomes and feelings.

O

Patient points to area just below scapula on left side to indicate area of pain
AROM: decrease left lateral flexion of thoracic spine with mild discomfort, sharp local pain with inspiration
Cardiac auscultation WNL, no shortness of breath, diaphoresis, no NTW in arms or chest
(-) Sternal compression, rib expansion: equal bilaterally
Prone rib palpation: 7th left rib sits more posterior, pt indicated pain with 7th rib palpation associated local myospasm and tenderness
Palp of right gastrosoleus shows focal tenderness & trigger points over injury

A

A// CC#1 Back Pain
WDx: L 7th rib subluxation
Pert (+): left 7th rib sits more posterior, localized pain over left 7th rib, decreased left lateral flexion, pain with inspiration
Pert (-): sternal compression –ve, rib expansion bilaterally, no provocation of pain after meals, no hx of pancreatitis, no signs of cardiovascular dysfunction

P

P// - 1. Hydroculator application over thoracic spine for 10 minutes prior to adjustment
2. Supine Rib Adjustment over L 7th rib, cavitation noted, well tolerated - patient noted significant pain reduction after adjustment "I can take a deep breath again"
3. Provided patient with home care instructions (hydrotherapy, light stretching)
4. Continue IASTM and acupuncture over lateral right gastrosoleus

Sample SOAP note #2

S "neck is feeling much better", ↓ HA frequency (1 in 2 weeks), pain scale = 1/10

O tight & tender +1/4 R >L suboccipital, MFTP referral over right eye

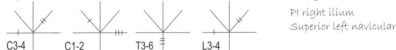

C3-4   C1-2   T3-6   L3-4

Pl right ilium
Superior left navicular

A hot pack (15 min) posterior cervical spine & upper shoulders, iSTM of suboccipitals region, stretch of upper trapezius & splenius, osseous manipulation of above motion restrictions

P ↓ Pain following Tx, continue home stretching, ↑ H₂O intake. return: 1 wk

Signature: Dr. Emma Wroids   Date: 2018/12/15

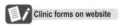 Clinic forms on website   prohealthsys.com

Free sample charts for all body region can be downloaded from **prohealthsys.com**

Star Diagram: used to record AROM & PROM information in an efficient format

Spinal Joint

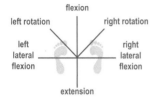

Peripheral Joint

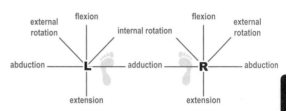

Spinal Listings

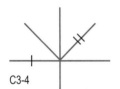

C3-4

- The star diagram may be modified to show spinal joint listings (restriction or malposition depending on clinician preference)
- | = mild, || = moderated, ||| = severe
- Example demonstrates a C3-4 moderate right rotation, mild left lateral flexion restriction

Text equivalent: shoulder
- Right shoulder flexion both active & passive is limited to ~50% (~90°) into flexion with pain at end ROM
- Shoulder active adduction is limited to ~50% (~15°) with pain at mid PROM
- All other ROM is WNL (AROM < PROM)

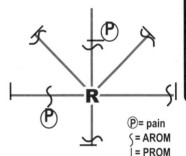

(P) = pain
S = AROM
| = PROM

- Each line represents 100% motion in that direction, therefore a mark half way on a line indicates 50% ROM ability; examiner should record any pain, abnormal movements or clunks & location within ROM
- Hypermobility would be noted as greater than 100% ROM (off the end of the line representing motion)

Joint Assessment

Treatment Frequency

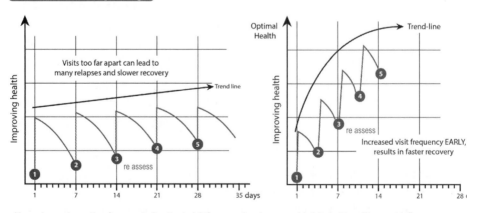

Above is a schematic of suggested patient visit frequencies, in general treatment has the most influence on healing early in the process. This influenced by a number of specific individual prognostic factors (positive mind-set, support, sleep, age, nutrition, activity, tissue type, genetics, etc. Fore more details see p vii)

1. Vizniak, NA. Human Cadaver Dissections. 1999-2018
2. Boal RW, Gillette RG. Central Neuronal Plasticity, Low Back Pain and Spinal Manipulative Therapy. JMPT 27(5):314-326, 2004.
3. Bodgduk N, Tynan W, Wilson AS. The nerve supply to the human intervertebral discs. J Anat 1981;132:39-56.
4. Bogduk N, Jull G. The theoretical pathology of acute locked back: a basis for manipulative therapy. Man Med 1985;1:78-82.
5. Boline PD, Haas M, Meyer JJ, Kassak K, Nelson C, Keating JC., Jr Interexaminer reliability of eight evaluative dimensions of lumbar segmental abnormality: Part II. JMPT. 1993 Jul–Aug;16(6):363–374.
6. Boline PD, Haas M, Meyer JJ, Kassak K, Nelson C, Keating JC., Jr Interexaminer reliability of eight evaluative dimensions of lumbar segmental abnormality: Part II. JMPT. 1993 Jul–Aug;16(6):363–374.
7. Bolton PS. Reflex Effects of Vertebral Subluxations: The Peripheral Nervous system. An Update. JMPT 23(2):101-103, 2000.
8. Bolton PS. The Somatosensory System of the Neck and Its Effects on the Central Nervous System. JMPT 21(8): 553-563, 1998.
9. Brennan PC, Cramer GD, Kirstukas SJ, Cullum ME. Basic science research in chiropractic: state-of-the-art and recommendations for a research agenda. JMPT 1997;20(3).
10. Brennan PC, Triano JJ, McGregor M, Kokjohn K, Hondras MA, Brennan DT. Enhanced neutrophil respiratory burst as a biological marker for manipulation forces: duration of the effect and association with substance P and tumor necrosis factor. JMPT 1992;15:83-9.
11. Brodeur R. The audible release associated with joint manipulation. JMPT 1995;18:155-64.
12. Budgell B, Igarashi Y. Response of Arrhythmia to Spinal Manipulation: Monitoring by ECG With Analysis of Heart-Rate Variability. JNMS 9(3):97-102, 2001.
13. Budgell B, Polus B. The Effects of Thoracic Manipulation on Heart Rate Variability: A Controlled Crossover Trial. JMPT 29(8):603-610, 2006.
14. Budgell BS, Sato A. The Cervical Subluxation and Regional Cerebral Blood Flow. JMPT 20(2):103-107, 1997
15. Budgell BS. Reflex Effects of Subluxation: The Autonomic Nervous System.
16. Buerger AA. Experimental neuromuscular models of spinal manual techniques. Man Med 1983;1:10-17.
17. Bugdell BS, et al. Reflex Responses of Bladder Motility After Stimulation of Interspinous Tissues in the Anesthetized Rat. JMPT 21(9):593-599, 1998.
18. Carrick FR. Changes in Brain Function Afrter Manipulation of the Cervical Spine.
19. Cassidy JD, Lopes AA, Yong-Hing K. The immediate effect of manipulation versus mobilization on pain and range of motion in the cervical spine: a randomized controlled trial. JMPT. 1992 Nov–Dec;15(9):570–575.
20. Cavalcanti FS, de Freitas GG. Alternative medicine in a patient with juvenile chronic arthritis. J Rheumatol. 1992 Nov;19(11):1827–1828.
21. Cherkin DC, MacCornack FA. Patient evaluations of low back pain care from family physicians and chiropractors. West J Med. 1989 Mar;150(3):351–355.
22. Christensen HW, Vach W, et al. Palpation of the Upper Thoracic Spine: An Observer Reliability Study. JMPT 25(5):285-292, 2002.
23. Christian GH, Stanton GJ, Sissons D, How HY, Jamison J, Alder B, Fullerton M, Funder JW. Immunoreactive ACTH, beta-endorphin and cortisol levels in plasma following spinal manipulative therapy. Spine 1988:13:1411-7.
24. Clarke, Judy MA ; van Tulder, Maurits PhD; Blomberg, Stefan MD, PhD, et al. Traction for Low Back Pain With or Without Sciatica: An Updated Systematic Review Within the Framework of the Cochrane Collaboration. Spine. 31(14):1591-1599, June 15, 2006.
25. Coderre TJ, Katz J, Vaccarino AL, Melzack R. Contribution of central neuroplasticity to pathological pain: review of clinical and experimental studies. Pain 1993;52:259-85.
26. Collaca JC, et al. Neurophysiological Responses to Intraoperative Lumbosacral Spinal Manipulation. JMPT 23(7):447-457, 2000.
27. Conway PJW, Herzog W, Zhang Y, et al. Forces required to cause cavitation during spinal manipulation in the thoracic spine. Clin Biomech 1993;8:210-4.
28. Cornwall MW, et al. The Effect of Physical Activity on Ligamentous Strength. J Orth Sports Phys Ther 5(5):275-277, 1984.
29. Cox JM, Fromelt KA, Shreiner S. Chiropractic statistical survey of 100 consecutive low back pain patients. JMPT. 1983 Sep;6(3):117–128.
30. Cox JM, Shreiner S. Chiropractic manipulation in low back pain and sciatica: statistical data on the diagnosis, treatment and response of 576 consecutive cases. JMPT. 1984 Mar;7(1):1–11.
31. Cox JM. Patient benefits of attending a chiropractic low back wellness clinic. JMPT. 1994 Jan;17(1):25–28.
32. Deboer KF, Harmon R, Jr, Tuttle CD, Wallace H. Reliability study of detection of somatic dysfunctions in the cervical spine. JMPT. 1985 Mar;8(1):9–16.
33. DeVocht JW, Pikar JG, Wilder DG. Spinal Manipulation Alters Electromyographic Activity of Paraspinal Muscles: A Descriptive Study. JMPT 28(7):465-471, 2005.
34. Deyo, Richard A. MD, MPH; Mirza, Sohail K. MD, MPH; Martin, Brook I. MPH. Back Pain Prevalence and Visit Rates: Estimates From U.S. National Surveys, 2002. Spine. 31(23):2724-2727, 2006.
35. Dishman JD, Ball KA, Burke J. Central Motor Excitability Changes After Spinal Manipulation: A Transcranial Magnetic Stimulation Study. JMPT 25(1):1-9, 2002.
36. Dishman JD, Cunningham BM, Burke J. Comparison of Tibial Nerve H-Reflex Excitability After Cervical and Lumbar Manipulation. JMPT 25(5):318-325, 2002.
37. Donatelli R, Owens-Burkhart H. Effects of Immobilization on the Extensibility of Periarticular Connective Tissue.J Ortho Sports Phys Ther 3(2):67-72, 1981.
38. Downey BJ, Taylor NF, Niere KR. Manipulative physiotherapists can reliably palpate nominated lumbar spinal levels. Man Ther. 1999 Aug;4(3):151–156.
39. Driscoll MD, Hall MJ. Effects of Spinal Manipulative Therapy on Autonomic Activity and the Cardiovascular System: A Case Study Using the Electrocardiogram and Arterial Tonometry. JMPT 23(8):545-550, 2000.
40. Ernst E, Canter PH. "A systematic review of systematic reviews of spinal manipulation". J R Soc Med 99 (4): 192–6. 2006.
41. Eskelund Hansen B, Simonsen T, Leboeuf-Yde C. Motion Palpation of the Lumbar Spine – A Problem With The Test or the Tester? JMPT 29(3):208-212, 2006.
42. Fjellner A, Bexander C, Faleij R, Strender LE. Interexaminer reliability in physical examination of the cervical spine. JMPT. 1999 Oct;22(8):511–516.
43. Frach JP, Osterbauer PJ, Fuhr AW. Treatment of Bell's palsy by mechanical force, manually assisted chiropractic adjusting and high-voltage electrotherapy. JMPT. 1992 Nov–Dec;15(9):596–598.
44. French SD, Green S, Forbes A. Reliability of chiropractic methods commonly used to detect manipulable lesions in patients with chronic low-back pain. JMPT. 2000 May;23(4):231–238.
45. Fryer G, Morris T, Gibbons P, Briggs A. The Electromyographic Activity of the Thoracic Paraspinal Muscles Identified as Abnormal With Palpation. JMPT 29(6):437-447, 2006.
46. Frymann VM, Carney RE, Springall P. Effect of osteopathic medical management on neurologic development in children. J Am Osteopath Assoc. 1992 Jun;92(6):729–744.
47. Gagnier, Joel J. ND, MSc, PhD(cand.); van Tulder, Maurits W. PhD; Berman, Brian MD]; Bombardier, Claire MD Herbal Medicine for Low Back Pain: A Cochrane Review. Spine. 32(1):82-92, January 1, 2007.
48. Gal JM, Herzog W, Kawchuk GN, Conway PJ, Zhang Y-T. Forces and relative vertebral movements during SMT to unembalmed post-rigor human cadavers: peculiarities associated with joint cavitation. JMPT 1995;18:4-9.
49. Giesen JM, Center DB, Leach RA. An evaluation of chiropractic manipulation as a treatment of hyperactivity in children. JMPT. 1989 Oct;12(5):353–363.
50. Giles LGF, Harvey AR. Immunohistochemical demonstration of nociceptors in the capsule and synovial folds of human zygapophyseal joint capsule and synovial fold innervation. Br J Rheumatol 1987;26:993-8.
51. Giles LGF. Mechnisms of Neurovascular Compression Within the Spinal and Intervertebral Canals. JMPT 23(2):107-111, 2000.
52. Gillette RG, Kramis RC, Roberts WJ. Spinal Neurons Likely to Mediate Low Back and Referred Leg Pain. Society for Neuroscience Abstracts Vol 16, 294-7.
53. Gillette RG. Spinal cord mechanisms of referred pain and neuroplasticity. In Gatterman MI (ed). Foundations of Chiropractic: Subluxation. St. Louis, MO: Mosby, 1995.
54. Gonnella C, Paris SV, Kutner M. Reliability in evaluating passive intervertebral motion. Phys Ther. 1982 Apr;62(4):436–444.
55. Gonnella C, Paris SV, Kutner M. Reliability in evaluating passive intervertebral motion. Phys Ther. 1982 Apr;62(4):436–444.
56. Good CJ, Mikkelsen GB. Intersegmental sagittal motion in the lower cervical spine and discogenic spondylosis: a preliminary study. JMPT. 1992 Nov–Dec;15(9):556–564.
57. Gotlib, A & Rupert R. Chiropractic manipulation in pediatric health conditions – an updated systematic review. Chiropractic & Osteopathy 2008, 16:11
58. Grice AS. Muscle tonus changes following manipulation. J Can Chiropr Assoc 1974;18:29-31.
59. Haas M. How to evaluate intraexaminer reliability using an interexaminer reliability study design. JMPT. 1995 Jan;18(1):10–15.
60. Haas M. Statistical methodology for reliability studies. JMPT. 1991 Feb;14(2):119–132.
61. Haas M. The reliability of reliability. JMPT. 1991 Mar–Apr;14(3):199–208.
62. Haldeman S. Neurologic Effects of the Adjustment. JMPT 23(2):112-114, 2000.
63. Hammer WI, Pfefer MT. Treatment of Subacute Lumbar Compartment Syndrome Using the Graston Technique. JMPT 28(3):199-204, 2005.
64. Hartvigsen, Jan DC, PhD; Christensen, Kaare MD, PhD Active Lifestyle Protects Against Incident Low Back Pain in Seniors: A Population-Based 2-Year Prospective Study of 1387 Danish Twins Aged 70-100 Years. Spine. 32(1):76-81, January 1, 2007.
65. Hawk C, Phongphua C, Bleecker J, Swank L, Lopez D, Rubley T. Preliminary study of the reliability of assessment procedures for indications for chiropractic adjustments of the lumbar spine. JMPT. 1999 Jul–Aug;22(6):382–389.
66. Hawk C, Phongphua C, Bleecker J, Swank L, Lopez D, Rubley T. Preliminary study of the reliability of assessment procedures for indications for chiropractic adjustments of the lumbar spine. JMPT. 1999 Jul–Aug;22(6):382–389.
67. HEILIG D. Principles of vertebral manipulation in the cervical area. J Am Osteopath Assoc. 1952 Oct;52(2):109–114.
68. Herzog W, Conway P, Kawchuk G, et al. Forces exerted during spinal manipulative therapy. Spine 1993a;18:1206-12.
69. Herzog W, Conway PJ, Zhang YT, et al. Reflex responses associated with manipulative treatments on the thoracic spine. JMPT 1995;18:233-6.
70. Herzog W, Scheele D, Conway PJ. Electromyographic Responses of Back and Limb Muscles Associated With Spinal Manipulative Therapy. Spine 24(2):146-153, 1999.
71. Herzog W, Zhang YT, Conway PJ, et al. Cavitation sounds during spinal manipulative treatments. JMPT 1993b;16:523-26.
72. Herzog W. Biomechanical studies of spinal manipulative therapy. J Can Chiropr Assoc 1991 (Invited review paper);35:156-64.
73. Herzog W. Mechanical, physiologic and neuromuscular considerations of chiropractic treatments. In Lawrence D, et al. (eds). Advances in Chiropractic, Vol 3. Chicago, IL: Mosby Year Book, 1996.
74. Hessel BW, Herzog W, Conway PJW, et al. Experimental measurement of the force exerted during spinal manipulation using the Thompson technique. JMPT 1990;13:448-53.
75. Hession EF, Donald GD. Treatment of multiple lumbar disk herniations in an adolescent athlete utilizing flexion distraction and rotational manipulation. JMPT. 1993 Mar–Apr;16(3):185–192.
76. Hestbaek L, Leboeuf-Yde C. Are chiropractic tests for the lumbo-pelvic spine reliable and valid? A systematic critical literature review. JMPT. 2000 May;23(4):258–275.
77. Hsieh CY, Hong CZ, Adams AH, Platt KJ, Danielson CD, Hoehler FK, Tobis JS. Interexaminer reliability of the palpation of trigger points in the trunk and lower limb muscles. Arch Phys Med Rehabil. 2000 Mar;81(3):258–264.
78. Hsieh CY, Hong CZ, Adams AH, Platt KJ, Danielson CD, Hoehler FK, Tobis JS. Interexaminer reliability of the palpation of trigger points in the trunk and lower limb muscles. Arch Phys Med Rehabil. 2000 Mar;81(3):258–264.
79. Hu JW, Yu XM, Vernon H, Sessle BJ. Excitatory effects on neck and jaw muscle activity of inflammatory irritant applied to cervical paraspinal tissues. Pain 1993;55:243-50.
80. Hubka MJ, Phelan SP. Interexaminer reliability of palpation for cervical spine tenderness. JMPT. 1994 Nov–Dec;17(9):591–595.
81. Jadad AR, Moore RA, Carroll D, Jenkinson C, Reynolds DJ, Gavaghan DJ, McQuay HJ. Assessing the quality of reports of randomized clinical trials: is blinding necessary? Control Clin Trials. 1996 Feb;17(1):1–12.
82. Jamison JR, McEwen AP, Thomas SJ. Chiropractic adjustment in the management of visceral conditions: a critical appraisal. JMPT. 1992 Mar–Apr;15(3):171–180.
83. Jensen Stochkendahl M, Christensen HW, Hartvigsen MJ, Vach W, Haas M, et al. Manual Examination of the Spine: A Systematic Critical Review of Reproducability. JMPT 20(6):475-485, 2006.
84. Johnston WL, Allan BR, Hendra JL, Neff DR, Rosen ME, Sills LD, Thomas SC. Interexaminer study of palpation in detecting location of spinal segmental dysfunction. J Am Osteopath Assoc. 1983 Jul;82(11):839–845.
85. Johnston WL, Beal MC, Blum GA, Hendra JL, Neff DR, Rosen ME. Passive gross motion testing: Part III. Examiner agreement on selected subjects. J Am Osteopath Assoc. 1982 Jan;81(5):309–313.
86. Johnston WL, Elkiss ML, Marino RV, Blum GA. Passive gross motion testing: Part II. A study of interexaminer agreement. J Am Osteopath Assoc. 1982 Jan;81(5):304–308.
87. Johnston WL, Hill JL, Elkiss ML, Marino RV. Identification of stable somatic findings in hypertensive subjects by trained examiners using palpatory examination. J Am Osteopath Assoc. 1982 Aug;81(12):830–836.
88. Johnston WL, Hill JL, Sealey JW, Sucher BM. Palpatory findings in the cervicothoracic region: variations in normotensive and hypertensive subjects. A preliminary report. J Am Osteopath Assoc. 1980 Jan;79(5):300–308.
89. Johnston WL. Interexaminer reliability studies: spanning a gap in medical research--Louisa Burns Memorial Lecture. J Am Osteopath Assoc. 1982 Aug;81(12):819–829.
90. Karason A, Drysdale IP. Somatovisceral Response Following Osteopathic HVLAT: A Pilot Syudy on the Effect of Unilateral lumbosacral High-Velocity Low-Amplitude Thrust Technique on the Cutaneous Blood Flow in the Lower Limb. JMPT 26(4):220-225, 2003.
91. Kawchuk GN, Herzog W, Hasler EM. Forces generated during spinal manipulative therapy of the cervical spine: a pilot study. JMPT 1992;15:275-8.
92. Kawchuk GN, Herzog W. Biomechanical characterization (finger printing) of five novel methods of cervical spinal manipulation. JMPT 1993;16:573-7.
93. Keating JC, Jr, Bergmann TF, Jacobs GE, Finer BA, Larson K. Interexaminer reliability of eight evaluative dimensions of lumbar segmental abnormality. JMPT. 1990 Oct;13(8):463–470.
94. Kellet J. Acute Soft Tissue Injuries - A Review of the Literature. Medicine and Science in Sports and Exercise 18(5):489-500, 1986.
95. Kemler MA, et al. Which Patients With Chronic RSD Are Most Likely to Benefit From Physical Therapy? J Manipulative & Physiol Ther 24(4):272-278, 2001.
96. Kessinger RC, Boneva DV. Vertigo, Tinnitus, and Hearing Loss in the Geriatric Patient.
97. Koes BW, Assendelft WJ, van der Heijden GJ, Bouter LM. Spinal manipulation for low back pain. An updated systematic review of randomized clinical trials. Spine. 1996 Dec 15;21(24):2860–2873.
98. Korr IM. Proprioceptors and somatic dysfunction. J Amer Osteopath Assoc 1975;74:638-50.
99. Kowal MA. Review of Physiological Effects of Cryotherapy. J Ortho Sports Phys Ther 5(2):66-73, 1983.
100. Lantz CA. Application and evaluation of the kappa statistic in the design and

Assessment Quiz (answer page)

1. What does the acronym o-HIPMNRS stand for? (46) ____________________
2. What are the parts of a fracture screen? (47)
   ____
3. List red flags for more serious pathology (48)
4. Give a list of potential outcome markers (50)
5. Give a sample 0-10 pain scale (51) ______
6. Differentiate tissue specific injuries (muscle, vs. ligament, vs. bone, vs joint) (53) ______
7. List 10 factors affecting posture (54) ______
8. What structures should a plumb line fall through during a postural assessment? (55)
9. Give examples of 5 postural variations (57)
10. What is an upper and lower cross syndrome? (58)
11. Give examples of pathologic gaits (59)
12. What are the parts of a normal gait cycle (61)
13. Give 5 tips for better palpation (64)
14. Explain 1-5 subjective palp. pain scale (65)
15. List factor that can affect ROM (67)
16. Give examples of pathologic and non-pathologic joint end-feels (68) ________
17. Define the 0-5 muscle strength grading scale (71)
18. How do you use a goniometer? (75)
19. What is the spectrum of joint dysfunctions? (77)
20. How do you chart spinal and extremity joint mobilizations? (83) ________________

Bonus: How many joints are in the body? (72)

Learning Objectives

After completing this chapter, students will be able to:

1. Perform a regional exam and recognize common pathologies of the region

2. Identify and palpate body region bony landmarks, ligaments and muscles

3. Discuss regional kinematics and joint organ biomechanics/function

4. Recognize and execute steps of effective mobilization and joint-play including indications, position, contact, force and relevant clinical notes

5. Perform side-lying, prone & supine assessment and mobilizations of

   - Iliac extension restriction (PI ilium/posterior tilt)
   - Iliac flexion restriction (AS ilium/anterior tilt)
   - Sacral counter-nutation restriction (nutated)
   - Sacral nutation restriction (counter-nutated)
   - Superior/inferior sacral glide restriction
   - Anterior/posterior ilium glide restriction
   - Anterior SI compression & distraction
   - Anteriorly displace coccyx
   - Pelvic blocking
   - SI contract relax

Most doctors and therapists have never actually seen inside a SI joint in real life as the dissection is quite challenging & the process is NOT covered in many anatomy programs! - if they have been among the fortunate few it was likely on a geriatric donor rather than their standard patient population

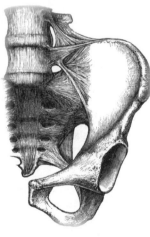

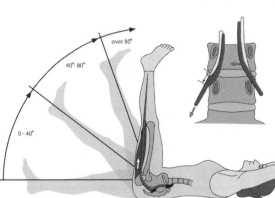

Video on website

SI & Pelvis

Special history questions

- Specific mechanism of injury & forces involved? - lifting & twisting?
- Any numbness, tingling or weakness?
- Coughing, sneezing or straining make it worse?
- Type of work, typical posture, sleeping posture?
- Prior injuries or treatments?
- What makes it better or worse?
- Review of systems (GI, urinary, cardiovascular)

Inspection

- Asymmetry, bruising, bumps, color, swelling, iliac crest height
- Posture

Palpation (may be done after ROM assessment)

Abdominal palpation	TFL
Inguinal lymph nodes	Greater trochanter
Femoral pulse	Piriformis
Pubic symphysis	Sacrotuberous lig.
ASIS	Sacroiliac joint
Iliac crest	Sacrospinous lig.
Paraspinal muscles	Gluteus maximus
Quadratus lumborum	Iliopsoas
Iliolumbar ligaments	Quadriceps
PSIS	Gastrosoleus
Ischial tuberosities	Spinous processes
Hamstrings	Lower ribs

Functional assessment (ADLs)

- Squat & rise

AROM

Flexion/Extension........0-10°
Int./external rotation ...0-10°

PROM & Joint Play (if indicated)

Myotomes (resisted isometric movements)

- Trunk rotation (T6-L2, segmental nn.)
- Trunk lateral flexion (T6-L2, segmental nn.)
- Trunk flexion/extension (T6-L2, segmental n.)
- Hip flexion (L1-L3, femoral n.)
- Knee extension (L3-L4; femoral n.)
- Knee flexion (L4-S2, sciatic n.)
- Ankle dorsiflexion (**L4**, L5 - deep peroneal),
- Ankle inversion (L4, **L5** - tibial & deep peron.)
- Ankle eversion (L5, **S1** - sup. peroneal)
- Big toe extension, (**L5**, S1; deep peroneal)
- Big toe flexion (L5-S1, tibial nerve)

Leg length measurements

- Greater trochanter to lateral malleolus
- Pubic symphysis to medial malleolus
- Umbilicus to medial malleolus
- Prone leg length evaluation

Abdominal exam (if indicated)

- Observe, auscultate, percuss, palpate, sit-up (abdominal strength & Beevor's sign)

Neurovascular screen

Sensory: Light touch, sharp/dull Vibration (DIP, 3rd digit)
UMNL: Babinski (L1 & above)
DTR's: Patella (L3, L4), hamstring (L5), Achilles (L5, S1)
Vascular: femoral, popliteal, dorsal pedal pulses, nail bed blanching

Special tests (if indicated)

Screening
- Minor's sign
- Belt test, Gillette Test (SI step test)
- Flamingo test, Fortin finger test
- Allis test (sky-line)
- SI joint anesthetic injection

SI joint dysfunction
- SI motion palpation test (step test)
- Sit-up leg length test (long sit test)
- Static palpation

SI sprain/strain
- Motion palpation
- Sacral shear
- Sacrotuberous stress test

Iliopsoas contracture
- Gaenslen's test
- Lewin-Gaenslen's test
- Thomas test

Lumbar spine & Hip Screen

Diagnostic imaging (if indicated)

 Video on website

Follow HIP-MNRS (see 'Physical Assessment' or 'Spinal Manual' texts for specific details or review)
History, Inspection, Palpation - Motion, Neurovascular screen, Referred pain, Special tests

SI & Pelvis

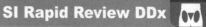
Condition	Clinical notes
Ankylosing spondylitis	*Hx:* 20-35 yrs old, M > F; insidious onset of vague LBP & stiffness worse with waking better with motion *SSx:* loss of lumbar/SI ROM, (+) blood tests HLA-B27, ↑ ESR *DDx:* progressive sclerosis of SI joints, expands up the spine visible on x-ray
Cauda equina syndrome	*Hx:* **bilateral** neurologic symptoms, saddle anesthesia, loss of bladder control *SSx:* gait abnormalities; ↓ DTRs, motor strength; (+) Babinski *DDx:* visible on MRI, spinal canal stenosis
Disc herniation	*Hx:* **unilateral** L4-S1 neurologic signs (numbness, weakness); antalgic posture *SSx:* ↑ pain with flexion; ↓ DTRs, motor strength; (+) SLR *DDx:* visible on MRI, IVF osteophyte encroachment, cauda equina syndrome
Lumbar (DJD) osteoarthrosis	*Hx:* local central pain, worse in morning, better with mild activity *SSx:* possible crepitus with motion; decreased AROM & PROM *DDx:* visible on x-ray: ↓ joint space, osteophyte formation
Lumbar joint dysfunction	*Hx:* insidious onset of local pain or discomfort *SSx:* tender to palpation; limited joint play; local myospasm; bone out of place *DDx:* lumbar sprain/strain, facet syndrome, meniscoid entrapment
Lumbar sprain/ strain	*Hx:* history of trauma, local pain with motion *SSx:* no neurologic signs; decreased AROM & PROM, RROM due to pain *DDx:* lumbar joint dysfunction often coexist
Pelvic fracture	*Hx:* significant trauma, severe pain *SSx:* gait abnormalities; (+) SI compression, distraction stress test *DDx:* visible on x-ray or CT, severe SI sprain
SI instability	*Hx:* chronic SI pain, possible repeatable "clunk" of SI joint; may occur during or shortly after pregnancy *SSx:* (+) sacral glide test for increased motion *DDx:* SI joint dysfunction, lumbar instability
Spinal stenosis	*Hx:* M > F (2:1), chronic low back pain, worse with prolonged standing *SSx:* decreased AROM & PROM; confirm with x-ray ↓ spinal canal diameter *DDx:* vascular claudication
SI joint dysfunction	*Hx:* insidious onset of local pain or discomfort (may be due to fall on sacrum) *SSx:* tender to palpation; limited joint play; local myospasm; bone out of place *DDx:* lumbar sprain/strain, PI ilium or AI (nutated) sacrum are most common
Piriformis syndrome	*Hx:* possible pain down back of leg, worse when sitting on hard surface *SSx:* tender to palpation, (+) SLR, sign of the buttock, (+) piriformis test *DDx:* lumbar radiculopathy, disc herniation, lumbar sprain/strain, stenosis

↑ = increase, ↓ = decrease, Hx = history, SSx = signs & symptoms, DDx = differential diagnosis

SI & Pelvis

The male pelvis is designed for strength and stability and female for childbirth and mobility

Pelvis	Male ♂	Female ♀
General	narrow & thick	wide & shallow
Pelvic inlet	heart shaped	circular shaped
Pelvic outlet	relatively small	relatively large
Pubic arch	< 70°	> 90°
Obturator foramen	round	oval
Acetabulum	large	small
Wing of ilium	less flared	more flared

Sacrum & Coccyx

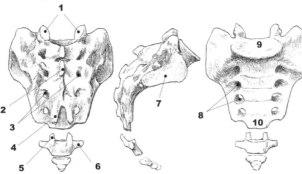

1. Superior articular facet
2. S2 tubercle
3. Posterior sacral foramen
4. Cornu of sacrum
5. Cornu of coccyx
6. Transverse process
7. Articular surface for ilium
8. Anterior sacral foramen
9. Sacral base (superior)
10. Sacral apex (inferior)

SI Joint Levels

Lumbosacral angle range: 26-57°
↑ angle = more lumbar lordosis

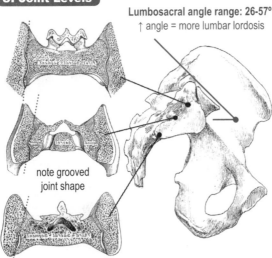

note grooved
joint shape

SI joints (~1-2mm wide synovial joint)
- **Hyaline cartilage sacral surface** (glossy, smooth, white)
- **Fibrocartilage iliac surface** (dull, striped, bluish, thin)
- Has 6x more resistance to lateral forces than lumber spine
- Joint is very strong, with limited motion due to the amount of ligamentous support & uneven joint surfaces (often fused in geriatrics)

Most doctors and therapists have never seen an SI joint in real life - it is NOT part of the standard dissection process (and if they have it was likely on a geriatric donor - video of 28 yr old SI joint dissection on website)

SI & Pelvis

prohealthsys

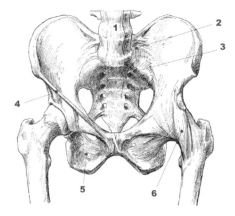

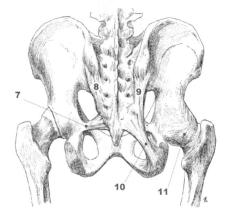

1. Anterior longitudinal ligament
2. Iliolumbar ligaments
3. Anterior sacroiliac ligaments
4. Inguinal ligament
5. Obturator membrane
6. Iliofemoral ligament
7. Sacrospinous ligament
8. Posterior sacroiliac ligament
9. Long posterior sacroiliac ligament
10. Sacrotuberous ligament
11. Acetabulofemoral joint capsule

Ligament	Attaches (origin/insertion)	Function
Iliolumbar	Transverse process of L4-5 to iliac crest	Resists lumbar flexion & rotation
Inguinal	ASIS to pubic tubercle	Attachment point of abdominal muscle and fascia lata of thigh
Sacrotuberous	Sacrum to ischial tuberosity	Resists sacral nutation
Sacrospinous	Sacrum to ischial spine	Resists sacral nutation & lateral flexion
Sacroiliac (ant/post)	Sacrum to ilium	Resists sacral nutation, holds SI joint together

SI & Pelvis

SI Motion with Breathing

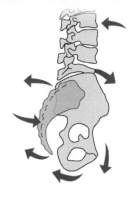

Inspiration

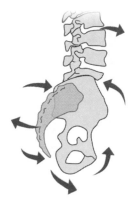

Expiration

prohealthsys

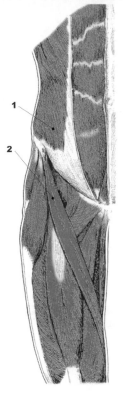

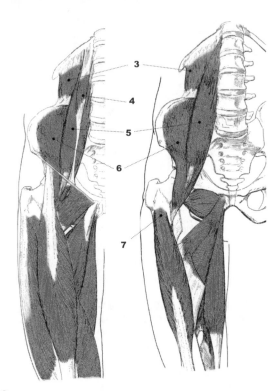

1
2
3
4
5
6
7

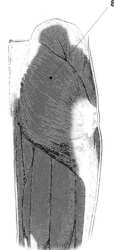

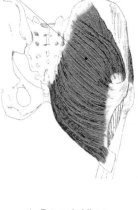

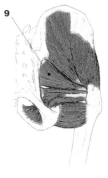

8

9

1. External oblique
2. Sartorius
3. Quadratus lumborum
4. Psoas minor
5. Psoas major

6. Iliacus
7. Vastus intermedius
8. Gluteus maximus
9. Piriformis

 Printable quizzes

Joint types:
- **SI:** gliding (synovial & syndesmosis regions)
- **Pubic symphysis:** cartilagenous (syndesmosis)

Articular surfaces
- **Sacrum:** concave
- **Ilium:** convex (rough sections)
- **Sacroiliac:** facets oriented ~45° from sagittal
- Fibrocartilage on ilium & hyaline cartilage on sacrum (FISH - fibro ilium, sacrum hyaline)
- Cartilage is ~2-3x thicker on the sacrum
- After ~60 yrs most males have fused SI joints

Active range of motion (sacroiliac)
Flexion/Extension........0-10°
Int./external rotation ...0-10°

Resting position: neutral

Close packed position: full nutation (SI flexion)

Capsular pattern of restriction
- Pain with torsion or shearing of joint

Normal end feel: firm ligamentous tissue stretch

Coupled motions
- Sacral motion is also coupled with lumbar motion
  - Lumbar extension (or hyperlordosis) is coupled with sacral *nutation* (anterior sacral tilting or "nod")
  - Lumbar flexion (or hypolordosis) is coupled with sacral *counter-nutation* (posterior sacral tilting)
  - Rotation of the SI joint follows the lumbar pattern

Pelvis
Lower
Vertebrae

 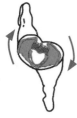 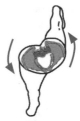

During gait the hip, the pelvis rotates forward around the stance leg (called Pelvic Step)

> **The farther from midline the center of gravity the greater force muscles (active stabilizers) and ligaments (passive stabilizers) have to resist (↑ injury risk)**

Among the strongest ligaments in the body, the **sacroiliac, sacrotuberous and sacrospinous ligaments** act as passive support cables to prevent the sacrum from falling forward (nutation) with the force of gravity pushing down from the lordotic lumbar spine

Piriformis may also assist with this lifting force on the sacrum (may also induce lateral forces on sacrum)

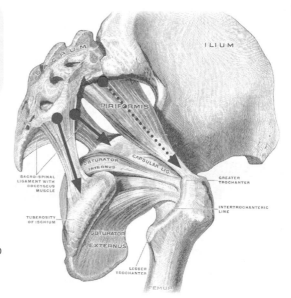

SI & Pelvis

PI ilium (flexion malposition) - more common

- Low iliac crest & PSIS when standing
- Short leg (supine functional assessment)
- Possible lumbar scoliosis to same side
- PSIS more pronounced
- ASIS high when standing
- ↓ thigh extension ROM
- Lower greater trochanter & gluteal fold (standing)
- Pain in lower 1/2 of SI joint or inguinal ligament
- Gillette's test: ↓ motion with *ipsilateral* hip flexion
- ↓ motion with prone SI flexion mobilization

AS ilium (extension malposition)

- High iliac crest & PSIS
- Long leg (supine assessment)
- Possible lumbar scoliosis to opposite side
- PSIS less pronounced
- ASIS low when standing
- High greater trochanter & gluteal fold (standing)
- ↑ thigh extension ROM
- Pain in lower 1/2 of SI joint or inguinal ligament
- Gillette's test: ↓ motion with *contralateral* hip flexion
- ↓ motion with prone SI extension mobilization

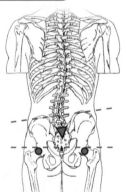

PI (flexion)   **AS** (extension)

Given the rough articular surfaces of the SI joint it is somewhat common for it to get 'stuck' out of optimal position

▶ Video on website

Leg Length & Pelvic Malposition

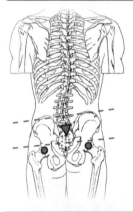

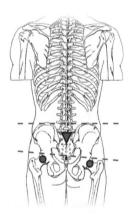

Anatomical Leg Inequality	Functional Leg Inequality	Functional Pelvic Torsion
• Right leg is anatomically long • Lifts right ilium & femoral head • Causes compensatory scoliosis	• *Right AS ilium* causing a functionally *long right leg* OR • *Left PI ilium* causing a functionally *short left leg*	• Left PI & right AS compensation of the pelvis to induce a level sacral base & neutral spine

Sacral Motion

Sacral Nutation (SI flexion)	Sacral Counter-Nutation (SI extension)
• Sacral base moves **Anterior Inferior (AI)** • Induces lumbar **hyperlodosis** • PSIS is *more* prominent to palpation	• Sacral base moves **Posterior Superior (PS)** • Induces lumbar **hypolordosis** • PSIS is *less* prominent to palpation

Sacral Motion with the Ilium (innominate) in Static Position

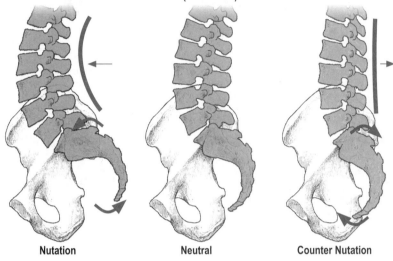

Nutation   Neutral   Counter Nutation

Ilium (innominate) Motion

PI (SI flexion) - more common	AS Ilium (SI extension)
• Ilium PSIS moves **Posterior Inferior (PI ilium)** • **Low iliac crest** when standing • PSIS become *more* prominent to palpation	• Ilium PSIS moves **Anterior Superior (AS ilium)** • **High iliac crest** when standing • PSIS become *less* prominent to palpation

Ilium (innominate) Motion with the Sacrum in Static Position and Equal Leg Length

Iliac crest level

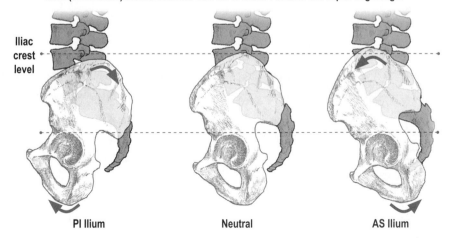

PI Ilium   Neutral   AS Ilium

SI & Pelvis

Anterior Tilt

Erector spinae
Multifidi

Gravity
Iliopsoas
hip joint capsule

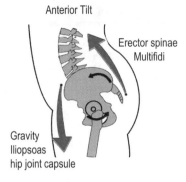

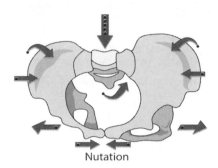

Nutation

Posterior Tilt

Rectus abd.
Obliques

Short lateral
rotators (piriformis)

Glut. max
Hamstrings

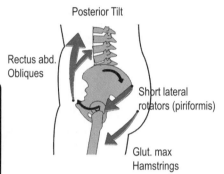

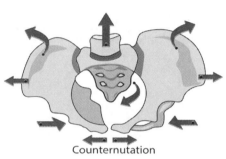

Counternutation

Trunk Extension & Flexion

Realize the same muscles are involved in both
flexion (eccentric) & extension (concentric)
from a bent to standing position when upright

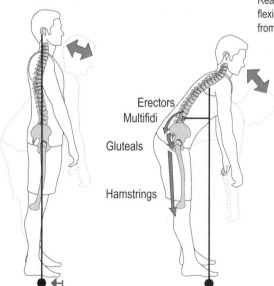

Erectors
Multifidi

Gluteals

Hamstrings

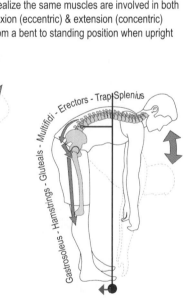

Gastrosoleus - Hamstrings - Gluteals - Multifidi - Erectors - Trap Splenius

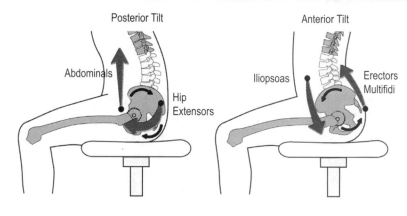

Posterior Tilt — Abdominals, Hip Extensors

Anterior Tilt — Iliopsoas, Erectors Multifidi

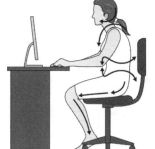 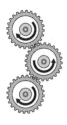 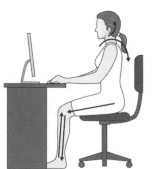 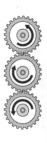

SI & Pelvis

Sit-up Leg Length / Long Sit Test

Procedure

Patient supine with leg straight, examiner at foot of examination table places one ankle in each hand & evaluates leg length by comparing side to side (malleoli length), examiner then instructs patient perform a sit-up (which induces flexion of hip)

Interpretation

(+) Leg that was shorter supine becomes longer when the patient sits up → Sacroiliac joint dysfunction (PI ilium on the leg that went from short supine to long sitting, or an AS ilium on opposite side)

Clinical notes

(RELIABILITY: 0.19-0.4 SENSTIVITY: 42-62 SPECIFICITY: 64-83 +LR: 1.4-3.6 -LR: 0.46-0.9)[12, 33, 41, 42]

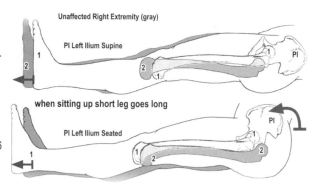

Unaffected Right Extremity (gray)
PI Left Ilium Supine
when sitting up short leg goes long
PI Left Ilium Seated

prohealthsys

All palpation methods involve tactile movement of soft tissues & osseous structures to evaluate **variations in elasticity, tone, motion from side to side, pain and/or discomfort.** - clinical style & preference will determine which specific methods clinicians use (use what works best for you)

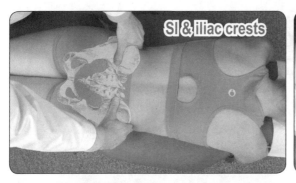

SI & iliac crests

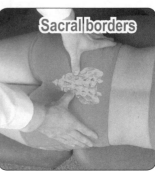

Sacral borders

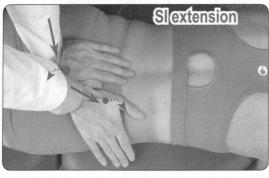

SI extension

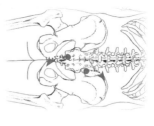

~90% of SI lesions are extension restrictions (PI ilium or nutated sacrum) due to the gravitational force pushing down on a the sacrum & normal lumbar lordotic curvature

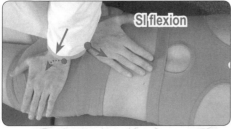

SI flexion

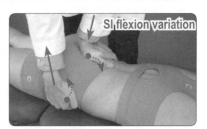

SI flexion variation

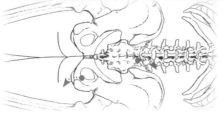

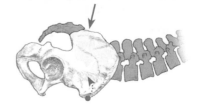

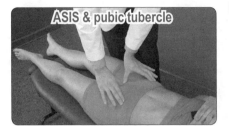

ASIS & pubic tubercle

Supine & Side-Posture Variations

Side-posture palpation is performed by the clinician moving the patient's thigh & hip (abducting, adducting, flexing and/or extending) to induce SI motion - if the clinician is likely going to choose side-posture mobilization or manipulation as a treatment method then by using side posture assessment one can improve their clinical efficiency & avoid unnecessary changes in patient position.

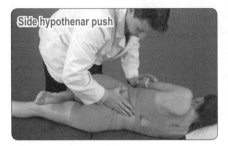

Side hypothenar push

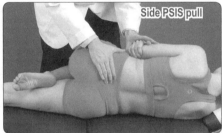

Side PSIS pull

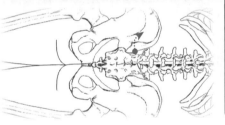

SI & Pelvis

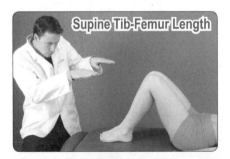

Supine Tib-Femur Length

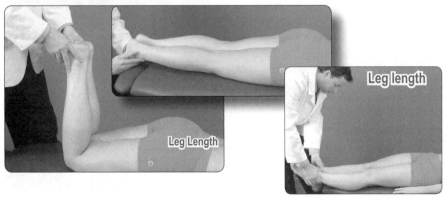

Leg length

Leg Length

Belt Test

Procedure

Standing patient is instructed to bend forward & touch toes with knees straight & return to standing; examiner then stabilizes the patient's pelvis bilaterally over the ASISs with hands & patient's sacrum with examiner's lateral thigh, then patient is instructed to repeat motion of touching toes

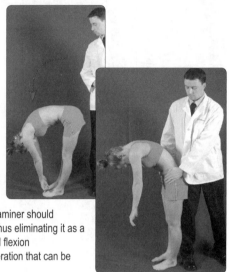

Interpretation

(+) Pain with both supported & unsupported flexion → Lumbar spine pathology

(+) No pain with support, pain without support → Sacroiliac joint pathology

Clinical notes

By supporting the patient's pelvis & sacrum the examiner should effectively prevent motion at the sacroiliac joint, thus eliminating it as a potential pain generator during supported forward flexion

An excellent differential for SI vs. lumbar pain generation that can be performed during active ROM assessment

SI Compression or Squish Test

Procedure

Patient side-lying, examiner places hands on superior ilium & applies downward pressure (compressing pelvis)

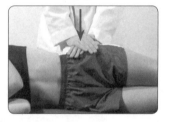

Interpretation

(+) Pain → Sacroiliac sprain/strain, fracture, SI joint dysfunction

Clinical notes

Test demonstrates good reliability & specificity
(R: 0.64-0.79 SN: 25-69 SP: 63-100 +LR: 1.6-2.2 -LR: 0.4-0.63)[10, 13, 25, 27, 28, 29, 41]

Jackson's One-Legged Hyperextension ★ ★ ★ ★

Procedure

Patient stands on one leg & extends back; examiner stands ready to support patient & observes for signs of pain & discomfort, test is repeated on other side

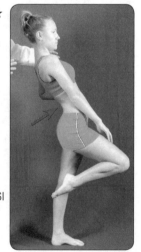

Interpretation

(+) Low back pain on right side when standing on left foot → right sided lumbar pathology, facet impaction, impending pars fracture

(+) Pain in SI on support leg → SI pathology (SN: 7-19 SP: 98-100 +LR: 3.5 -LR: 0.95)[26]

Clinical notes

By standing on one leg the SI joint is loaded on the ipsilateral side; thus when contra-lateral pain is felt it is possible to rule out the elevated leg SI joint as a primary cause

SI & Pelvis

Gaenslen's Test

Procedure

Patient supine, examiner flexes knee & thigh of affected leg to patient's abdomen, then examiner slowly hyperextends the opposite leg & observes the patient for signs of discomfort or pain, the test is then repeated on the opposite extremity

Interpretation

(+) Sacroiliac or anterior thigh pain → sacroiliac joint pathology (ligamentous sprain, instability) (R: 0.6-0.72 SN: 50-71 SP: 26-77 +LR: 1-2.2 -LR: 0.65-1.1)[21, 27, 28, 29]

(+) Elevation of extended hip → iliopsoas contracture

(-) No sacroiliac pain → possible lumbar or hip pain origination (if the leg hanging off the table starts to straighten look for iliopsoas contracture)

Clinical notes

Clinician's option: examiner may have patient bring the knee to chest & hyperextend the straight leg off the lateral edge of the examination table

Lewin-Gaenslen's Test - patient side-lying on unaffected side & brings unaffected knee towards chest, examiner then applies gentle over pressure attempting to hyperextended the affected thigh

Thomas Test / Knee to Shoulder Test - patient supine, examiner flexes affected knee & hip to 90°, then examiner pushes flexed knee toward the opposite shoulder (+) Elevation of the straight leg → hip contracture, tight iliopsoas or rectus femoris

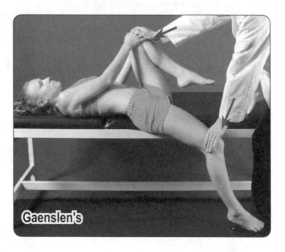

Gaenslen's

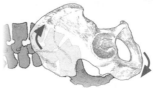

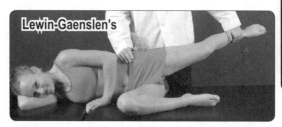

Lewin-Gaenslen's

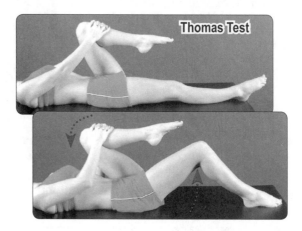

Thomas Test

Sacroiliac Marching Test

Synonyms: Gillette Test, SI motion palpation, Step Test, Sacral Fixation Test

Procedure

1. Patient standing with arm against wall, examiner palpates the PSIS & S4 tubercle (spinous process)

2. Patient is instructed to flex *ipsilateral* hip to 90°, examiner observes/palpates motion of PSIS relative to S4 (normally PSIS moves closer to S4 tubercle)

3. Examiner then instructs the patient to flex *contralateral* hip to 90°, examiner observes/palpates motion of S4 relative to PSIS (normal motion should move S4 away from PSIS)

4. Repeat test on contralateral SI joint

Interpretation

(+) Pain → Sacroiliac or pubic joint sprain, pelvic fracture

(+) Excess motion → hypermobility, joint dysfunction

(+) Decreased ROM → ipsilateral SI joint dysfunction

Clinical notes

Occasionally patients will have a repeatable 'click' or 'snap' with this maneuver, this finding is most likely due to a tendon snapping over a tubercle

Some clinicians further modify this test by palpating the PIIS & sacral apex or S4 tubercle & ischial tuberosity to evaluate the "lower SI" joint separately (given that these variations still involve contact on the same two bones as the above method, it is questionable if they really offer any additional clinical assessment information)

Clinician's option (other SI motion maneuvers): Patient prone, examiner applies force over the sacral base & ischial tuberosity to check SI flexion; test repeated with force applied over the sacral apex & PSIS to check SI extension

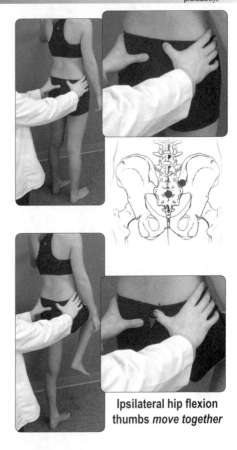

Ipsilateral hip flexion thumbs *move together*

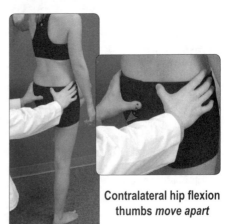

Contralateral hip flexion thumbs *move apart*

Lack of thumb movement indicates joint fixation

S = stabilization (indifferent hand), ● = contact, ⟶ = examiner force, ┈┈┈▶ = patient motion

SI & Pelvis

Basic procedure - have patient take **deep relaxing breathes** through the entire process
1. Gently stretch patient into direction of restriction or decreased range of motion
2. Patient gently (~50% of maximum) contracts in exact opposite motion
3. Clinician resists contraction for ~7 seconds, then patient completely relaxes
4. On relaxation, clinician moves to new resistive barrier; repeat 3-5 times & reassess

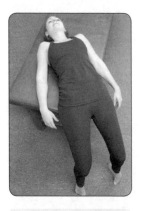

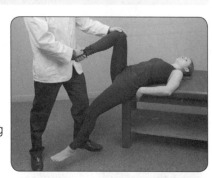

Clinician anchors patient's foot into their pelvis or shoulder (this allow clinician biomechanical advantage of using body weight)

Have patient angled on treatment table to allow for maximum SI joint motion while maintaining balance - sacrum balanced on corner

Always start with one knee/hip flexed before laying down to reduce lumbar loads

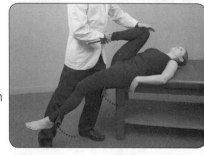

Clinician leans body toward patient (note left sided hip flexion and knee extension on this patient)

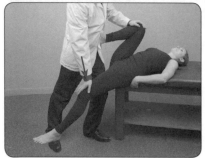

Clinician applies over pressure to the hanging leg to lengthen the left iliopsoas

The sequence demonstrated in this page is one of the best SI mobilization techniques this author has used (excellent results, easy on the clinician's body - it just works!)

Clinician also apply over pressure on patient's hand ankle to further stretch (go slow and make sure you have good balance)

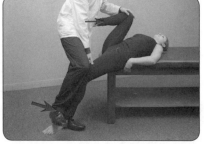

S = stabilization (indifferent hand), ● = contact, ⟶ = examiner force, ┈┈┈▶ = patient motion

SI & Pelvis

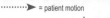

SI & Pelvis

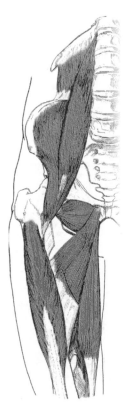

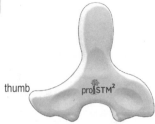

thumb — pro STM²

Save your thumbs -
91% of physios using massage
had to modify treatment because of
thumb pain
(Snodgrass SJ. Thumb pain in physiotherapists: potential
risk factors and proposed prevention strategies. J of
Manual and Manipulative Therapy 2002;10(4):206-217)

Start with hip
flexed to shorten
muscle - slowly
proceed with
gradual increase
in pressure (note
biomechanically
solid position of the
clinician's wrist)

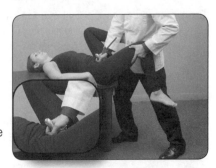

With pressure on
iliopsoas, slowly
lower the patient's
hip into extension
- make sure the
patient is breathing
deeply (people
have a tendency to
hold their breath)

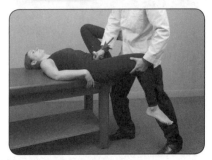

Push hip into
extension and
apply over
pressure on knee

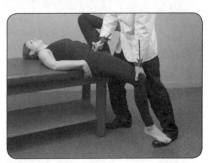

Apply over
pressure on
patient's ankle

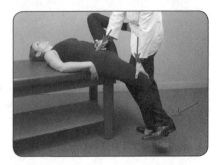

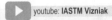
youtube: **IASTM Vizniak**

Do NOT over treat

Excessive treatment may exacerbate the patient's condition if using too many treatment modalities,
excessive pressure or excessive time spent on one specific restriction or lesion for too long

S = stabilization (indifferent hand),　● = contact,　⟶ = examiner force,　••••••▷ = patient motion

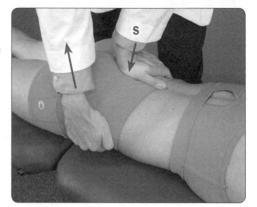

Ilium Posterior Glide

Indications: posterior glide restriction of ilium, anterior glide restriction of sacrum

Position: patient prone; clinician at side of table

Contact: clinician stabilizes sacrum and pulls ilium posteriorly

Force: pull ASIS posteriorly & instruct patient take in a deep breath; with exhalation mobilize the pull up on the ASIS

Clinical notes: same force may be induced by using a unilateral contact & simply pushing sacrum anteriorly - lifting of the ilium does put more strain on the clinician, rather than pushing down with weight and gravity on the sacrum

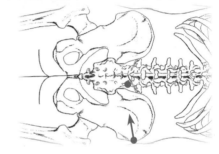

Posterior SI Distraction

Indications: SI hypomobility, pain

Position: patient prone; clinician at side of table

Contact: clinician's bilaterally places thenar or hypothenar eminences over patient's PSISs

Force: tissue pull **M-L, slightly P-A** & instruct patient take in a deep breath; with exhalation mobilize the SI joints laterally

Clinical notes: may be performed with a unilateral contact pushing the PSIS laterally

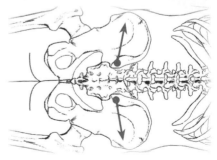

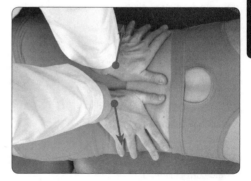

S = stabilization (indifferent hand),　● = contact,　——▶ = examiner force,　┈┈┈▶ = patient motion

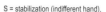

Superior Sacral Glide/Shear

Indications: superior glide restriction

Position: patient prone

Force: examiner stabilizes the patient's pelvis over the PSIS, & applies an **I-S force** over the sacrum; compare bilaterally & repeat as needed

Clinical notes: method may also help correct ilium up-slip

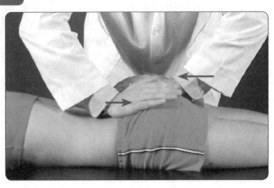

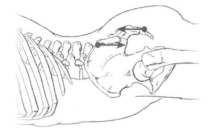

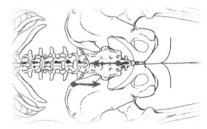

Inferior Sacral Glide/Shear

Indications: inferior glide restriction

Position: patient prone

Force: examiner stabilizes the patient's pelvis over the ischial tuberosity & applies a **S-I force** over the base of the sacrum; compare bilaterally & repeat as needed

Clinical notes: method may also help correct ilium down-slip

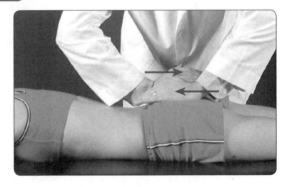

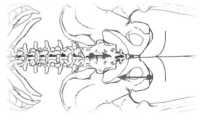

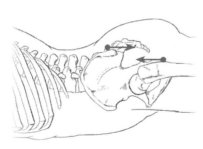

S = stabilization (indifferent hand), ● = contact, ⟶ = examiner force, ┈┈┈▷ = patient motion

Anterior SI Compression

Indications: out-flare of ilium

Position: patient supine; clinician at side of table

Contact: clinician's thenar or hypothenar eminence bilaterally contact the patient's ASISs

Force: tissue pull **L-M & instruct patient take in a deep breath;** with exhalation mobilize the ilium medially; repeat as needed

Clinical notes: ASIS contacts can be sensitive, use a soft hand; a side posture set-up may also be used to compress the ilium

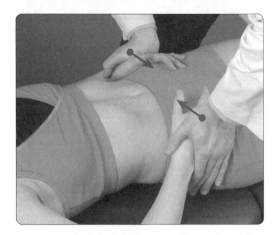

Anterior SI Distraction

Indications: inflare of ilia

Position: patient supine; clinician at side of table

Contact: clinician's thenar or hypothenar eminence bilaterally contacts the patient's ASISs

Force: tissue pull **M-L & instruct patient take in a deep breath**; with exhalation mobilize the ilium laterally; repeat as needed

Clinical notes: ASIS contacts can be sensitive, use a soft hand

Patient may cover their own ASIS with their hands to soften the contact and help avoid incidental contact

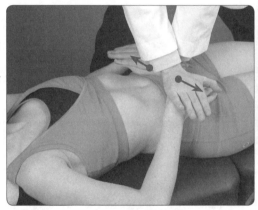

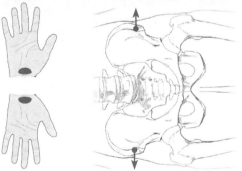

SI & Pelvis

S = stabilization (indifferent hand),   ● = contact,   ——→ = examiner force,   ·········▷ = patient motion

Indications: flexion malposition or extension restriction (PI ilium or nutated sacrum)

Position: patient prone; clinician at side of table

Contact: clinician's thenar or hypothenar eminence over patient's sacral apex & PSIS

Force: tissue pull **sacral apex contact S-I & PSIS contact I-S & M-L**; instruct patient take in a deep breath with exhalation mobilize the SI joint into extension; repeat as needed

Clinical notes: due to the sacral base angle and constant force of gravity when standing, nutation of the sacrum is very common

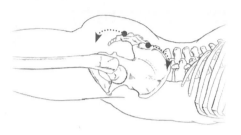

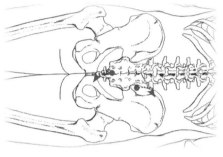

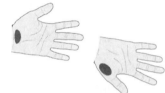

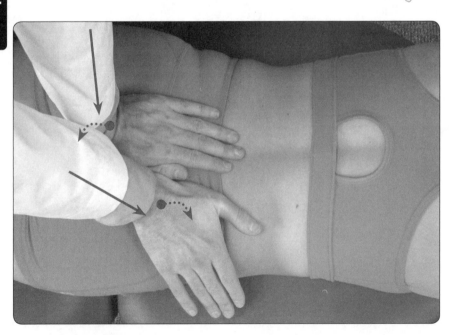

S = stabilization (indifferent hand), ● = contact, ➤ = examiner force, ┄┄➤ = patient motion

Indications: flexion restriction or extension malposition (AS ilium or counter-nutated sacrum)

Position: patient prone; clinician at side of table

Contact: clinician's thenar or hypothenar eminence over patient's sacral base & ischial tuberosity

Force: tissue pull **sacral base contact I-S & ischial tuberosity contact S-I & M-L**; instruct patient take in a deep breath with exhalation mobilize the SI joint into flexion; repeat as needed

Clinical notes: use soft hand contacts

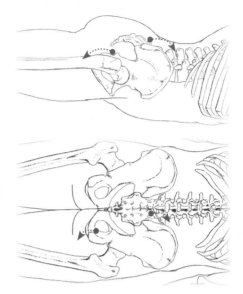

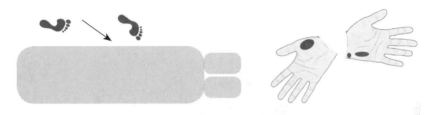

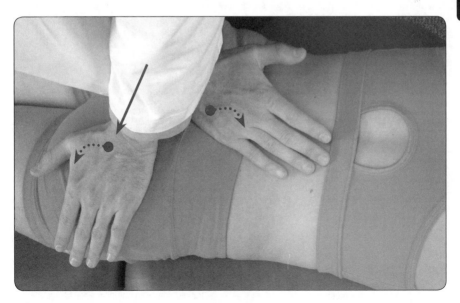

S = stabilization (indifferent hand),   ● = contact,   ➞ = examiner force,   ┈┈▸ = patient motion

Hypothenar PSIS Push

Indication: PI ilium (ilium flexion malposition or extension restriction)

Position: patient side posture with hip flexed 60°-80° & clinician in ~45° fencer thigh to thigh or side posture straddle stance

Contact: clinician's inferior hand hypothenar eminence over the medial edge of patients superior PSIS; stabilization over the patients shoulder or elbow

Force: tissue pull **M-L, I-S, P-A**; develop SI distraction by lowering body on patients thigh; mobilize or thrust by dropping body & pushing through contact hand

Clinical notes: clinician's upper stabilization hand should only develop a mild distraction force and not a rotational force

Rather than a hypothenar-PSIS contact clinician may choose to use a forearm-PSIS contact to reduce stress on wrist

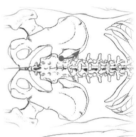

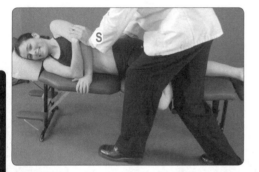

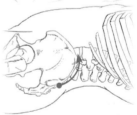

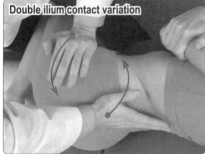

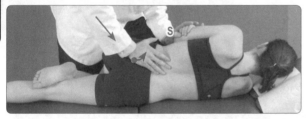

Double ilium contact variation

Contact over PSIS and AIIS, force is directed in a circular motion

Forearm contact variation

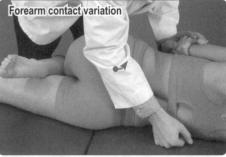

Contact over PSIS with forearm - contact recommended for clinicians with potential wrist issues

S = stabilization (indifferent hand), ● = contact, ➤ = examiner force, ┈┈➤ = patient motion

SI & Pelvis

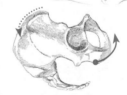
Hypothenar-Ischium Push

Indication: AS ilium (ilium extension malposition, flexion restriction)

Position: patient side posture with hip flexed > 90° & clinician in side posture straddle stance

Contact: clinician's inferior hand hypothenar eminence & palm over the medial inferior ischium; stabilization over the patients shoulder or elbow while maintaining spinal flexion

Force: tissue pull **P-A, M-L** ('J-shaped' scooping action); develop SI distraction by lowering body on patients thigh & hip; mobilize or thrust by dropping body & pushing through contact hand

Clinical notes: clinician's upper stabilization hand should only develop a mild distraction force and not a rotational force

Rather than a hypothenar-ischial contact clinician may choose to use a forearm-ischial contact to reduce stress on wrist

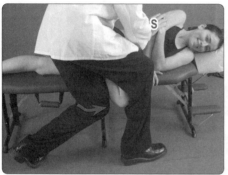

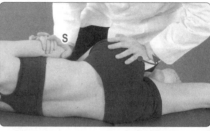

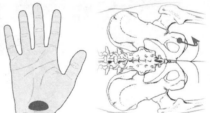

Flexion Sacroiliac (AS Ilium)
Hypothenar-inferior Ischium Contact
Forearm-Inferior Ischium Contact
Various Doctor/Patient Leg Positions
- Straddle flexed knee (low fencer)
- Straddle thigh
- Double thigh to shin
- Split leg (knee to popliteal fossa)

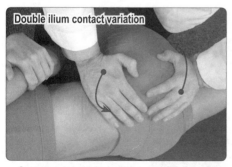

Double ilium contact variation

Contact over ischial tuberosity and ASIS, force is directed in a circular motion

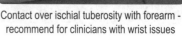

Forearm contact variation

Contact over ischial tuberosity with forearm - recommend for clinicians with wrist issues

S = stabilization (indifferent hand), ● = contact, ⟶ = examiner force, ┈┈▶ = patient motion

SI & Pelvis

Hypothenar Sacral Base Push

Indication: PS sacrum (unilateral posterior superior sacral malposition, sacral flexion restriction)

Position: patient side posture with hip flexed 60°-80° & clinician in ~45° fencer thigh to thigh or side posture straddle stance

Contact: clinician's inferior hand hypothenar eminence over the lateral edge of the superior sacral base (just medial to PSIS); stabilization over the patients shoulder or elbow

Force: tissue pull **I-S, P-A**; develop SI distraction by lowering body on patients thigh; mobilize or thrust by dropping body & pushing through contact hand

Clinical notes: clinician's upper stabilization hand should only develop a mild distraction force and not a rotational force

Clinician may choose to treat this condition with either the dysfunctional side up or the dysfunctional side down; all parameters are essentially the same with the clinician's contact either on the superior sacral base (affected side up) or the inferior sacral base (affected side down)

Note that there is **minimal lumbar rotation** to ensure the mobe/ manip is specific to the SI joint

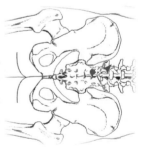

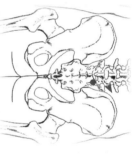

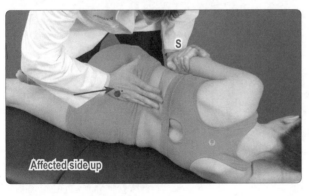

Affected side down

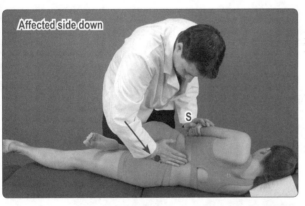

Affected side up

S = stabilization (indifferent hand),   ● = contact,   ——➤ = examiner force,   ·······➤ = patient motion

SI & Pelvis

Sacral Apex Push

Indication: AI sacrum (anterior inferior sacral malposition, SI extension restriction)

Position: patient side posture with hip flexed ~100° & clinician in side posture straddle stance

Contact: clinician's inferior hand hypothenar eminence & palm over the sacral apex; stabilization over the patients shoulder or elbow

Force: tissue pull slight **S-I, P-A** (a torquing/twisting motion can be added to the adjusting hand); develop distraction by lowering body on patients thigh; mobilize or thrust by dropping body & pushing through contact hand

Clinical notes: clinician's upper stabilization hand should only develop a mild distraction force and not a rotational force

Rather than a hypothenar-sacral contact clinician may choose to use a forearm-sacral contact

Note that there is **minimal lumbar rotation** to ensure the mobilization/manipulation is specific to the SI joint

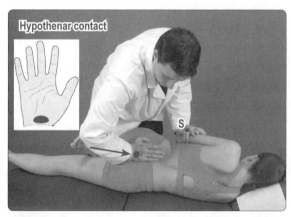

Hypothenar contact

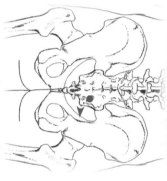

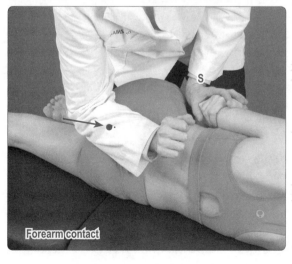

Forearm contact

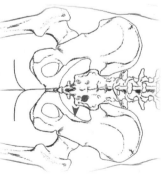

S = stabilization (indifferent hand),　● = contact,　———➤ = examiner force,　·········➤ = patient motion

Hypothenar PSIS Sacral Apex Push

Indication: PI ilium (ilium flexion malposition or extension restriction) or AI sacrum

Position: patient prone & clinician in facing stance on side opposite dysfunction

Contact: clinician places one hand over PSIS and other over sacral apex using hypothenar &/or palmar contacts

Force: tissue pull **PSIS (P-A, I-S, M-L), & Sacral apex (P-A, S-I)**; develop SI motion by lowering body and leaning into patient; mobilize or thrust by dropping body & pushing through both contact hands

Clinical notes: unilateral joint SI joint dysfunctions may be treated by modifying PSIS contacts

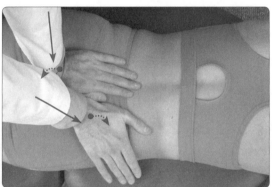

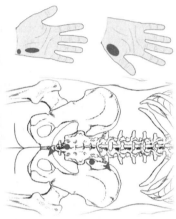

Knee Lift Ilium Push

Indication: PI ilium (ilium flexion malposition or extension restriction) or AI sacrum

Position: patient prone & clinician in fencer stance on side opposite dysfunction

Contact: clinician places superior hand hypothenar eminence & palm over PSIS and lifts the ipsilateral knee to induce hip/SI extension

Force: tissue pull P-A, I-S, M-L; develop SI motion by lowering body and leaning into patient; mobilize or thrust by dropping body & pushing through contact hand

Clinical notes: this technique may be used in combination with a drop table

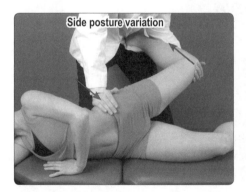

Side posture variation

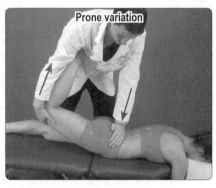

Prone variation

S = stabilization (indifferent hand), ● = contact, ➞ = examiner force, ┈┈┈▸ = patient motion

SI & Pelvis

Hypothenar Ischium Sacral Base Push

Indication: AS ilium (ilium extension malposition, flexion restriction) or PS sacrum

Position: patient prone & clinician in facing stance on side opposite dysfunction

Contact: clinician's places one hand over ischium and other over sacral base using hypothenar &/or palmar contacts

Force: tissue pull **P-A, S-I with ischial contact & P-A, I-S with sacral base contact;** develop SI motion by lowering body and leaning into patient; mobilize or thrust by dropping body & pushing through both contact hands

Clinical notes: unilateral joint SI joint dysfunctions may be treated by modifying sacral contacts

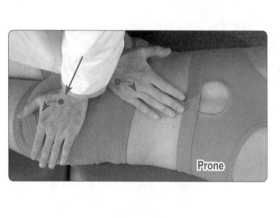

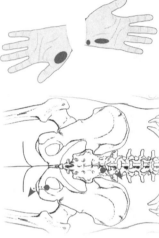

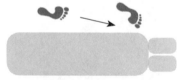

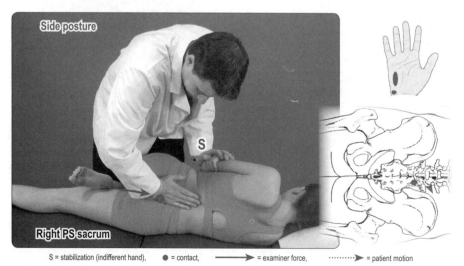

S = stabilization (indifferent hand), ● = contact, ——————▶ = examiner force, ·········▶ = patient motion

SI & Pelvis

Indication: PI ilium malposition or AS ilium malposition (rotated pelvis)

Position: patient prone (arrows below denote location of pelvic blocks)

Contact: clinician places blocks under ASIS & contralateral ischial tuberosity depending on the motion desired

Force: passive force of gravity is used to mobilize SI joints, over pressure may be applied by clinician - treatment time may be 30 sec up to ~10-15 minutes (start small to gage patient tolerance)

Clinical notes: this technique may be combined with gentle oscillatory movements applied to the posterior SI joint (PSIS, ischial tuberosity)

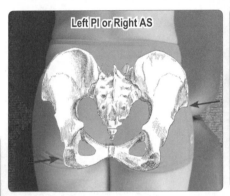

Left PI or Right AS

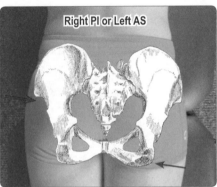

Right PI or Left AS

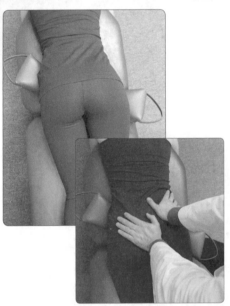

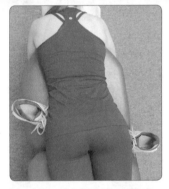

Consider pelvic blocking with a
rolled up towel or **patient's shoes**
(note this 5'5" female patient does not wear
size 10 men's shoes ☺)

Pelvic blocking and mobilization for a **right PI ilium or nutated sacrum** - a very common SI joint dysfunction

Pregnancy: if patient cannot lay prone or side lying, consider supine pelvic blocking (let the weight of the mom and baby do the work to stretch & mobilize the joint - most women will love it!

S = stabilization (indifferent hand), ● = contact, ➤ = examiner force, ┄┄➤ = patient motion

prohealthsys

Hypothenar Sacral Base

Indication: restricted posterior glide or anterior malposition of ilium

Position: patient supine with hip flexed 90° and knee bent; clinician stands on opposite side of table

Contact: clinician places one hand over the patient's knee and other hand just medial to patient's PSIS over the sacral base, clinician uses thenar eminence as contact

Force: clinician applies long axis compression down the patients thigh to the SI joint; a low amplitude P-A mobilize or thrust may be used

Clinical notes: can be grade 1-5 mobilization

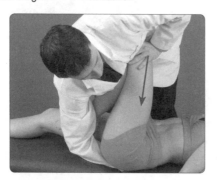

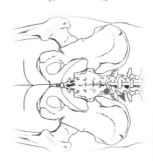

Hypothenar Ilium-Ischium

Indication: restricted superior glide or inferior malposition of pubic symphysis

Position: patient supine with involved side knee & hip fully flexed; clinician stands on contralateral side and reaches over patient

Contact: clinician places one hand over ASIS and other over ischium

Force: tissue pull **A-P with ASIS contact & P-A, S-I with ischial contact** (rotating the pelvis); at tension mobilize or thrust by dropping body & pushing/pulling through contact hands

Clinical notes: use soft contacts

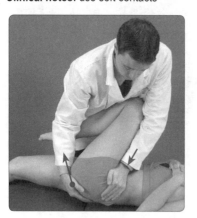

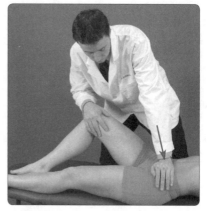

S = stabilization (indifferent hand),   ● = contact,   ➝ = examiner force,   ┈┈➤ = patient motion

SI & Pelvis

prohealthsys

Pubic Distraction

Indication: restriction or malposition of pubic symphysis

Position: patient supine with hips & knee flexed & feet close together; clinician stands at side of table

Contact: palmar contact bilaterally over patient's medial knees

Force: tissue pull M-L; ask patient to adduct thighs against resistance then after 2-3 seconds apply low amplitude M-L mobes in a pumping action

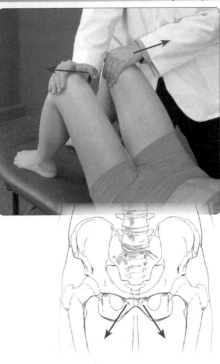

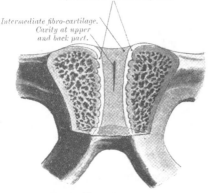

Hyaline cartilage covering bone.

Intermediate fibro-cartilage.
Cavity at upper
and back part.

Hypothenar Pubic Symphysis

Indication: restricted posterior glide or anterior malposition of pubic symphysis

Position: patient supine with uninvolved knee & hip flexed; clinician facing inferiorly on uninvolved side

Contact: clinician places one hand over ipsilateral pubic symphysis and other over patient's contralateral distal thigh (clinician may use a bilateral thenar contact on pubic symphysis)

Force: tissue pull S-I; at tension mobilize or thrust P-A

Clinical notes: technique may be combined with a pelvic drop table or activator

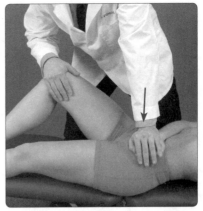

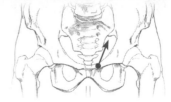

SI & Pelvis

S = stabilization (indifferent hand), ● = contact, ⟶ = examiner force, ┈┈┈▶ = patient motion

External Coccyx Push

Indication: restriction or malposition of coccyx

Position: patient prone; clinician in fencer stance

Contact: clinician place thumb with reinforced palm over coccyx

Force: tissue pull I-S; at tension mobilize or thrust by dropping body & pushing through contact hands

Clinical notes: increased success may be noted with direct physical skin contact

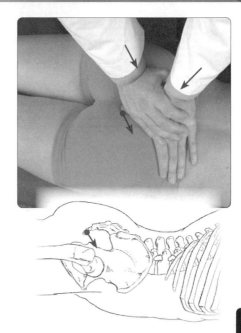

Internal Coccyx Pull

Indication: restriction or malposition of coccyx (usually secondary to hard fall on tail bone)

Position: patient side posture or prone, clinician stands at side of table

Contact: a *gloved*, lubricated finger is inserted into the rectum and contacts the patient's anterior coccyx, while the other hand stabilizes the sacrum

Force: gently tissue pull S-I, A-P; at tension apply a gentle mobilize or thrust (essentially distraction)

Clinical notes: before beginning maneuver be sure patient is fully aware of procedure (written consent is a must) - be sure you are within your scope of practice for your region

The first instinct of many clinicians is to find this manipulation disturbing, however in patients with coccygeal dysfunction this maneuver can drastically improve their quality of life

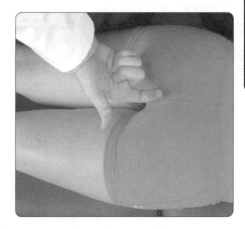

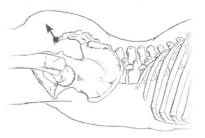

SI & Pelvis

S = stabilization (indifferent hand), ● = contact, ⟶ = examiner force, ┄┄┄▶ = patient motion

1. Vizniak, NA. Applied Human Cadaver Dissections. 1999-2018.
2. Abbott JH, McCane B, Herbison P, Moginie C, Chapple C, Hogarty T. Lumbar segmental instability: a criterion-related validity study of manual therapy assessment. BMC Musculoskelet Disord. 2005;6:56.
3. Abram SE. Treatment of lumbosacral radiculopathy with epidural steroids. Anesthesiology. Dec 1999;91(6):1937-41.
4. Akuthota V, Nadler SF. Core strengthening. Arch Phys Med Rehabil. Mar 2004;85(3 suppl 1):S86-92.
5. Albeck M. A critical assessment of clinical diagnosis of disc herniation in patients with monoradicular sciatica. Acta Neurochir. 1996;138:40.
6. Barr KP, Griggs M, Cadby T. Lumbar stabilization: a review of core concepts and current literature, part 2. Am J Phys Med Rehabil. Jan 2007;86(1):72-80.
7. Bertilson BC, Bring I, Sjoblom A, Sundell K, Strender LE. Inter-examiner reliability in the assessment of low back pain (LBP) using the Kirkaldy-Willis classification (KWC). Eur SpineJ. 2006; 1-9.
8. Binkley J, Stratford PW, Gill C. Interrater reliability of lumbar accessory motion mobility testing. Phys Ther. 1995;75(9):786-792.
9. Boal RW, Gillette RG. Central Neuronal Plasticity, Low Back Pain and Spinal Manipulative Therapy. JMPT 27(5):314-326, 2004.
10. Boline PD, Haas M, Meyer JJ, Kassak K, Nelson C, Keating JC., Jr Interexaminer reliability of eight evaluative dimensions of lumbar segmental abnormality: Part II. 1993 Jul–Aug;16(6):363–374.
11. Bono CM. Low-back pain in athletes. J Bone Joint Surg Am. Feb 2004;86-A(2):382-96.
12. Borg-Stein J, Wilkins A. Soft tissue determinants of low back pain. Curr Pain Headache Rep. Oct 2006;10(5):339-44.
13. Brown FW. Management of diskogenic pain using epidural and intrathecal steroids. Clin Orthop Relat Res. Nov-Dec 1977;129:72-8.
14. Charnley J. Orthopaedic signs in the diagnosis of disc protrusion with special reference to the straight-leg raising test. Lancet. 1951;1:186-192.
15. Chiradejnant A, Maher CG, Latimer J. Objective manual assessment of lumbar posteroanterior stiffness is now possible. J Manipulative Physiol Ther. 2003;26(1):34-39.
16. Cohen SP, Wenzell D, Hurley RW, et al. A double-blind, placebo-controlled, dose-response pilot study evaluating intradiscal etanercept in patients with chronic discogenic low back pain or lumbosacral radiculopathy. Anesthesiology. Jul 2007;107(1):99-105.
17. Cook C, Cook A, Fleming R. Rehabilitation for clinical lumbar instability in an adolescent diver with spondylolisthesis. 1 Man Manipulative Ther. 2004;1 2(2):91-99.
18. Cyteval C, Fescquet N, Thomas E, et al. Predictive factors of efficacy of periradicular corticosteroid injections for lumbar radiculopathy. AJNR Am J Neuroradiol. May 2006;27(5):978-82.
19. DePalma MJ, Bhargava A, Slipman CW. A critical appraisal of the evidence for selective nerve root injection in the treatment of lumbosacral radiculopathy. Arch Phys Med Rehabil. Jul 2005;86(7):1477-83.
20. Dishman JD, Cunningham BM, Burke J. Comparison of Tibial Nerve H-Reflex Excitability After Cervical and Lumbar Manipulation. JMPT 25(5):318-325, 2002.
21. Donelson R, Aprill C, Medcalf R, Grant W. A prospective study of centralization of lumbar and referred pain. A predictor of symptomatic discs & annular competence. Spine. 1997;22(10):1115-1122.
22. Downey BJ, Taylor NF, Niere KR. Manipulative physiotherapists can reliably palpate nominated lumbar spinal levels. Man Ther. 1999 Aug;4(3):151–156.
23. Eskelund Hansen B, Simonsen T, Leboeuf-Yde C. Motion Palpation of the Lumbar Spine – A Problem With The Test or the Tester? JMPT 29(3):208-212, 2006.
24. Friedly J, Chan L, Deyo R. Increases in lumbosacral injections in the Medicare population: 1994 to 2001. Spine. Jul 15 2007;32(16):1754-60.
25. Fritz JM, Piva S, Childs J. Accuracy of the clinical examination to predict radiographic instability of the lumbar spine. Eur Spine J. 2005;14(8):743-50.
26. Gurdjian E, Webster J, Ostrowski AZ, Hardy W, Lindner D, Thomas L. Herniated lumbar intervertebral discs: an analysis of 11 76 operated cases. J Trauma. 1961;1:158-176.
27. Hakelius A, Hindmarsh J. The comparative reliability of preoperative diagnostic methods in lumbar disc surgery. Acta Orthop Scand. 1972;43:234-238.
28. Hammer WI, Pfefer MT. Treatment of Subacute Lumbar Compartment Syndrome Using the Graston Technique. JMPT 28(3):199-204, 2005.
29. Hawk C, Phongphua C, Bleecker J, Swank L, Lopez D, Rubley T. Preliminary study of the reliability of assessment procedures for indications for chiropractic adjustments of the lumbar spine. JMPT. 1999 Jul–Aug;22(6):382–389.
30. Hession EF, Donald GD. Treatment of multiple lumbar disk herniations in an adolescent athlete utilizing flexion distraction and rotational manipulation. JMPT. 1993 Mar–Apr;16(3):185–192.
31. Keating JC, Jr, Bergmann TF, Jacobs GE, Finer BA, Larson K. Interexaminer reliability of eight evaluative dimensions of lumbar segmental abnormality. JMPT. 1990 Oct;13(8):463–470.
32. Kerr RSC, Cadoux-Hudson TA, Adams CBT. The value of accurate clinical assessment in the surgical management of the lumbar disc protrusion. J Neurol Neurosurg Psychiatr. 1988;51:169-173.
33. Knuttson B. Comparative value of electromyographic, myelographic, & clinical-neurological examinations in diagnosis of lumbar root compression syndrome. Acta Ortho Scand. 1961;(Suppl 49):1 9-49.
34. Kosteljanetz M, Bang F, Schmidt-Olsen S. The clinical significance of straight leg raising (Lasegue's sign) in the diagnosis of prolapsed lumbar disc. Spine. 1988;13:393-395.
35. Kosteljanetz M, Espersen 0, Halaburt H, Miletic T. Predictive value of clinical & surgical findings in patients with lumbago-sciatica: aprospective study (part 1). Acta Neurochirugica. 1984;73:67-76.
36. Kreitz BG, Cote P, Yong-Hing K. Crossed femoral stretching test: a case report. Spine. 1996;21(13):1584-1586.
37. Laslett M, Aprill CN, McDonald B, Oberg B. Clinical predictors of lumbar provocation discography: a study of clinical predictors of lumbar provocation discography. Eur Spine J. 2006;1-12.
38. Laslett M, Oberg B, Aprill CN, McDonald B. Centralization as a predictor of provocation discography results in chronic low back pain, and the influence of disability & distress on diagnostic power. Spine J. 2005;5(4): 370-380.
39. LauderTD, DillinghamTR,AndaryMl Kumar S, Pezzin LE, Stephens RT. Effect of history and exam in predicting electrodiagnostic outcome among patients with suspected lumbosacral radiculopathy. Am J Phys Med Rehabil.
40. Lehman GJ, McGill SM. The Influence of a Chiropractic Manipulation on Lumbar Kinematics and Electromyography During Simple and Complex Tasks. JMPT 22(9):576-581, 1999.
41. Lutz GE, Vad VB, Wisneski RJ. Fluoroscopic transforaminal lumbar epidural steroids: an outcome study. Arch Phys Med Rehabil. Nov 1998;79(11):1362-6.
42. Lyle MA, Manes 5, McGuinness M, Ziaei S, Iversen MD. Relationship of physical examination findings & self-reported symptom severity & physical function in patients with degenerative lumbar conditions. Phys Ther. 2005;85(2):1 20-1 33.
43. Maher C, Adams R. Reliability of pain & stiffness assessments in clinical manual lumbar spine examination. Phys Ther. 1994;74(9):801 -809.
44. Maher C, Adams R. Reliability of pain and stiffness assessments in clinical manual lumbar spine examination. Phys Ther. 1994 Sep;74(9):801–811.
45. Matyas T, Bach T. The reliability of selected techniques in clinical arthrometrics. Aust J Physio. 1985;31 :1 75-1 99.
46. McLain RF, Pickar JG. Mechanoreceptor Endings in Human Thoracic and Lumbar Facet Joints.
47. Memmo PA, Nadler SF, Malanga GA. Lumbar disc herniation: a review of surgical and non-surgical indications and outcomes. J Back Musculoskelet Rehabil. 2000;14(3):79-88.
48. Mootz RD, Keating JC, Jr, Kontz HP, Milus TB, Jacobs GE. Intra- and interobserver reliability of passive motion palpation of the lumbar spine. JMPT. 1989 Dec;12(6):440–445.
49. Padua L, Commodari I, Zappia M, Pazzaglia C, Tonali PA. Misdiagnosis of lumbar-sacral radiculopathy: usefulness of combination of EMG and ultrasound. Neurol Sci. Jun 2007;28(3):154-5.
50. Panzer DM. The reliability of lumbar motion palpation. JMPT. 1992 Oct;15(8):518–524.
51. Phillips DR, Twomey LT. A comparison of manual diagnosis with a diagnosis established by a uni-level lumbar spinal block procedure. Man Ther. 1996 Mar;1(2):82–87.
52. Phillips DR, Twomey LT. A comparison of manual diagnosis with a diagnosis established by a unilevel lumbar spinal block procedure. Man Ther. 1996; 1(2):82-87.
53. Porchet F, Fankhauser H, de Tribolet N. Extreme lateral lumbar disc herniation: clinical presentation in 178 patients. Acta Neurochir (Wien). 1994;1 27(3-4):203-209.
54. Potter L, McCarthy C, Oldham J. Interexaminer Reliability of Identifying a Dysfunctional Segment in the Thoracic and Lumbar Spine. JMPT. 1993; 203-207, 2006
55. Song XJ, et al. Spinal Manipulation Reduces Pain and Hyperalgesia After Lumbar Intervertebral Foramen Inflammation in the Rat. JMPT 29(1):5-13, 2006.
56. Spangfort EV. The lumbar disc herniation: a computer aided analysis of 2504 operations. Acta Orthop Scand. l972;11(Supl 142):1-93.
57. Stankovic R, Johnell 0, Maly P, Willner S. Use of lumbar extension, slump test, physical andneurological examination in the evaluation of patients with suspected herniated nucleus pulposus: a prospective clinical study. Man Ther. 1999;4(1):25-32.
58. Suseki K, et al. Innervation of the Lumbar Facet Joints: Origins and Function. Spine 22(5):477-485, 1997.
59. Tarulli AW, Raynor EM. Lumbosacral radiculopathy. Neurol Clin. May 2007;25(2):387-405.
60. Tsao B. The electrodiagnosis of cervical and lumbosacral radiculopathy. Neurol Clin. May 2007;25(2):473-94.
61. Vroomen PC, de Krom MC, Wilmink JT, Kester AD, Knottnerus JA. Diagnostic value of history and physical examination in patients suspected of lumbosacral nerve root compression. J Neurol Neurosurg Psychiatry. 2002; 72(5):630-634.
62. Willardson JM. Core stability training: applications to sports conditioning programs. J Strength Cond Res. Aug 2007;21(3):979-85.

2000;79:60-68.

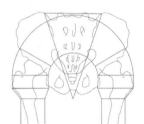

SI & Pelvis Joint Quiz (page reference)

1. What are the joint type classifications for this region? (91) _____

2. What are the joint surface shapes for the SI joint (convex/concave)? (91)

_____

3. What is the normal ROM for _____? (91)
   • SI Flexion/Ext.: _____, _____

4. Lumbosacral angle can range is _____? (88)

5. What is the SI joint tight packed position? (91)

_____

6. What ligaments resist nutation? (89)

_____

7. What muscles cause cross the SI joint? (90)

_____

8. What muscle cause anterior pelvic tilt? (94)

_____

9. Nutation causes lumbar _____? (93)

10. Can you palpate _____ ? (86)

S = stabilization (indifferent hand),   ● = contact,   ➡ = examiner force,   ┅┅➤ = patient motion

SI & Pelvis

Learning Objectives

After completing this chapter, students will be able to:

1. Perform a regional exam and recognize common pathologies of the region & indication for mobilization

2. Identify and palpate body region bony landmarks, ligaments and muscles

3. Discuss regional kinematics and joint organ biomechanics including lumbar disc kinesiology

4. Demonstrate regional AROM, PROM & inclinometry

5. Recognize and execute the steps of effective mobilization and joint-play including indications, position, contact, force and relevant clinical notes

6. Perform side-lying, supine, seated, prone assessment and mobilizations of

   - Rotation restrictions
   - Flexion, Lateral flexion restrictions
   - Extension restrictions
   - Lateral glides, P-A glides
   - Muscle Energy Technique
   - Lumbar IASTM

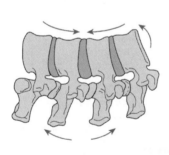

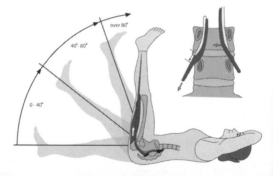

Lumbar Spine

Cluster for patients likely to benefit from SPINAL MANIPULATION

- Duration low back pain for ≤ 16 days
- No symptoms below the knee
- FABQ work subscale score 18 points or less
- Segmental mobility testing finding 1 or more hypomobile segments in the lumbar spine
- Hip internal rotation with at least one hip having at least 35 degrees of internal rotation
- 1-2 criteria met: -LR: 0.1
- 4-5 criteria met: +LR: 13.2

1. Childs JD, Fritz JM, Flynn TW, et al. "A clinical prediction rule to identify patients with low back pain most likely to benefit from spinal manipulation: a validation study." Ann Intern Med 2004; 141: 920-928. Web. 08/18/2017.

Cluster for patients likely to benefit from LUMBAR STABILIZATION EXERCISES

- Age < 40
- Avg Straight Leg Raise > 91 degrees
- Positive Prone Instability Test
- Aberrant movement present (found during lumbar ROM test) - often described as instability catch, painful arc of motion, Minor's sign, or a reversal of lumbopelvic motion
- 1 criteria met: -LR: 0.2 or 2 criteria met: -LR: .3
- 3 or 4 criteria met: +LR: 4.0

1. Hicks G, Fritz J, Delitto A, "Preliminary development of a clinical prediction rule for determining which patients w/ low back pain will respond to a stabilization exercises." Arch Phys Med Rehabil 2005; 86: 1753-1762. Web. 07/28/2017.

History special questions
- Specific mechanism of injury & forces involved? - lifting & twisting?
- Any numbness, tingling or weakness?
- Coughing, sneezing or straining make it worse?
- Type of work, typical posture, sleeping posture?
- Prior injuries or treatments?
- What makes it better or worse?
- Review of systems (GI, urinary, cardiovascular)

Inspection
- Asymmetry, bruising, bumps, color, swelling, iliac crest height
- Posture, gait analysis (limp)

Palpation (may be done after ROM assessment)

Abdominal palpation	TFL
Inguinal lymph nodes	Greater trochanter
Femoral pulse	Piriformis
Pubic symphysis	Sacrotuberous lig.
ASIS	Sacroiliac joint
Iliac crest	Sacrospinous lig.
Paraspinal muscles	Gluteus maximus
Quadratus lumborum	Iliopsoas
Iliolumbar ligaments	Quadriceps
PSIS	Gastro-soleus
Ischial tuberosities	Spinous process
Hamstrings	Lower ribs

Functional assessment (ADLs)
- Toe touch or squat & rise

AROM (lumbar)
Flexion ....40-60° (Adam's sign)
Extension ....20-35°
Lateral Flexion ....15-20°
Rotation ....5-20°

PROM & Joint Play (if indicated)

Myotomes (resisted isometric movements)
- Trunk rotation (T6-L2, segmental nn.)
- Trunk lateral flexion (T6-L2, segmental nn.)
- Trunk flexion/extension (T6-L2, segmental n.)
- Hip flexion (L1-L3, femoral n.)
- Knee extension (L3-L4; femoral n.)
- Knee flexion (L4-S2, sciatic n.)

- Ankle dorsiflexion (**L4**, L5 - deep peroneal),
- Ankle inversion (L4, **L5** - deep peroneal)
- Ankle eversion (L5, **S1** - sup. peroneal)
- Big toe extension, (L4, **L5**, S1; deep peron.)
- Big toe flexion (L5-S1, tibial nerve)

Leg length measurements
- Greater trochanter to lateral malleolus
- Pubic symphysis to medial malleolus
- Umbilicus to medial malleolus
- Prone leg length evaluation

Abdominal exam (if indicated)
- Observe, auscultate, percuss, palpate, sit-up (abdominal strength & Beevor's sign)

Neurovascular screen
Sensory: Light touch, sharp/dull
Vibration (DIP, 3rd digit)
UMNL: Babinski (L1 & above)
DTR's: Patella (L3, L4), hamstring (L5), Achilles (L5, S1)
Vascular: femoral, popliteal, dorsal pedal pulses, nail bed blanching

Orthopedic tests (if indicated)
Screening
- Dejerine's triad, Minor's sign
- Heel walk, toe walk, squat & rise
- Kemp's test, Goldwait's test, Farfan's test

Lumbar sprain/strain
- ROM & Palpation
- Kemp's Test, Nachlas test
- Sign of the buttock

Lumbar Radiculopathy
- Straight leg raise (SLR), Well leg raise
- Bowstring sign, Bragard's test
- Femoral nerve traction test, Piriformis test

SI joint lesion
- Belt test, Lasège's test, Nachlas test
- Motion palpation

Instability
- Segmental instability test
- P-A glide test
- Lumbar flexion/extension test

Thoracic spine, SI joints & Hip Screen

Diagnostic imaging (if indicated)

 youtube: **Lumbar Exam Brief Vizniak**

Lumbar Spine

Condition	Clinical notes
Abdominal aortic aneurysm (AAA)	*Hx:* smoker, hypertension, first degree family connection, > 50 years old, M>F (atherosclerosis, CT disorders – Marfan's & Ehler danlos Syndrome) *SSx:* most are asymptomatic until rupture - possible low back pain *DDx:* kidney stone, DJD, appendicitis, constipation
Ankylosing spondylitis	*Hx:* 20-35 yrs old, M > F; insidious onset of vague LBP & stiffness worse with waking better with motion *SSx:* loss of lumbar/SI ROM, (+) blood tests HLA-B27, ↑ ESR *DDx:* progressive sclerosis of SI joints, expands up the spine visible on x-ray
Cauda equina syndrome	*Hx:* **bilateral** neurologic symptoms, saddle anesthesia, loss of bladder control *SSx:* gait abnormalities; ↓ DTRs, motor strength; (+) Babinski *DDx:* visible on MRI, spinal canal stenosis
Disc herniation	*Hx:* **unilateral** L4-S1 neurologic signs (numbness, weakness); antalgic posture *SSx:* ↑ pain with flexion; ↓ DTRs, motor strength; (+) SLR *DDx:* visible on MRI, IVF osteophyte encroachment, cauda equina syndrome
Lumbar (DJD) osteoarthrosis	*Hx:* local central pain, worse in morning, better with mild activity *SSx:* possible crepitus with motion; decreased AROM & PROM *DDx:* visible on x-ray: ↓ joint space, osteophyte formation
Lumbar joint dysfunction (subluxation)	*Hx:* insidious onset of local pain or discomfort *SSx:* tender to palpation; limited joint play; local myospasm; bone out of place *DDx:* lumbar sprain/strain, facet syndrome, meniscoid entrapment
Lumbar sprain/ strain	*Hx:* history of trauma, local pain with motion *SSx:* no neurologic signs; decreased AROM & PROM, RROM due to pain *DDx:* lumbar joint dysfunction often coexist
Pelvic fracture	*Hx:* significant trauma, severe pain (some can still ambulate) *SSx:* gait abnormalities; (+) SI compression, distraction stress test *DDx:* visible on x-ray or CT, severe SI sprain
Piriformis syndrome	*Hx:* possible pain down back of leg, worse when sitting on hard surface *SSx:* tender to palpation; (+) Hibb's test, Piriformis test *DDx:* lumbar disc herniation, spinal stenosis, lumbar sprain/strain
Sacroiliac instability	*Hx:* chronic SI pain, possible repeatable "clunk" of SI joint; may occur during or shortly after pregnancy *SSx:* (+) sacral glide test for increased motion *DDx:* SI joint dysfunction, lumbar instability
Spinal stenosis	*Hx:* M > F (2:1), chronic low back pain, worse with prolonged standing *SSx:* decreased AROM & PROM; confirm with x-ray ↓ spinal canal diameter *DDx:* vascular claudication
Spondylolisthesis	*Hx:* chronic low back pain, repetitive extension motions (e.g. rowing) *SSx:* possible hyperlordosis; repeatable 'clunk' or 'catch' with lumbar ROM *DDx:* confirm on x-ray with flexion/extension studies

↑ = increase, ↓ = decrease, Hx = history, SSx = signs & symptoms, DDx = differential diagnosis

Lumbar Spine

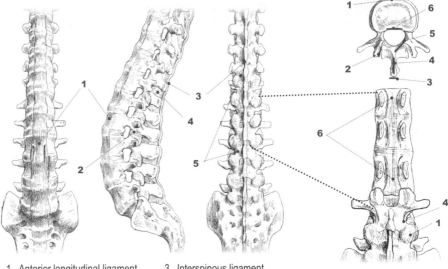

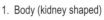

1. Anterior longitudinal ligament
1. Zygapophyseal joint capsule
2. Supraspinous ligament
3. Interspinous ligament
4. Ligamentum flavum
5. Posterior longitudinal ligament

posterior view L1-L5
(pedicles have been cut to show
posterior aspect of the lumbar
vertebral bodies)

Lumbar Vertebra

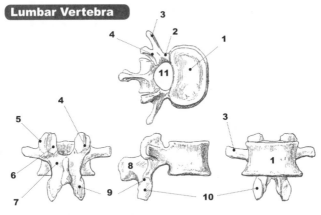

1. Body (kidney shaped)
2. Pedicles
3. Transverse process
4. Superior articular process
5. Mammillary process
6. Superior articular facet
7. Lamina
8. Spinous process
9. Inferior articular process
10. Inferior articular facet
11. Vertebral canal

Lumbar Spine Innervation

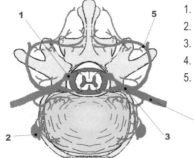

1. Dorsal root ganglion
2. Sympathetic ganglion
3. Spinal nerve
4. Ventral ramus
5. Dorsal ramus

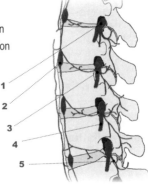

Intervertebral Disc

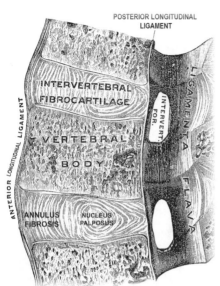

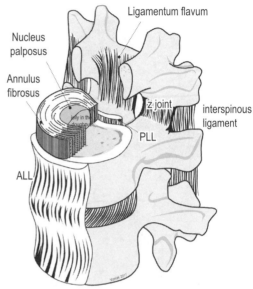

Ligament	Attaches (origin/insertion)	Function
Anterior longitudinal	Anterior vertebral body & disc to next vertebrae	Resists spinal extension
Annulus fibrosus	Vertebral bodies from C3-S1	Shock absorption, resists all spinal motions **strongest ligament of spine**
Posterior longitudinal	Posterior vertebral body & disc to next vertebrae	Resists spinal flexion
Z-joint capsule	Facet below to facet above	Resist flexion & lateral flexion of trunk
Ligamentum flavum	Laminae to laminae	Resists flexion of trunk, elasticity assists extension of trunk
Interspinous	Spinous process to spinous process	Resists flexion of trunk, & shear forces on vertebrae
Supraspinous	Spinous process to SP above	Resists trunk flexion & forward shear force on spine
Intertransverse	Transverse process to TP	Resists lateral flexion of trunk
Iliolumbar	Transverse process of L4-5 to iliac crest	Resists lumbar flexion, lateral flexion & rotation

Lumbar Spine

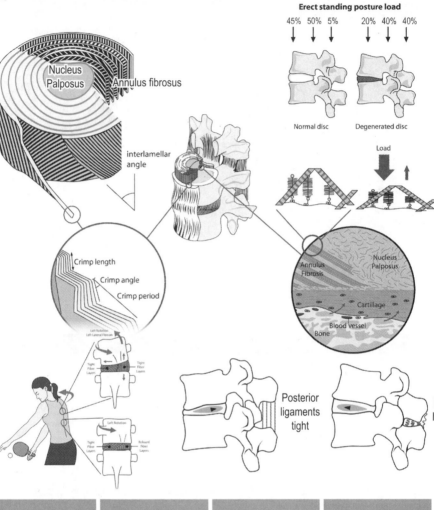

Erect standing posture load

45% 50% 5%   20% 40% 40%

Normal disc   Degenerated disc

Nucleus Palposus
Annulus fibrosus

interlamellar angle

Crimp length
Crimp angle
Crimp period

Load

Annulus Fibrosis
Nucleus Palposus
Cartillage
Blood vessel
Bone

Left Rotation
Left Lateral Flexion
Tight Fibro Layers
Tight Fibro Layers

Left Rotation
Tight Fibro Layers
Relaxed Fiber Layers

Posterior ligaments tight

Pos ligam la

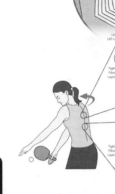
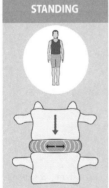

STANDING	FLEXION	EXTENSION	LATERAL FLEXION

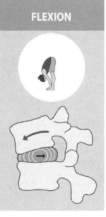
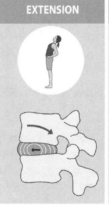
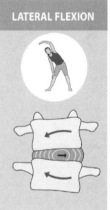

➡ Movement of vertebrae   ➡ Movement of nucleus pulposus

IVD composition:

- 60- 70% water,
- ~30% proteoglycans (PG) and collagen

PG is mainly consists of cell ground substances GAGs (Glysaminoglycan) which is primarily CS (Chondroitin sulfate) and KS (Keratan sulfate) with the high molecular weight complex proteins, disaccharides. This PG acts as the backbone of the HA (Hyaluronic acid). HA acts as the binding sites for CS and KS forming large brush like hydrophylic macromolecules inside the IVD cells

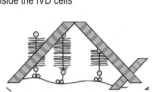

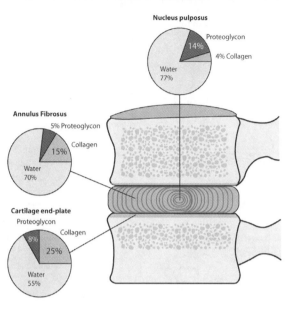

Nucleus pulposus
Proteoglycon 14%
4% Collagen
Water 77%

Annulus Fibrosus
5% Proteoglycon
Collagen 15%
Water 70%

Cartilage end-plate
Proteoglycon 8%
Collagen 25%
Water 55%

Component	Nucleus Palposus	Annulus fibrosus
Water	90 % at birth 80 % at age 20 70 % at older age	60-70 %, mild decrease with age (lower fluid movement with increased age)
Collagens (collagen I & II, collagen X (scar tissue) produced by the degenerated disc - very poor mechanical properties)	Only collagen I, 15-20 % with (dry weight) - mild change with age, decreased with herniation or degeneration	Only collagen II, 50-60 % with (dry weight) - little change with age
PGs (Proteoglycans)	65% with (dry weight) - little change with age	15-20 % with (dry weight) - little change with age
Non-collagenous proteins & elastin	20-45% with (dry weight) - little change with age	5-25% with (dry weight) (elastin content may decrease with age & loss of flexibility)

Extracellular enzymes, age pigments, cells are also present but make up only a minor portion.

(margin) Lumbar Spine

1. Le Maitre CL, Hoyland JA, Freemont AJ (2007) Catabolic cytokine expression in degenerate and herniated human intervertebral discs: IL-1beta and TNFalpha expression profile. Arthritis Res Ther 9:R77.
2. Farndale RW, Buttle DJ, Barrett AJ (1986) Improved quantitation and discrimination of sulphated glycosaminoglycans by use of dimethylmethylene blue. Biochim Biophys Acta 883: 173-177.
3. Holm S, Maroudas A, Urban JP, Selstam G, Nachemson A (1981) Nutrition of the intervertebral disc: solute transport and metabolism. Connect Tissue Res 8: 101-119.
4. Wallach CJ, Sobajima S, Watanabe Y, Kim JS, Georgescu HI, et al. (2003) Gene transfer of the catabolic inhibitor TIMP-1 increases measured proteoglycans in cells from degenerated human intervertebral discs. Spine (Phila Pa 1976) 28: 2331-2337.
5. Luoma K, Riihimaki H, Luukkonen R, Raininko R, Viikari-Juntura E, et al. (2000) Low back pain in relation to lumbar disc degeneration. Spine (Phila Pa 1976) 25: 487-492.
6. Le Maitre CL, Pockert A, Buttle DJ, Freemont AJ, Hoyland JA (2007) Matrix synthesis and degradation in human intervertebral disc degeneration. Biochem Soc Trans 35: 652-655.
7. Risbud MV, Izzo MW, Adams CS, Arnold WW, Hillibrand AS, et al. (2003) An organ culture system for the study of the nucleus pulposus: description of the system and evaluation of the cells. Spine (Phila Pa 1976) 28: 2652-2658.
8. MacLean JJ, Lee CR, Alini M, Iatridis JC (2005) The effects of short-term load duration on anabolic and catabolic gene expression in the rat tail intervertebral disc. J Orthop Res 23: 1120-1127.
9. Leitinger B, Kwan AP (August 2006). "The discoidin domain receptor DDR2 is a receptor for type X collagen". Matrix Biol. 25 (6): 355–64. doi:10.1016/j.matbio.2006.05.006. PMID 16806867.
10. Vizniak, NA. Unfixed-tissue Clinical Dissections. 1999-2018.

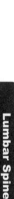

Degenerative Joint Disease (DJD)
- most common at L4-L5-S1 (greatest load stress, but can occur anywhere there is excess stress or prior injury)

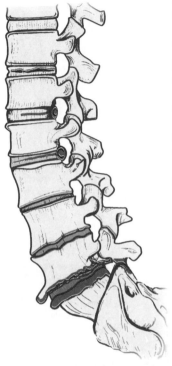

I – Dysfunctional phase:
- Purely **functional = HYPOmobility is the hallmark sign**
- Patient is typically young; minimal trauma (mild to moderate strain) "I should not have done that" or "I threw my back out playing golf or dead lifting etc."
- NO x-ray degenerative changes noted (possible on MRI)
- Circumferential tears or fissures in outer annulus, outer annulus is innervated → low back pain
- Nucleus pulposus loses water & proteoglycan content

II – Unstable phase (instability):
- Loss of mechanical integrity, multiple annular tears, internal disc disruption & resorption, or loss of disc space height
- Other changes include z-joint cartilage degenerates, capsule laxity & subluxation
- Leading to segmental instability& herniation
- Onset around 30s...radiographic evidence of traction spurs (response to excess motion) - disc herniations occur here
- Person who's back "goes out all the time" or changes ADL b/c of chance of pain - "I really would like to do that but last time I tried my back went out"

III – Stabilization phase:
- Structural **HYPOmobility is hallmark sign**
  - Further disc resorption - disc-space narrowing, end-plate destruction, fibrosis, reactive sclerosis & osteophyte formation ligamentum flavum thickening- increased force on z-joints
- Discogenic pain results, varies in patients (ankylosis or spinal DISH in sever cases)

20% 40% 40%

Degenerated disc

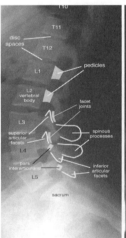

x-ray of normal lumbar spine anatomy (lateral view)

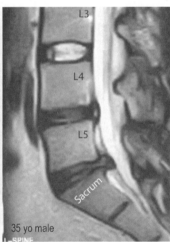

35 yo male

MRI of **disc herniation (L5-S1)**, disc bulge (L4-5), intact disc (L3-4) Degenerative Joint Disease

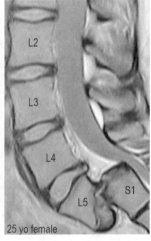

25 yo female

MRI of severe **lumbar instability** (L5-S1 spondylolisthesis) L3-4-5 disc bulges

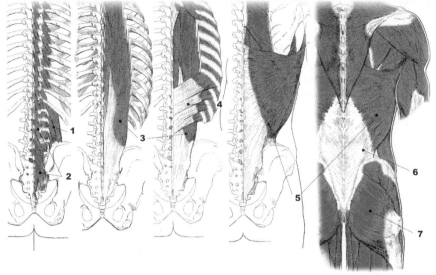

deep ──────────────────────────────────► superficial

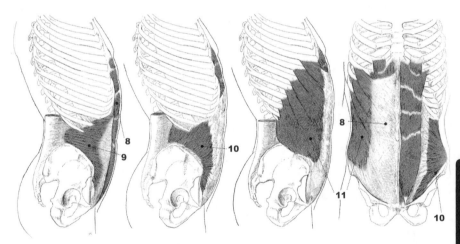

Lumbar Spine

1. Quadratus lumborum
2. Multifidi lumborum
3. Erector spinae
4. Serratus posterior inferior
5. Latissimus dorsi
6. Thoracolumbar fascia
7. Gluteus maximus
8. Rectus abdominis
9. Transversus abdominis
10. Internal oblique
11. External oblique

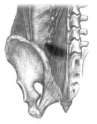
Mild Sprain/Strain

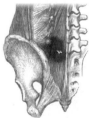
Moderate

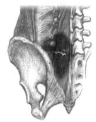
Severe

Joint types:
- Gliding (zygapophyseal joints)
- Fibrocartilaginous (intervertebral joints)

Articular surfaces
- Intervertebral discs oriented in horizontal plane
- **Lumbar:** facet oriented in sagittal plane
- Facets (z-joints) are for motion, discs are for weight bearing (~80% weight)
- **Sacroiliac:** facets oriented ~45°

Active range of motion (lumbar)
Flexion ....40-60°
Extension ....20-35°
Lateral Flexion ....15-20°
Rotation ....5-20°

Active range of motion (SI)
Flexion/Extension........0-10°
Int./external rotation ...0-10°

Main muscle actions

- **Flexion:** iliopsoas, rectus abdominis, internal/external oblique

- **Extension:** multifidi, erector spinae

- **Lateral flexion:** erector spinae, semispinalis, rectus abdominis, internal/external oblique, quadratus lumborum

- **Rotation:** rotatores, multifidi, semispinalis, erector spinae, internal/external oblique

Resting position: mid flexion & extension

Close packed position: full extension

Capsular pattern of restriction
- **L-spine:** lateral flexion = rotation, then extension

Normal end feel: soft tissue stretch (all motions)
- Rotation may be limited as a bony end-feel (facets)

Abnormal end feel
- **Early myospasm** → muscle/ligament tear
- **Late myospasm** → instability
- **Empty** → ligament rupture
- **Hard** → bone approximation (osteophyte)

Coupled motions - pure rotation and pure lateral flexion do not occur in the spine below C1-C2

T6-L5 vertebral segments*
- Left lateral flexion coupled with right rotation
- Right lateral flexion coupled with left rotation
- *this is the opposite coupling that occurs in the cervical & upper thoracic spine (rotation & lateral flexion occur to the same side)

Lumbar motion is coupled with sacral motion

- **Lumbar extension** (hyperlordosis) is coupled with sacral **nutation** (anterior sacral tilting or "nod")

- **Lumbar flexion** (hypolordosis) is coupled with sacral **counter-nutation** (posterior sacral tilting) when standing

Lumbar Spine

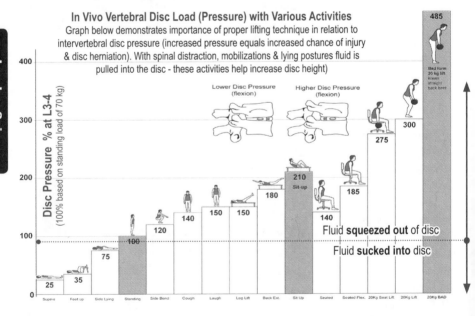

In Vivo Vertebral Disc Load (Pressure) with Various Activities
Graph below demonstrates importance of proper lifting technique in relation to intervertebral disc pressure (increased pressure equals increased chance of injury & disc herniation). With spinal distraction, mobilizations & lying postures fluid is pulled into the disc - these activities help increase disc height)

Disc Pressure % at L3-4 (100% based on standing load of 70 kg)

Lower Disc Pressure (flexion)   Higher Disc Pressure (flexion)

485 — Bad form 20 kg lift knees straight, back bent
300 — 20Kg Lift
275 — 20Kg Seat Lift
210 — Sit-up
185 — Seated Flex.
180 — Sit Up
150 — Back Ext.
150 — Leg Lift
140 — Seated
140 — Laugh
120 — Cough
100 — Standing
75 — Side Bend
35 — Side Lying
25 — Feet up / Supine

Fluid **squeezed out** of disc
Fluid **sucked into** disc

Introduction statement: "Try and move as far as possible, if any of the actions or movements are painful please let me know, do not do any action you feel will cause you further injury."

Flexion

Muscles Activated: *eccentric* contraction of erector spinae

Tissue Stretched: erector spinae, supraspinous & interspinous ligaments, posterior IVD, posterior facet joint capsule & intercostal muscles

Tissue Compressed: anterior thoracic structure, anterior longitudinal ligament, anterior IVD, lungs, heart, aorta, abdominal contents

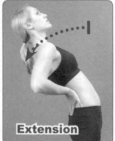

Flexion

Extension

Muscles Activated: *concentric* contraction of erector spinae, *eccentric* contraction of rectus abdominis & abdominal obliques

Tissue Stretched: rectus abdominis, anterior longitudinal ligament, aorta, lungs, anterior intercostal muscles

Tissue Compressed: erector spinae, supraspinous & interspinous ligaments, posterior IVD & IVF, z-joint capsule & posterior intercostal muscles

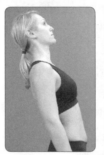

Extension

Lateral Flexion

Muscles Activated: *eccentric* contraction of *contralateral* erector spinae, transversospinalis

Tissue Stretched: *contralateral* erector spinae, transverso-spinalis, intercostal muscles, contralateral IVD & IVF, z-joints

Tissue Compressed: *ipsilateral:* erector spinae, transverso-spinalis, intercostal muscles, ipsilateral IVD & IVF, z-joints

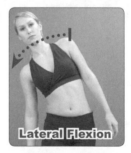

Lateral Flexion

Rotation

Muscles Activated: *contralateral* external oblique & transverso-spinalis, *ipsilateral* internal oblique

Tissue Stretched: *ipsilateral* external oblique & transverso-spinalis, *contralateral* internal oblique

Tissue Compressed: abdominal contents, ipsilateral intervertebral foramen

* T-spine & L-Spine are usually assessed together; to remove lower extremity influence consider performing in a seated position

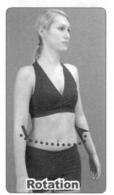

Rotation

Lumbar Spine

Compare bilaterally; if possible palpate joint during PROM & use the shortest level possible, apply over pressure at end ROM; introduction statement:
"If any of the actions or movements are painful or uncomfortable please let me know."

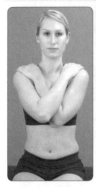 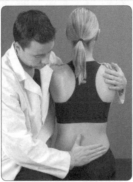 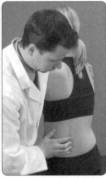 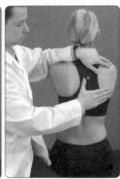

| Starting position Patient arms crossed | Thenar spinous contact to assess motion | Alternate finger-tip spinous contact | Alternate patient contact with forearm-shoulder stabilization |

Flexion (> 70°-90°)

Tissue Stretched: erector spinae, supraspinous & interspinous ligaments, posterior IVD, posterior facet joint capsule

Tissue Compressed: anterior lumbar structures, anterior longitudinal ligament, anterior IVD, intestines, aorta

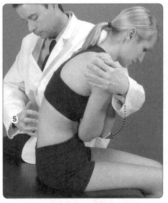

Extension (> 20°-30°)

Tissue Stretched: rectus abdominis, anterior longitudinal ligament, aorta, abdominal obliques

Tissue Compressed: erector spinae, supraspinous & interspinous ligaments, posterior IVD, posterior facet joint capsule

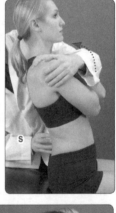

Lateral Flexion (> 25°-35°)

Tissue Stretched: *contralateral* erector spinae, transverso-spinalis, QL, IVD, z-joints

Tissue Compressed: *ipsilateral:* erector spinae, transverso-spinalis, QL, IVD, z-joints

Rotation (> 15°-30°)

Tissue Stretched: *ipsilateral* external oblique & transverso-spinalis, *contralateral* internal oblique

Tissue Compressed: abdominal contents

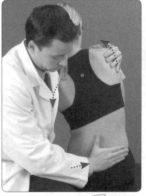 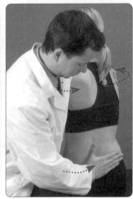

Lumbar Spine

Patient instructions for assessing general muscle strength:
"I am going to try and move you in _____ direction, don't let me do it" or "resist my force"

Flexion
Muscles Activated: *isometric or eccentric* contraction of erector spinae, multifidi & transversospinalis

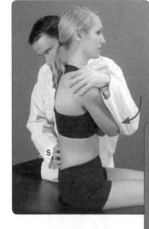

Extension
Muscles Activated: *isometric or eccentric* contraction of rectus abdominis & abdominal obliques

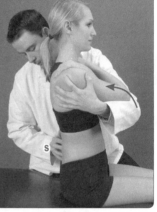

Lateral Flexion
Muscles Activated:
eccentric contraction of *contralateral* erector spinae, transversospinalis & quadratus lumborum, & abdominal muscles

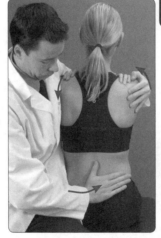

Rotation
Muscles Activated: *contralateral* external oblique & transversospinalis, *ipsilateral* internal oblique

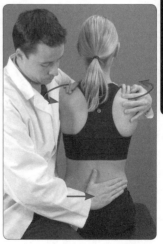

Lumbar Spine

Flexion (normal 40-60º)
- Patient standing
- Zero inclinometers over T12 & sacrum
- Ask patient to flex trunk, subtract T12 inclination from sacrum inclination = ROM

Extension (normal: 20º-35º)
- Same as flexion except patient extends trunk

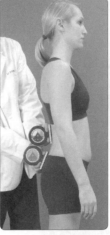

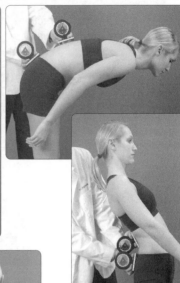

Lateral flexion (normal: 15-20º)
- Patient seated or standing
- Zero inclinometers over T12 & sacrum
- Ask patient to laterally flex trunk, subtract T12 inclination from sacrum inclination = ROM
- Repeat on contralateral side

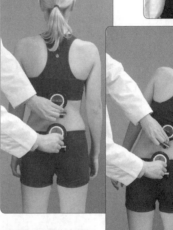

Rotation (normal: 5-20º)
- Patient standing with trunk flexed 90º
- Zero inclinometers over T12 & sacrum
- Ask patient to turn spine to one side, subtract T12 inclination from sacrum inclination = ROM
- Repeat on contralateral side

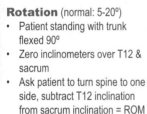

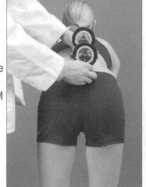

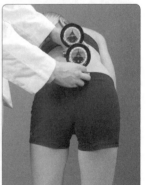

Lumbar Spine

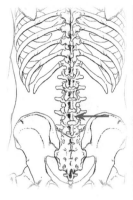

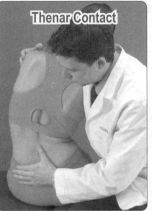

Thenar Contact

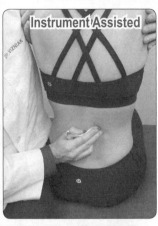

Instrument Assisted

Side-Posture Palpation Assessment

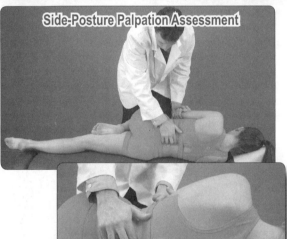

- Side-posture palpation is performed by the clinician moving the patient's thigh & hip (abducting, adducting, flexing and/or extending) to induce lumbar & SI motion

- If the clinician is likely going to choose side-posture mobilization or manipulation as a treatment method then by using side posture assessment one can improve their clinical efficiency & avoid unnecessary changes in patient position.

Lumbar Spine

Goldthwait's Test

Procedure

Patient supine, examiner slowly raises the patient's affected leg with one hand while palpating motion at the lumbar spine with the other hand; the test is then repeated on the opposite side

Interpretation

(+) Pain before lumbar spine motion is felt → Sacroiliac joint pathology (ligamentous sprain, arthritis)

(+) Pain beginning when lumbar spine motion is felt → Lumbosacral pathology (sprain/strain, possible disc syndrome)

Clinical notes

Sacroiliac joint involvement should be suspected if the unaffected leg can be elevated higher than the affected leg

Consider placing one finger to palpate SI joint (just medial to PSIS) and other to palp lumbar spine to better asses motion

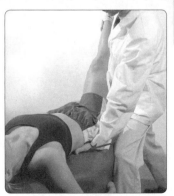

All palpation methods involve tactile movement of soft tissues & osseous structures to evaluate **variations in elasticity, tone and motion from side to side, pain or discomfort.** - clinical style & preference will determine which specific methods clinicians choose (use what works best for you)

Prone Variations

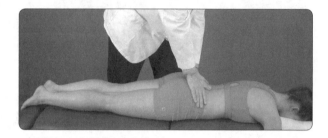

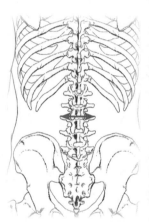

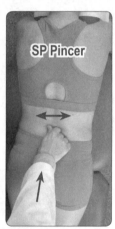

SP Pincer

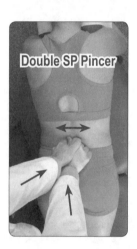

Double SP Pincer

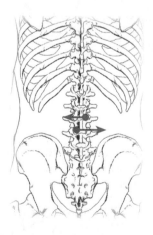

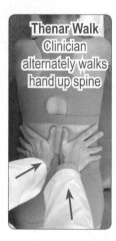

Thenar Walk
Clinician alternately walks hand up spine

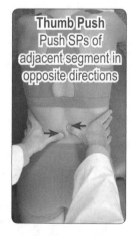

Thumb Push
Push SPs of adjacent segment in opposite directions

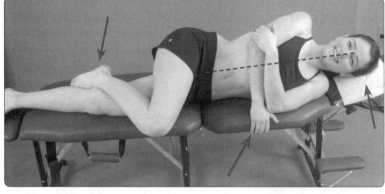

Head piece
up or pillow
to save neck-
spine should
be relatively
neutral

Basics - Ask patient to lay on side facing you

1. Head & neck in relatively neutral position, adjust head piece as they roll over

2. Upside hip flexed ~80° (increased hip flexion will cause hypolordosis of the lumbar spine if needed)

3. Knee flexed with foot hooked over down-side straight leg

4. Patient's arm crossed so upside arm is closer to body and hand can hold edge of table for stability

5. Down-side arm crossed over chest with hand over contralateral elbow

• Exact positioning will vary depending on patient size, table height and individual practitioner style

Increased hip flexion results in increased lumbar spine flexion (z-joint gapping), allowing greater specificity of the mobilization force to higher lumbar segments

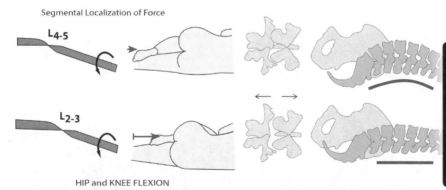

Segmental Localization of Force

L4-5

L2-3

HIP and KNEE FLEXION

Lumbar Spine

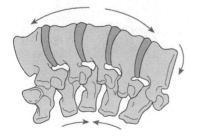

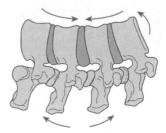

Indication: restricted rotation &/or lateral flexion or rotation or lateral flexion malposition

Position: patient in side posture with legs straight; clinician in square stance or modified fencer

Contact:

Inferior contact: clinician places forearm in to patients ASIS & first 3 fingers of inferior hand on the up-side of the patient's SP;

Superior contact: clinicians forearm/ arm over posterior shoulder, with the clinician's finger tips contacting the down-side spinous process on the segment directly above the inferior contact hand

Force: tissue pull L-M for the superior hand & L-M for the inferior hand, develop tension by rotating the patient's upper body anteriorly & distracting (lengthening) the spine; at tension mobilize by dropping body & pulling through lumbar contact hand - also consider using breathing technique to lengthen spine and use as a mild stretching mobilization

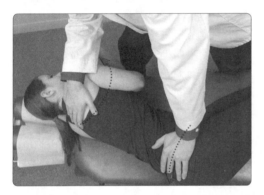

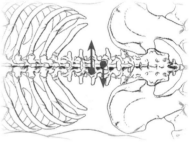

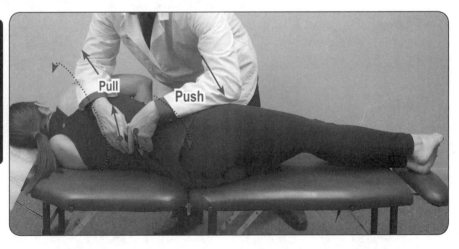

Lumbar Spine

Indication: restricted rotation &/or lateral flexion or rotation or lateral flexion malposition

Position: patient in side posture hip flexed ~90°; clinician in square stance or fencer

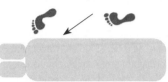

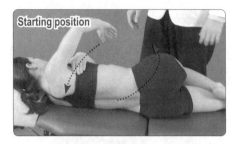

Starting position

Contact:

Inferior contact: clinician places fingers of inferior hand on the down-side of the patient's SPs with the clinician's forearm over the patient's posterior PSIS/glutes;

Superior contact: clinicians forearm/arm is interlaced through the patient's axilla/anterior shoulder, with the clinician's finger tips contacting the up-side spinous process on the segment directly above the inferior contact hand

Force: push first then pull - tissue pull L-M for the superior hand & L-M for the inferior hand, develop tension by rotating the patient's upper body posteriorly & distracting (lengthening) the spine; at tension mobilize by lowering body & pulling through lumbar contact hand

Clinical notes: this is an extremely powerful & controlled mobilization position that allows for maximal & specific distractive, rotation and/or lateral flexion forces to be developed

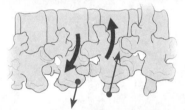

Use a **soft or gentle end range pressure to reduce guarding and discomfort**. When learning do NOT hold people in a hard end-ROM - relax your hands/body for more effective application.

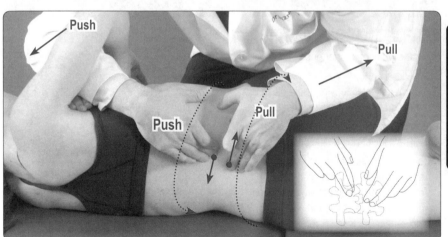

Push
Pull
Pull
Push

Lumbar Spine

The push-pull setup provides the clinician with the maximum amount of force and specificity of location when applying joint mobilization or manipulation in the lumbar spine, and may also be used as an excellent myofascial stretch, contract relax, IASTM or spinal traction technique.

Quadratus Lumborum Stretch

Indications: tight or shortened QL, erector spinae & abdominal obliques

Position: patient side-lying with upside arm over head & pillow under side, clinician at side of table

Contact: clinician's places hand over patient's iliac crest & lower lateral rib cage

Force: stabilize iliac crest, tissue I-S over ribs; instruct patient take in a deep breath; with inspiration apply I-S force over the lower ribs; repeat as necessary & take up slack with each breath

Clinical notes: use a 'soft' contact, classically this is thought of as a QL stretch however when one performs numerous cadaver dissections & correlates this to real life anatomy the fibers of the abdominal obliques will be preferentially stretched in this position

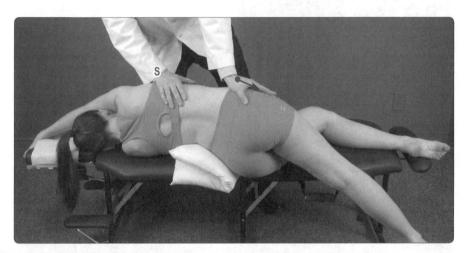

QL Contract Relax Stretch

Indications: tight or shortened QL & erector spinae

Position: patient side-lying with upside leg hanging off table, clinician fencer stance

Contact: clinician places hand over patient's lower ribs & iliac crest

Force: have patient 'hike hip' & apply resistive force (isometric contraction) for ~5 seconds; with patient exhalation mobilize iliac crest inferiorly & hold for ~7 sec; repeat 3-5 times & reassess

Clinical notes: use a 'soft' contact, classically thought of as a QL stretch, but also stretches abdominal obliques & erector spinae

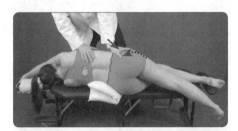

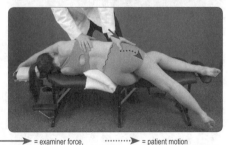

S = stabilization (indifferent hand), ● = contact, ——➤ = examiner force, ·········➤ = patient motion

Lumbar Spine

Lumbar Extension Restriction

Indications: ↓ lumbar extension, hypolordosis

Position: patient seated or standing

Contact: clinician contacts patient's facet joint with thumb (patient crosses arms in front of body)

Force: tissue pull I-S & passively extend & laterally flex the patient's trunk to the contact side until the facet stops moving; instruct patient to bend forward against resistance for ~5 seconds; with relaxation take up the slack into initial passive movement; repeat 3-5 times & reassess

Clinical notes: demonstrate the procedure to the patient prior to application

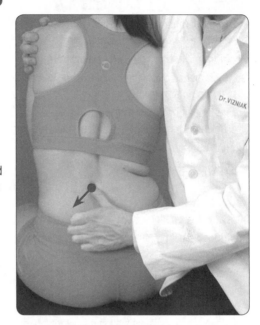

Lumbar Flexion Restriction

Indications: ↓ lumbar flexion, hyperlordosis

Position: patient seated or standing

Contact: clinician contacts patient's facet joint with thumb (patient crosses arms in front of body)

Force: tissue pull I-S & passively flex & laterally flex the patient's trunk away from the contact hand until the facet stops moving; instruct patient to straighten up against resistance for ~5 seconds; with relaxation take up the slack into initial passive movement; repeat 3-5 times & reassess

Clinical notes: demonstrate the procedure to the patient prior to application

Save your thumbs - use instruments.
91% of physios using massage had to modify treatment because of thumb pain
(Snodgrass SJ. Thumb pain in physiotherapists: potential risk factors and proposed prevention strategies. J of Manual and Manipulative Therapy 2002;10(4):206-217)

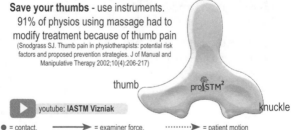

thumb

proISTM²

knuckle

▶ youtube: **IASTM Vizniak**

Lumbar Spine

S = stabilization (indifferent hand), ● = contact, ⟶ = examiner force, ┈┈▶ = patient motion

Lumbar Paraspinal Release

Indications: thoracolumbar fascia restriction, paraspinal myospasm, low back pain

Position: patient prone, clinician at side of table

Contact: thenar, digital, thumb or forearm contact over patient's paraspinal muscle

Force: tissue pull into direction of soft tissue restriction & hold until tissue release is felt; repeat as required

Clinical notes: clinician should stand close to the patient & use good body biomechanics

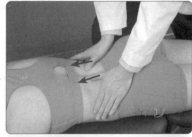

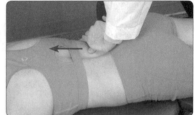

Distraction

Indications: hyperlordosis, hypomobility, pain

Position: patient prone with pillow under abdomen; clinician in fencer stance facing inferiorly

Contact: clinician bilaterally places thenar eminences over patient's PSISs

Force: tissue pull S-I, P-A & instruct patient take in a deep breath; with exhalation push inferiorly & hold; repeat 3-5 times or as necessary

Clinical notes: use good biomechanics and transfer body weight to apply force

Use of a flexion distraction table will greatly improve this mobilization

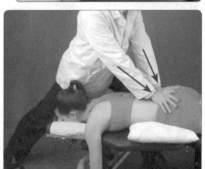

Flexion Mobilization

Indications: ↓ flexion, assess for joint dysfunction

Position: patient prone with lumbar spine predisposed to flexion; clinician in fencer stance

Contact: clinician places thenar eminences over patients spinolaminar junction

Force: tissue pull I-S, P-A & instruct patient take in a deep breath; with exhalation mobilize superior & slightly anterior; repeat as necessary

Clinical notes: the lumbar spine may be predisposed to flexion by placing a pillow/towels under the patient's abdomen or using a flexion-distraction table

Lower image shows supine alternate variation for flexion mobilization (may be difficult to perform on some patients)

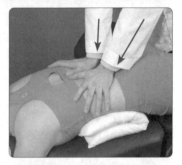

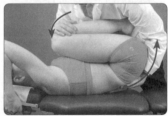

Lumbar Spine

S = stabilization (indifferent hand),   ● = contact,   ⟶ = examiner force,   ·········▷ = patient motion

prohealthsys

Anterior Glide

Indications: ↓ extension, assess for joint dysfunction

Position: patient prone; clinician in fencer stance

Contact: clinician grasps patient's SP with thumb & index finger middle phalanx

Force: push into lamina until tissue resistance and stretch is felt; repeat up & down the spine noting mobility differences at various segments

Clinical notes: a reinforced contact may be used

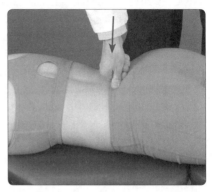

Extension (P-A) Mobilization

Indications: ↓ extension, lateral flexion or rotation

Position: patient prone; clinician in fencer stance

Contact: clinician places hypothenar eminence or thumb over patients spinolaminar junction & extends patient's hip & pelvis

Force: tissue pull I-S, P-A & instruct patient take in a deep breath; with exhalation mobilize anterior & superior; repeat as necessary

Clinical notes: use a 'soft' contact to avoid tissue aggravation

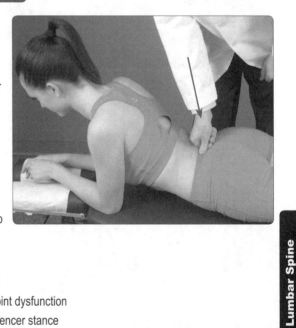

Rotation Mobilization

Indications: ↓ rotation, assess for joint dysfunction

Position: patient prone, clinician in fencer stance

Contact: clinician places one thumb on SP of a segment & other thumb on contralateral side of segment above or below

Force: clinician mobilizes both contacts L-M (creating a counter rotation force) until tissue resistance is felt; repeat up & down the spine noting mobility differences at various segments

Clinical notes: use a 'soft' contact

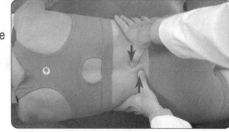

S = stabilization (indifferent hand), ● = contact, ——▶ = examiner force, ·········▶ = patient motion

Lumbar Spine

Indication: restricted rotation &/or lateral flexion; or rotation or lateral flexion malposition

Position: patient in side posture with slight lumbar flexion; clinician in fencer stance (thigh to thigh or straddle) stabilizing patient

Contact: clinician places hypothenar region over patient's up-side transverse or mammillary process, stabilization/traction hand contacts the patients upside shoulder or elbow

Force: varies depending on specific joint dysfunction

Rotation: tissue pull M-L, P-A, develop tension by rotating the patient's upper body posteriorly; at tension thrust by dropping body & pushing through lumbar contact hand

Lateral flexion: tissue pull M-L & P-A, develop tension by pre-setting the patient in a laterally flexed position; at tension mobilize by dropping body & pushing through lumbar contact

Clinical notes: the more inferior the lumbar segmented contacted, the more shoulder rotation required to generate pre-adjustive tension (i.e. more shoulder rotation for L4-L5 than L1-L2)

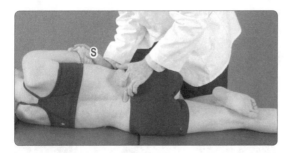

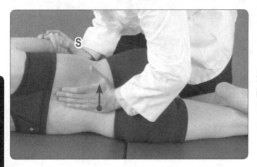

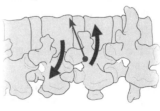

Start of tissue pull on opposite side of SP

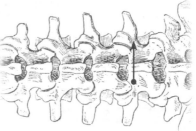

End of tissue pull & tension; ready for mobilization or HVLA thrust with contact on upside of spine

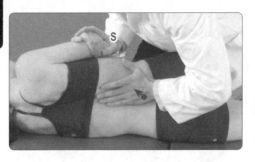

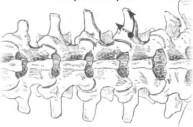

S = stabilization (indifferent hand), ● = contact, ⟶ = examiner force, ┈┈┈▶ = patient motion

Lumbar Spine

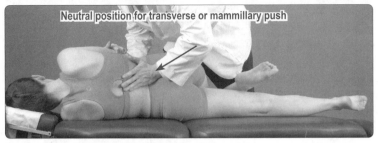

Neutral position for transverse or mammillary push

Convex Mammillary/Transeverse Push

Note pillow placed under lateral lumbar spine
to help predispose patient to lateral flexion
toward the table

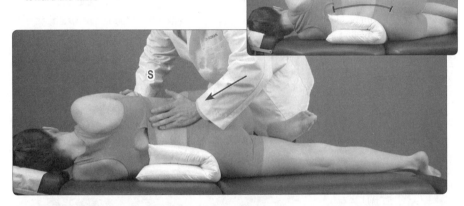

Concave Mammillary/Transverse Push

Note pillow placed under lateral ilium and
greater trochanter to help predispose patient
to lateral flexion away from the table

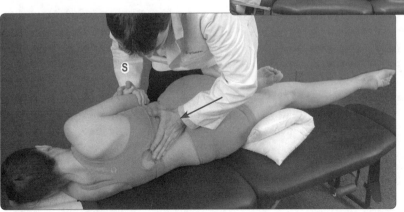

Lumbar Spine

S = stabilization (indifferent hand),　● = contact,　——▶ = examiner force,　·······▶ = patient motion

Indication: restricted rotation, lateral flexion, extension, flexion or corresponding malposition

Position: patient in side posture; clinician in fencer stance (thigh to thigh or straddle) stabilizing patient

Contact: clinician places hypothenar or thenar region over patient's spinous process of the upper vertibrae, stabilization/traction hand contacts the patients upside shoulder or elbow

Force: varies depending on specific joint dysfunction treated

Rotation: tissue pull M-L, develop tension by rotating the patient's upper body posteriorly; at tension thrust by dropping body & pushing through lumbar contact hand

Lateral flexion: tissue pull M-L, develop tension by pre-setting the patient in a laterally flexed position; at tension thrust by dropping body & pushing through lumbar contact hand

Flexion: tissue pull S-I, develop tension by pre-setting the patient in a flexed position; at tension thrust by dropping body & pushing superiorly through lumbar contact hand

Extension: tissue pull I-S, P-A, develop tension by pre-setting the patient in an extended position; at tension mobilize by dropping body & pushing through lumbar contact hand

Clinical notes: spinous process contacts can be painful, as such pre-adjustive tension force over the SP must be made as soft as possible with either the thenar or hypothenar eminence and maximized only at the apex of the thrust

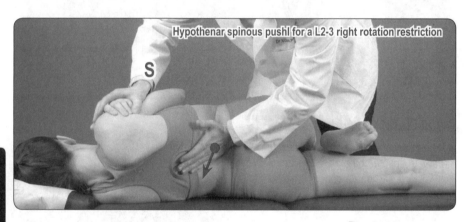

Hypothenar spinous pushl for a L2-3 right rotation restriction

S

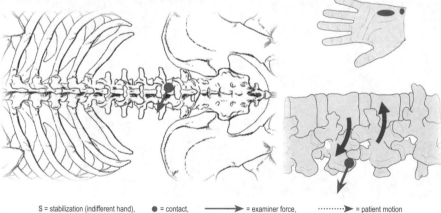

S = stabilization (indifferent hand),   ● = contact,   ——▶ = examiner force,   ·········▶ = patient motion

Lumbar Spine

prohealthsys

Indication: restricted rotation &/or lateral flexion or rotation or lateral flexion malposition

Position: patient in side posture; clinician in square stance or kick-start

Contact: clinician places first 3 fingers on the down-side of the patient's spinous process of the lower vertebrae & place forearm over the patient's posterior lateral gluteal region; stabilization/traction hand contacts the patient's upside shoulder or elbow

Force: tissue pull M-L, develop tension by rotating the patient's upper body posteriorly; at tension mobilize by dropping body & pulling through lumbar contact hand

Clinical notes: the more inferior the lumbar segment contacted, the more shoulder rotation required to generate pre-adjustive tension (more shoulder rotation for L4-L5 than L1-L2)
This method may also be applied to SI manipulation by using the PSIS as a contact

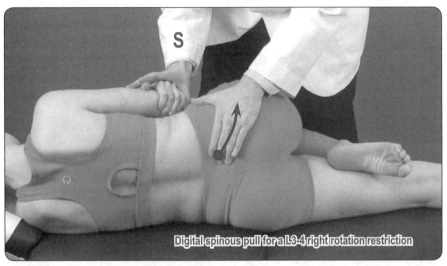

Digital spinous pull for a L3-4 right rotation restriction

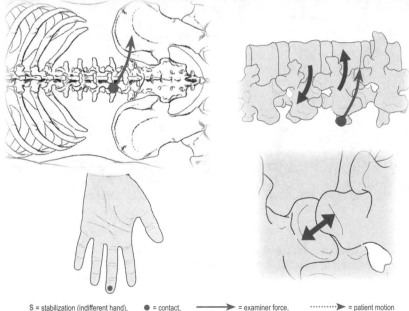

S = stabilization (indifferent hand),　● = contact,　———▶ = examiner force,　••••••••▶ = patient motion

Lumbar Spine

Indication: restricted rotation &/or lateral flexion

Position: patient in side posture hip flexed ~90°; clinician in square stance or modified fencer

Contact: same as Push Pull (million dollar roll) except an instrument is used

Force: push first then pull instrument along soft tissue line - tissue pull L-M for the superior hand & L-M for the inferior hand, develop tension by rotating the patient's upper body posteriorly & distracting (lengthening) the spine; at tension mobilize by lowering body & pulling through lumbar contact hand

Clinical notes: this is an extremely powerful & controlled mobilization position that allows for maximal & specific distractive, rotation and/or lateral flexion forces to be developed while still permitting relatively easy soft tissue mobilization

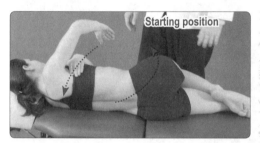
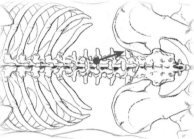

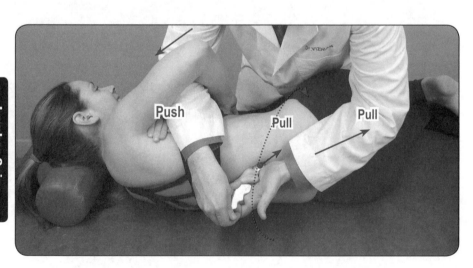

The push-pull setup provides the clinician with the maximum amount of force and specificity of location when applying joint mobilization or manipulation in the lumbar spine, and may also be used as an excellent myofascial stretch, contract relax, IASTM or spinal traction technique.

S = stabilization (indifferent hand),   ● = contact,   ⟶ = examiner force,   ·········▷ = patient motion

Lumbar Spine

Indication: restricted rotation or lateral flexion (rotation or lateral flexion malposition)

Position: patient seated with legs straddling table & arms crossed over chest; clinician seated behind patient

Contact: clinician places thenar or hypothenar eminence over mammillary processes (spinous contact may also be used) and other hand & shoulder pulling patient's upper body in desired direction

Force: rotate or laterally flex body, tissue pull P-A & M-L; at tension mobilize by pushing through contact hand & mildly rotating or laterally flexing with upper stabilization arm

Clinical notes: these mobilizations are very similar to basic seated assessment methods and as the clinician's experience increases assessment may be simultaneously followed with treatment at a given segment (developing this skill greatly increases clinical efficiency)

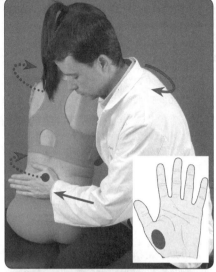

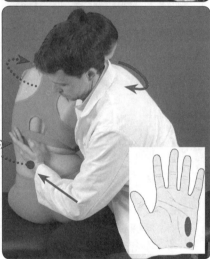

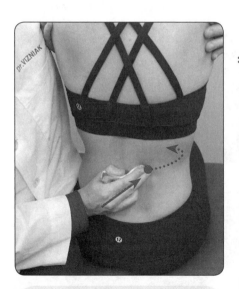

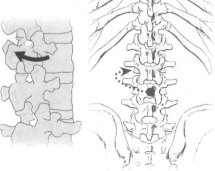

Instrument assisted mobilization and manipulation is a great way to get solid, efficient patient results and reduce wear & tear on the practitioners body

S = stabilization (indifferent hand),　● = contact,　——▶ = examiner force,　•••••••▶ = patient motion

Lumbar Spine

Bilateral Thenar Mammillary Push

Indication: restricted extension or flexion (extension or flexion malposition)

Position: patient prone; clinician in fencer stance

Contact: clinician bilaterally places thenar eminences over mammillary processes (clinician may also choose to use a *crossed bilateral hypothenar mammillary* contact)

Force: varies with specific joint dysfunction & desired treatment action

> **Extension:** place pillow under patient's ASIS or lower lumbar drop section of table to predispose to an extension position; tissue pull P-A & slightly S-I; at tension thrust by dropping body & pushing through contact hands

> **Flexion:** place pillow under patient's abdomen or raise thoracolumbar table section to predispose to flexion; tissue pull P-A & slightly I-S; at tension mobilize by dropping body & pushing through contact hands

Clinical notes: these manipulations may also be done with a flexion distraction table, drop table or activator

> A ***unilateral hypothenar mammillary push*** or ***hypothenar spinous*** may be used in a similar method as above if there is a combination flexion/extension restriction coupled with rotational restrictions or malpositions

Extension mobilization	Flexion mobilization
note pillow under pelvis to help predispose patient to extension	note pillow under abdomen to help predispose patient to flexion

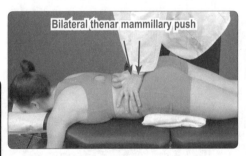
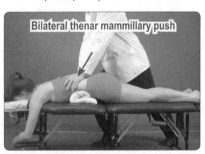

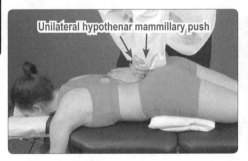
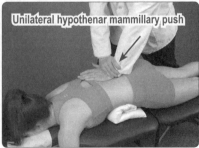

S = stabilization (indifferent hand), ● = contact, ——▶ = examiner force, ·····▶ = patient motion

Lumbars From the Rear

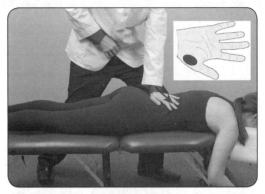

Indication: restricted rotation, lateral flexion or extension

Position: patient prone; clinician in fencer stance

Contact: clinician places thenar eminence over spinous processes (clinician may also choose to use a *hypothenar mammillary* contact); opposite hand pulls posterior on far side ASIS

Force: clinician pulls upward on patient's ASIS while applying M-L & P-A force over the patient's spine with contact hand

Clinical notes: ensure to use a soft contact when using a spinous process contact & feel a solid lock out prior to any attempted mobilization or thrust

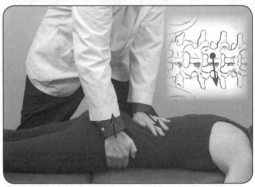

Knee-Chest Table Push

Indication: restricted extension, flexion or rotation (extension, flexion or rotation malposition)

Position: patient prone kneeling position with chest supported & hips flexed 90°-100°; clinician in square or fencer stance

Contact: clinician bilaterally places thenar eminences over mammillary processes (clinician may also choose to use a *crossed bilateral hypothenar mammillary* contact)

Force: varies with specific joint dysfunction & desired treatment action
  Extension: tissue pull P-A & slightly S-I; at tension thrust by dropping body & pushing through contact hands
  Flexion: tissue pull P-A & slightly I-S; at tension thrust by dropping body & pushing through contact hands
  Rotation: use a unilateral contact or thrust with one side more when using a bilateral contact

Clinical notes: *unilateral hypothenar mammillary push* or *hypothenar spinous* may be used in a similar method as above if there is a combination flexion/extension restriction coupled with rotational restrictions

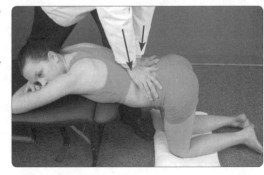

S = stabilization (indifferent hand), ● = contact, ➤ = examiner force, ┈┈┈➤ = patient motion

Lumbar Spine

1. Vizniak NA. Applied Human Cadaver Dissections. 1999-2017
2. Abbott JH, McCane B, Herbison P, Moginie C, Chapple C, Hogarty T. Lumbar segmental instability: a criterion-related validity study of manual therapy assessment. BMC Musculoskelet Disord. 2005;6:56.
3. Abram SE. Treatment of lumbosacral radiculopathy with epidural steroids. Anesthesiology. Dec 1999;91(6):1937-41.
4. Akuthota V, Nadler SF. Core strengthening. Arch Phys Med Rehabil. Mar 2004;85(3 suppl 1):S86-92.
5. Albeck M. A critical assessment of clinical diagnosis of disc herniation in patients with monoradicular sciatica. Acta Neurochir. 1996;138:40.
6. Barr KP, Griggs M, Cadby T. Lumbar stabilization: a review of core concepts and current literature, part 2. Am J Phys Med Rehabil. Jan 2007;86(1):72-80.
7. Bertilson BC, Bring I, Sjoblom A, Sundell K, Strender LE. Inter-examiner reliability in the assessment of low back pain (LBP) using the Kirkaldy-Willis classification (KWC). Eur SpineJ. 2006; 1-9.
8. Binkley J, Stratford PW, Gill C. Interrater reliability of lumbar accessory motion mobility testing. Phys Ther. 1995;75(9):786-792.
9. Boal RW, Gillette RG. Central Neuronal Plasticity, Low Back Pain and Spinal Manipulative Therapy. JMPT 27(5):314-326, 2004.
10. Boline PD, Haas M, Meyer JJ, Kassak K, Nelson C, Keating JC., Jr Interexaminer reliability of eight evaluative dimensions of lumbar segmental abnormality: Part II. JMPT. 1993 Jul–Aug;16(6):363–374.
11. Bono CM. Low-back pain in athletes. J Bone Joint Surg Am. Feb 2004;86-A(2):382-96.
12. Borg-Stein J, Wilkins A. Soft tissue determinants of low back pain. Curr Pain Headache Rep. Oct 2006;10(5):339-44.
13. Brown FW. Management of diskogenic pain using epidural and intrathecal steroids. Clin Orthop Relat Res. Nov-Dec 1977;129:72-8.
14. Charnley J. Orthopaedic signs in the diagnosis of disc protrusion with special reference to the straight-leg raising test. Lancet. 1951;1:186-192.
15. Chiradejnant A, Maher CG, Latimer J. Objective manual assessment of lumbar posteroantenor stiffness is now possible. J Manipulative Physiol Ther. 2003;26(1):34-39.
16. Cohen SP, Wenzell D, Hurley RW, et al. A double-blind, placebo-controlled, dose-response pilot study evaluating intradiscal etanercept in patients with chronic discogenic low back pain or lumbosacral radiculopathy. Anesthesiology. Jul 2007;107(1):99-105.
17. Cook C, Cook A, Fleming R. Rehabilitation for clinical lumbar instability in an adolescent diver with spondylolisthesis. 1 Man Manipulative Ther. 2004;1 2(2):91-99.
18. Cyteval C, Fescquet N, Thomas E, et al. Predictive factors of efficacy of periradicular corticosteroid injections for lumbar radiculopathy. AJNR Am J Neuroradiol. Aug 2006;27(5):978-82.
19. DePalma MJ, Bhargava A, Slipman CW. A critical appraisal of the evidence for selective nerve root injection in the treatment of lumbosacral radiculopathy. Arch Phys Med Rehabil. Jul 2005;86(7):1477-83.
20. Dishman JD, Cunningham BM, Burke J. Comparison

of Tibial Nerve H-Reflex Excitability After Cervical and Lumbar Manipulation. JMPT 25(5):318-325, 2002.
21. Donelson R, Aprill C, Medcalf R, Grant W. A prospective study of centralization of lumbar and referred pain. A predictor of symptomatic discs & annular competence. Spine. 1997;22(10):1115-1122.
22. Downey BJ, Taylor NF, Niere KR. Manipulative physiotherapists can reliably palpate nominated lumbar spinal levels. Man Ther. 1999 Aug;4(3):151–156.
23. Eskelund Hansen B, Simonsen T, Leboeuf-Yde C. Motion Palpation of the Lumbar Spine – A Problem With The Test or the Tester? JMPT 29(3):208-212, 2006.
24. Friedly J, Chan L, Deyo R. Increases in lumbosacral injections in the Medicare population: 1994 to 2001. Spine. Jul 15 2007;32(16):1754-60.
25. Fritz JM, Piva S, Childs J. Accuracy of the clinical examination to predict radiographic instability of the lumbar spine. Eur Spine J. 2005;14(8):743-50.
26. Gurdjian E, Webster J, Ostrowski AZ, Hardy W, Lindner D, Thomas L. Herniated lumbar intervertebral discs: an analysis of 11 76 operated cases. J Trauma. 1961;1:158-176.
27. Hakelius A, Hindmarsh J. The comparative reliability of preoperative diagnostic methods in lumbar disc surgery. Acta Orthop Scand. 1972;43:234-238.
28. Hammer WI, Pfefer MT. Treatment of Subacute Lumbar Compartment Syndrome Using the Graston Technique. JMPT 28(3):199-204, 2005.
29. Hawk C, Phongphua C, Bleecker J, Swank L, Lopez D, Rubley T. Preliminary study of the reliability of assessment procedures for indications for chiropractic adjustments of the lumbar spine. JMPT. 1999 Jul–Aug;22(6):382–389.
30. Hession EF, Donald GD. Treatment of multiple lumbar disk herniations in an adolescent athlete utilizing flexion distraction and rotational manipulation. JMPT. 1993 Mar–Apr;16(3):185–192.
31. Keating JC, Jr, Bergmann TF, Jacobs GE, Finer BA, Larson K. Interexaminer reliability of eight evaluative dimensions of lumbar segmental abnormality. JMPT. 1990 Oct;13(8):463–470.
32. Kerr RSC, Cadoux-Hudson TA, Adams CBT. The value of accurate clinical assessment in the surgical management of the lumbar disc protrusion. J Neurol Neurosurg Psychiatr. 1988;51:169-173.
33. Knuttson B. Comparative value of electromyographic, myelographic, & clinical-neurological examinations in diagnosis of lumbar root compression syndrome. Acta Ortho Scand. 1961;(Suppl 49):1 94-99.
34. Kosteljanetz M, Bang F, Schmidt-Olsen S. The clinical significance of straight leg raising (Lasegue's sign) in the diagnosis of prolapsed lumbar disc. Spine. 1988;13:393-395.
35. Kosteljanetz M, Espersen O, Halaburt H, Miletic T. Predictive value of clinical & surgical findings in patients with lumbago-sciatica: aprospective study (part 1). Acta Neurochirurgica. 1984;73:67-76.
36. Kreitz BG, Cote P, Yong-Hing K. Crossed femoral stretching test: a case report. Spine. 1996;21(13):1584-1586.
37. Laslett M, Aprill CN, McDonald B, Oberg B. Clinical predictors of lumbar provocation discography: a study of clinical predictors of lumbar provocation discography. Eur Spine J. 2006;1-12.
38. Laslett M, Oberg B, Aprill CN, McDonald B. Centralization as a predictor of provocation discography results in chronic low back pain, and the influence of disability & distress on diagnostic power. Spine J. 2005;5(4): 370-380.
39. LauderTD, DillinghamTR,AndaryMI Kumar S, Pezzin LE, Stephens RT. Effect of history and exam in predicting electrodiagnostic outcome among patients with suspected lumbosacral radiculopathy. Am J Phys Med Rehabil. 2000;79:60-68.
40. Lehman GJ, McGill SM. The Influence of a Chiropractic

Manipulation on Lumbar Kinematics and Electromyography During Simple and Complex Tasks. JMPT 22(9):576-581, 1999.
41. Lutz GE, Vad VB, Wisneski RJ. Fluoroscopic transforaminal lumbar epidural steroids: an outcome study. Arch Phys Med Rehabil. Nov 1998;79(11):1362-6.
42. Lyle MA, Manes S, McGuinness M, Ziaei S, Iversen MD. Relationship of physical examination findings & self-reported symptom severity & physical function in patients with degenerative lumbar conditions. Phys Ther. 2005;85(2):1 20-1 33.
43. Maher C, Adams R. Reliability of pain & stiffness assessments in clinical manual lumbar spine examination. Phys Ther. 1994;74(9):801 -809.
44. Maher C, Adams R. Reliability of pain and stiffness assessments in clinical manual lumbar spine examination. Phys Ther. 1994 Sep;74(9):801–811.
45. Matyas T, Bach T. The reliability of selected techniques in clinical arthrometrics. Aust J Physio. 1 985;31 :1 75-1 99.
46. McLain RF, Pickar JG. Mechanoreceptor Endings in Human Thoracic and Lumbar Facet Joints.
47. Memmo PA, Nadler SF, Malanga GA. Lumbar disc herniation: a review of surgical and non-surgical indications and outcomes. J Back Musculoskelet Rehabil. 2000;14(3):79-88.
48. Mootz RD, Keating JC, Jr, Kontz HP, Milus TB, Jacobs GE. Intra- and interobserver reliability of passive motion palpation of the lumbar spine. JMPT. 1989 Dec;12(6):440–445.
49. Padua L, Commodari I, Zappia M, Pazzaglia C, Tonali PA. Misdiagnosis of lumbar-sacral radiculopathy: usefulness of combination of EMG and ultrasound. Neurol Sci. Jun 2007;28(3):154-5.
50. Panzer DM. The reliability of lumbar motion palpation. JMPT. 1992 Oct;15(8):518–524.
51. Phillips DR, Twomey LT. A comparison of manual diagnosis with a diagnosis established by a uni-level lumbar spinal block procedure. Man Ther. 1996 Mar;1(2):82–87.
52. Phillips DR, Twomey LT. A comparison of manual diagnosis with a diagnosis established by a unilevel lumbar spinal block procedure. Man Ther. 1996;1(2):82-87.
53. Porchet F, Fankhauser H, de Tribolet N. Extreme lateral lumbar disc herniation: clinical presentation in 178 patients. Acta Neurochir (Wien). 1994;1 27(3-4):203-209.
54. Potter L, McCarthy C, Oldham J. Interexaminer Reliability of Identifying a Dysfunctional Segment in the Thoracic and Lumbar Spine. JMPT 29(3):203-207, 2006
55. Song XJ, et al. Spinal Manipulation Reduces Pain and Hyperalgesia After Lumbar Intervertebral Foramen Inflammation in the Rat. JMPT 29(1):5-13, 2006.
56. Spangfort EV. The lumbar disc herniation: a computer aided analysis of 2504 operations. Acta Orthop Scand. 1972;11(Supl 142):1-93.
57. Stankovic R, Johnell O, Maly P, Willner S. Use of lumbar extension, slump test, physical andneurological examination in the evaluation of patients with suspected herniated nucleus pulposus: a prospective clinical study. Man Ther. 1999;4(1):25-32.
58. Suseki K, et al. Innervation of the Lumbar Facet Joints: Origins and Function. Spine 22(5):477-485, 1997.
59. Tarulli AW, Raynor EM. Lumbosacral radiculopathy. Neurol Clin. May 2007;25(2):387-405.
60. Tsao B. The electrodiagnosis of cervical and lumbosacral radiculopathy. Neurol Clin. May 2007;25(2):473-94.
61. Vroomen PC, de Krom MC, Wilmink JT, Kester AD, Knottnerus JA. Diagnostic value of history and physical examination in patients suspected of lumbosacral nerve root compression. / Neurol Neurosurg Psychiatry. 2002; 72(5):630-634.
62. Willardson JM. Core stability training: applications to sports conditioning programs. J Strength Cond Res. Aug

Lumbar Quiz (answer page)

1. What are the joint type classifications for this region - z joint & disc? (128) _____

2. What is the orientation of the lumbar facet joints? (128)

   _____

3. What is the normal ROM for _____? (128)
   • Flexion/Ext.: _____, _____
   • Lateral flexion: _____
   • Rotation _____

4. What is the joint resting position? _____

5. What is the joint tight packed position? (128)

   _____

6. What ligaments resist flexion? (123)

   _____

7. What muscles cause extension to occur? (128)

   _____

8. Lumbar disc pressure is greatest with ___? (128)

9. Can you palpate _____ ? (120)

S = stabilization (indifferent hand), ● = contact, ➤ = examiner force, ⋯⋯➤ = patient motion

Learning Objectives

After completing this chapter, students will be able to:

1. Perform a regional exam and recognize common pathologies of the region

2. Identify and palpate body region bony landmarks, ligaments and muscles

3. Discuss regional kinematics and joint organ biomechanics including rib/vertebrae kinesiology

4. Demonstrate regional AROM, PROM & inclinometry

5. Recognize and execute the steps of effective mobilization and joint-play including indications, position, contact, force and relevant clinical notes

6. Perform supine, prone, seated assessment and mobilizations of spine and rib

   - Rotation, flexion restrictions
   - Lateral flexion restrictions
   - Extension restrictions
   - Lateral glides, P-A & A-P glides
   - Diaphragm release
   - Muscle Energy Technique
   - Upper rib motion restrictions
   - CT junction motion restrictions

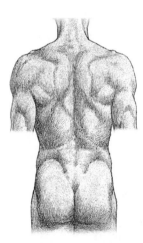
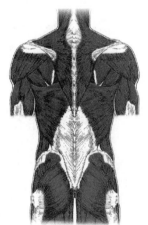
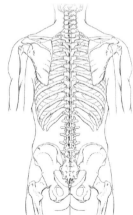

Realize that any mobilization (grade 1-4) can be made into a manipulation (grade 5) with the addition of a high velocity low amplitude (HVLA) thrust & vise versa with the lack of a HVLA thrust

Conversely any technique can be adapted to use IASTM where indicated - save your hands...

T-Spine & Ribs

Follow HIP-MNRS (see Yellow "Physical Assessment" text for specific details or review)
History, Inspection, Palpation - Motion, Neurovascular screen, Referred pain, Special tests

Special history considerations
- Specific mechanism of injury & forces involved?
- Pain with breathing or rib motion?
- Any numbness, tingling or weakness?
- Scoliosis? Family history?
- Type of work, typical posture? (sitting at desk)
- Review of systems (cardiovascular, GI, pulmonary)

Standing or sitting

Inspection
- Asymmetry, bruising, bumps, color, swelling, height
- Posture (hyperkyphosis/military spine)

Palpation (may be done after ROM assessment)

Erector spinae	Sternum
Upper ribs	Clavicle
Lower ribs	Supraclavicular fossa
Scapulae	Axilla
Spinous process	Lymph nodes
Trapezius	Pectoralis major
Rhomboids	Upper abdominals
Sternoclavicular joint	Sternocostal joints
Z-Joints & SPs	Costovertebral joints

Spinal percussion (C7-L3)

Functional assessment (ADL)
- Bend forward to touch toes

AROM
Flexion..............60° *(Adam's test)*
Extension..........25°
Lateral flexion...35°
Rotation.............50°

PROM & Joint Play (if lacking AROM in any motion)
- P-A glide
- Rotation (x2)
- Lateral flexion (x2)
- Costovertebral joints (rib springing)

Myotomes (resisted isometric movements)
- Shoulder elevation (C4, XI)
- Deltoid (**C5**, C6 - axillary)
- Brachioradialis (C5, C6 - radial)
- Biceps (C5, **C6** - musculocutaneous)
- Triceps (C6, **C7**, C8, T1 - radial)
- Wrist extensors (**C6**, C7, C8 - radial)
- Wrist flexors (C6, **C7** - median/ulnar)
- Finger flexors (C7, **C8**, T1 - ulnar/median)
- Interossei (C7, C8, **T1** - ulnar)
- Trunk rotation (T1-T12)
- Trunk lateral flexion (T1-T12)
- Trunk flexion/extension (T1-T12)

Heart & Lung Auscultation (if indicated)

Neurovascular screen
- *Sensory:*
  - Light touch
  - Two point discrimination
  - Vibration (3rd digit)
- *DTR's:*
  - Biceps (C5)
  - Brachioradialis (C6)
  - Triceps (C7)
- Grip strength (Dynamometer)
- Radial & brachial pulse, blanching, temperature

Orthopedic tests (as indicated)

Thoracic outlet syndrome
- Adson's
- Roo's/EAST
- Wright's test

Nerve compression
- SLR
- Slump test
- Brudzinski's test
- Passive scapular adduction test

Tissue contracture
- AROM, PROM
- Chest expansion test
- Rib motion test

Cervical, lumbar & shoulder screen

Diagnostic imaging (if indicated)

T-Spine & Ribs

152 | Joint Mobilization

	Condition	History	Physical exam	Diagnostic tests
Cardiovascular disorders	Angina pectoris	Substernal pressure Lasts 2-3 min Exertion/emotional Relieved: rest/nitroglycerine	Usually transient SSx Tachycardia, hypertension Systolic murmur	Stress ECG, Coronary arteriogram
	Mycardial infarction	Substernal pain or pressure on chest, lasts a few seconds Radiates left neck & arm	Patient may be pale, sweating or anxious Increased or irregular heart rate	ECG exercise stress test Ultrasound PET scan
	Mitral valve prolapse	Young F>M, non-exertional Unpredictable	Mid-systolic click Late systolic murmur	ECG
Chest wall disorders	Rib fracture	Sharp, local pain following trauma or prolonged cough	Palpable crepitus Possible edema & or discoloration Pain with chest motion	x-ray
	Rib subluxation	Sharp local pain on near spine with inspiration	Palpatory tenderness & local myospasm	Joint play & passive ROM
	Breast disorder	Tender mass Family history breast CA Large breasts Vague chest wall pain	Palpable, unilateral mass Non-supportive bra	Mammogram, biopsy
Abdominal disorders	Esophagitis	Burning, substernal pain ↑ by lying & eating ↓ by antacids	Usually WNL Possible: thrush or herpetic lesions	CBC, endoscope, barium swallow
	Peptic ulcer	Burning, epigastric pain, Dietary indiscretions ↑ by fasting, stress ↓ by food & antacids	Usually WNL	Barium swallow
	Biliary colic	Epigastric ache, nausea, vomiting, restlessness ↑ by fatty meals	Usually WNL	Oral cholecysto-gram, ultrasound
Respiratory	Pleuritis	Sharp, lateral chest pain, Increased inspiratory effort Precipitated by cough Relieved by analgesics	Possible: fever, dull percussion, bronchial breath sounds, friction rub	Chest x-ray, CBC
	Bronchitis/ Asthma/ COPD	Vague recurrent chest pain Prolonged coughing Asthma/infection	Possible: rales, rhonchi, wheezing, ↑ with chest motion, cough, respiration	Chest x-ray
Other	Herpes Zoster (Hx: dermatomal pain, prolonged duration, PE: rash) Biomechanical, Myofascial Trigger Points, Thoracic outlet syndrome			

↑ = increase pain, ↓ = decrease pain   -   **Scoliosis - see page 194**

T-Spine & Ribs

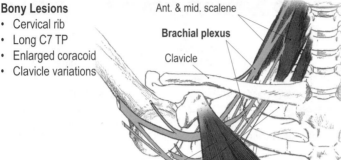

Bony Lesions
- Cervical rib
- Long C7 TP
- Enlarged coracoid
- Clavicle variations

Ant. & mid. scalene

Brachial plexus

Clavicle

Pectoralis minor

1st rib

Soft tissue lesions
- Scalenus minimus
- Costoclavicular lig.
- Fibrous bands
- Pectoralis minor

Neurologic SSx (90%)
- Pain
- Numbness, tingling
- Weakness
- Atrophy
- Raynaud's (sympathetic)

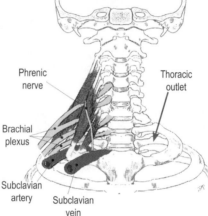

Phrenic nerve

Brachial plexus

Subclavian artery

Subclavian vein

Thoracic outlet

Vascular SSx (~10%)
- Subclavian artery
  - loss of pulse
  - motor weakness
  - claudication
- Subclavian vein
  - Edema
  - Cyanosis
  - Venous distension

Rib Subluxation ('Heart attack rib')
- Usually sudden, onset of local back or mid scapula **pain with a deep breath**, cough, sneeze or trunk movement, patient may have history of chronic poor posture
- Pain may be described as sharp with motion, then a dull ache & is usually **localized to posterior thorax**, but may radiate to anterior chest wall
- Pain with respiration, restriction of thoracic movement & sleep may be affected
- Difficulty breathing due to pain & may be associated with active trigger points or myospasm

Physical
- Tenderness over costotransverse joint & rib angle
- Ribs may be prominent to palpation, have local tenderness or muscle spasm
- Motion palpation will show decreased tissue compliance (springiness) over affected segments
- Must DDx from cardiac event or fracture

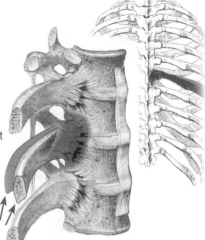

Image shows right 7th rib Subluxation
(Often associated with local pain, myospasm & biomechanical thoracic vertebral joint dysfunction)

T-Spine & Ribs

prohealthsys

All palpation methods involve tactile movement of soft tissues & osseous structures to evaluate **variations in elasticity, tone, motion from side to side, pain and/or discomfort.** - clinical style & preference will determine which specific methods clinicians use (use what works best for you)

Luke 'Spine Walker'

Procedure
> Patient prone, examiner palpates TP & ribs; examiner then alternately applies P-A force to body - walks hands up & down the spine & ribs
> Some describe this as a cat alternating paw pressure or kneading dough

Interpretation
> (+) Nonuniform motion → joint dysfunction, malposition or restriction of motion

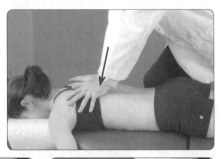

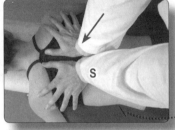
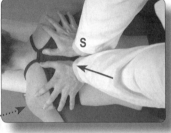

Force Vectors

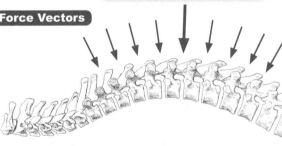

General vectors (line of drive) varies depending on the segment assessed and shape of the patients spine

Segmental Rotational Assessment

Procedure - patient prone, examiner palpates SPs; examiner then alternately applies L-M force - walks hands up & down the spine

Interpretation - (+) Nonuniform motion → joint dysfunction, malposition or restriction of motion

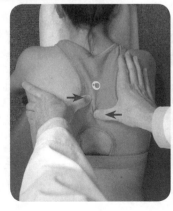
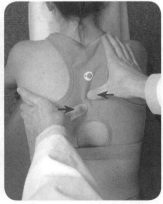

T-Spine & Ribs

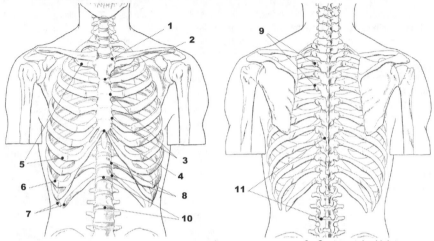

1. Sternoclavicular joint
2. Sternomanubrial joint
3. Sternocostal joint
4. Xiphisternal joint

5. True ribs (1-7)
6. False ribs (8-12)
7. Floating ribs (11-12)

8. Costovertebral joint
9. Transverse costovertebral
10. Intervertebral joint
11. Zygapophyseal joint

Thoracic Vertebrae

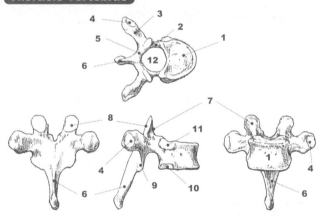

1. Body
2. Pedicle
3. Transverse process
4. Transverse costal facet
5. Lamina
6. Spinous process
7. Superior articular process
8. Superior articular facet
9. Inferior articular process
10. Inferior costal facet
11. Superior costal facet
12. Vertebral canal

Ribs (costals)

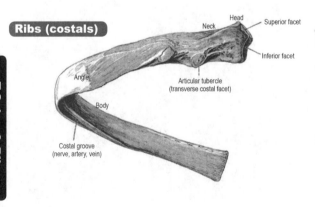

Head
Neck
Superior facet
Inferior facet
Angle
Articular tubercle
(transverse costal facet)
Body
Costal groove
(nerve, artery, vein)

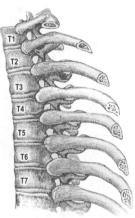

T1
T2
T3
T4
T5
T6
T7

T-Spine & Ribs

prohealthsys

Realize that normal anatomical variation in bone size & shape may alter exact spinal levels being palpated

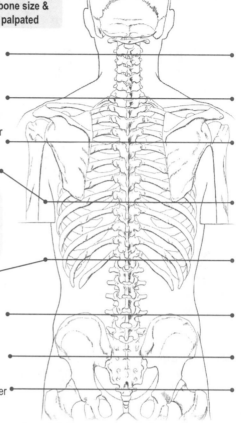

- **C2** - first palpable SP below the occipital bone

- **C7 or T1** - most prominent SP at base of neck (C7 will usually move from a palpating finger with cervical flexion/extension or rotation)

- **T4** - level with the root of the spine of scapula or apex of axillary fold

- **T7-T8** - level with the inferior angle of scapula

  Thoracic TP palpation Rule of 3s
  - **T1-T3 TPs:** at level of corresponding SP
  - **T4-T6 TPs:** ~½ segment *above* SP
  - **T7-T9 TPs:** ~1 segment *above* SP
  T10-T12 have TP's that project from a position similar to T9 & rapidly regress until T12 is like T1

- **T12** - level with the head of the 12ᵗʰ rib

- **L4** - level with the superior border of the iliac crest

- **PSIS & S2** - level with the most inferior portion of the PSIS

- **Sacral Apex** - level with upper greater trochanter (rotate patient's hip to locate trochanter)

Structure	Location
EOP	midline of occipital base
C1 TP	~1 cm (½" inch) anterior & inferior to mastoid process (under ear lobe)
C2 SP	1st prominent SP below EOP
C4 SP	hyoid bone
C5 SP	thyroid cartilage
C7 SP	usually second most prominent SP, spins with cervical rotation
T1 SP	most prominent SP (usually)
T7-T8 SP	inferior angle of scapula with patient standing (~T7 SP, T8 body)
L4 SP	level of iliac crest
S2 SP	level of the most inferior portion of PSIS
PSIS	follow iliac crest to dimples on back (usually ~2-3 cm long)
Sciatic notch	~5 cm (2") inferior, ~2.5 cm (1") lateral to PSIS
Ischial tub.	~5 cm (2") inferior & lateral to apex of coccyx (covered by glut. max standing)

TP = transverse process, SP = spinous process, thoracic TP palpation rule of 3s is a guideline more than a strict rule

T-Spine & Ribs

anterior view   lateral view   posterior view

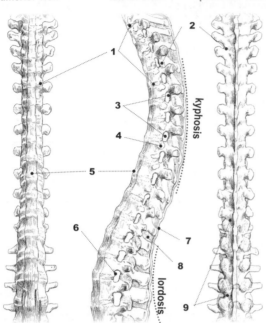

kyphosis

lordosis

1. Intervertebral joint (disc)
2. Zygapophyseal joint
3. Intervertebral foramen
4. Costal facet (for rib head)
5. Anterior longitudinal ligament
6. Posterior longitudinal ligament
7. Supraspinous ligament
8. Interspinous ligament
9. Ligamentum flavum

IVFs (intervertebral foramen) are made of pedicles of the vertebrae above and below and the intervertebral discs and Z-joints - IVFs are the pathway for spinal nerves

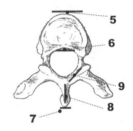

Nucleus Palposus
Annulus Fibrosis
INTERARTICULAR LIGAMENT
Costovertebral Joint
ANTERIOR COSTO-TRANSVERSE LIGAMENT DIVIDED
MIDDLE COSTO-TRANSVERSE OF INTEROSSEOUS
POSTERIOR COSTO-TRANSVERSE LIGAMENT
Costotransverse Joint
Vertebral Foramen (spinal cord)
Neck of Rib
Transverse Process
Transverse Process
Tuberosity

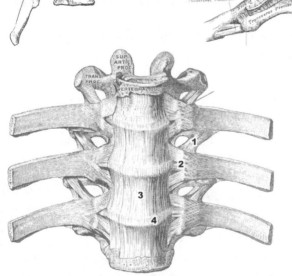

SUP. ARTIC. PROC.
TRANS. PROC.
VERTEBRAL BODY

1. Superior costotransverse lig.
2. Radiate ligament
3. Anterior longitudinal ligament
4. Intervertebral disc

T-Spine & Ribs

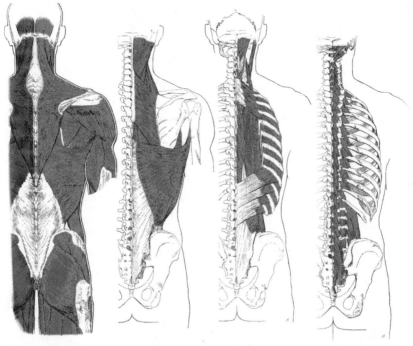

Ligament	Attaches (origin/insertion)	Function
Anterior longitudinal	Anterior vertebral body & disc to next vertebrae	Resists spinal extension
Annulus fibrosus	Vertebral bodies from C3-S1	Shock absorption, resists all spinal motions
Posterior longitudinal	Posterior vertebral body & disc to next vertebrae	Resists spinal flexion
Z-joint capsule	Facet to facet	Resist flexion & lateral flexion of trunk
Ligamentum flavum	Laminae to laminae	Resists flexion of trunk, elasticity assists extension of trunk
Interspinous	Spinous process to SP	Resists flexion of trunk, & shear forces on vertebrae
Supraspinous	Spinous process to SP above on tips	Resists trunk flexion & forward shear force on spine
Intertransverse	Transverse process to TP	Resists lateral flexion of trunk
Costotransverse	Tubercles of ribs to transverse process of vertebrae	Supports rib attachment to thoracic vertebrae
Radiate	Head of ribs to body of vertebrae	Maintains ribs to thoracic vertebrae

T-Spine & Ribs

Joint types:
- Gliding (zygapophyseal/facet joints)
- Gliding (costal & transverse costal)
- Fibrocartilaginous (intervertebral joints)

Articular surfaces
- **Thoracic:** facets are oriented in coronal plane

Active range of motion (thoracic)
Flexion...............20-45° *(Adam's sign scoliosis)*
Extension..........25-45°
Lateral flexion...20-40°
Rotation.............35-50°

Main muscle actions
- **Flexion:** rectus abdominis, internal/external oblique, iliopsoas, pec major, lats
- **Extension:** erector spinae, multifidi
- **Lateral flexion:** erector spinae, semispinalis, rectus abdominis, internal/external oblique
- **Rotation:** internal/external oblique, rotatores, multifidi, semispinalis, erector spinae

Resting position
- **T-spine:** mid way between flexion & extension

Close packed position
- **T-spine:** full extension

Capsular pattern of restriction
- **T-spine:** lateral flexion = rotation, then extension

Normal end feel
- **Flexion:** tissue stretch
- **Extension:** tissue stretch
- **Lateral flexion:** tissue stretch
- **Rotation:** tissue stretch

Abnormal end feel
- **Early myospasm** → muscle/ligament tear
- **Late myospasm** → instability
- **Empty** → ligament rupture
- **Hard** → bone approximation (osteophyte)

Coupled motions - pure rotation and pure lateral flexion do not occur in the spine below C1-C2

~T7-L5 vertebral segments*
- Left lateral flexion coupled with right rotation
- Right lateral flexion coupled with left rotation
- *this is the opposite coupling that occurs in the **cervical & upper thoracic spine (rotation & lateral flexion occur to the same side)**

Rotation, and especially rotation with lateral flexion increases the tensile (stretching load onto the intervertebral discs - heavy loads associated with rotation & lateral flexion cause disc injuries

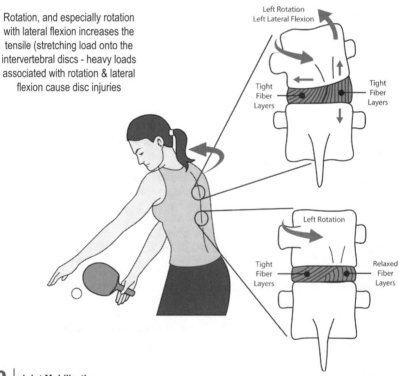

Left Rotation
Left Lateral Flexion

Tight Fiber Layers

Tight Fiber Layers

Left Rotation

Tight Fiber Layers

Relaxed Fiber Layers

T-Spine & Ribs

prohealthsys

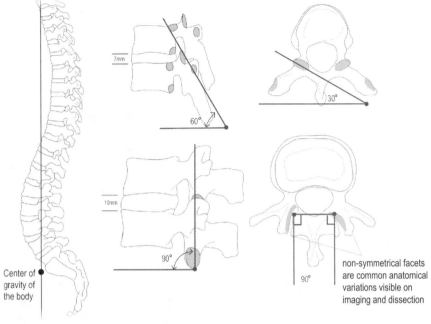

7mm

60°

30°

10mm

90°

90°

Center of
gravity of
the body

non-symmetrical facets
are common anatomical
variations visible on
imaging and dissection

Rib motion

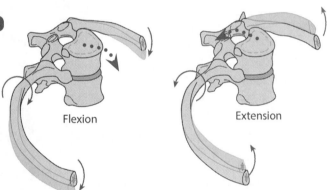

As thoracic vertebrae move,
they alter rib biomechanics
and vise versa - in practice
**correct the foundational
axis of the vertebrae first**,
then evaluate rib motion
(correcting the spine motion
often corrects rib issues)

Flexion

Extension

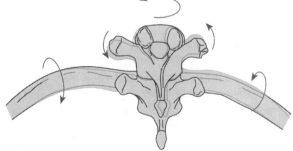

As the thoracic vertebrae rotates
or laterally flexes to the left, the
left rib rotates posteriorly, and
the right rib rotates anteriorly

Lateral Flexion/Rotation

T-Spine & Ribs

Adapted from: White, A & Panjabi, M. Clinical Biomechanics of the Spine. Lippincott, 1978. Hoppenfeld, S. Physical Examination of the Spine
& Extremities. New York: Appleton-Century Crofts, 1976. Kapandji, LA. Physiology of the Joints. Vols. 1& 2, second edition. Demeter et al.
Disability Evaluation. American Medical Association, Mosby 2003. American Academy of Orthopedic Surgeons 2018.

Introduction statement: "Try and move as far as possible, if any of the actions or movements are painful please let me know, do not do any action you feel will cause you further injury."

Flexion

Muscles Activated: *eccentric* contraction of erector spinae

Tissue Stretched: erector spinae, supraspinous & interspinous ligaments, posterior IVD, posterior facet joint capsule & intercostal muscles

Tissue Compressed: anterior thoracic structure, anterior longitudinal ligament, anterior IVD, lungs, heart, aorta, abdominal contents

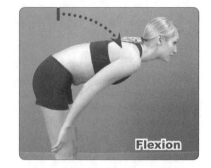

Flexion

Extension

Muscles Activated: *concentric* contraction of erector spinae, *eccentric* contraction of rectus abdominis & abdominal obliques

Tissue Stretched: rectus abdominis, anterior longitudinal ligament, aorta, lungs, anterior intercostal muscles

Tissue Compressed: erector spinae, supraspinous & interspinous ligaments, posterior IVD & IVF, z-joint capsule & posterior intercostal muscles

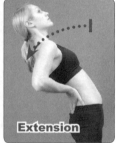

Extension

Lateral Flexion

Muscles Activated: *eccentric* contraction of *contralateral* erector spinae, transversospinalis

Tissue Stretched: *contralateral* erector spinae, transverso-spinalis, intercostal muscles, contralateral IVD & IVF, z-joints

Tissue Compressed: *ipsilateral:* erector spinae, transverso-spinalis, intercostal muscles, ipsilateral IVD & IVF, z-joints

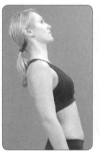

Lateral Flexion

Rotation

Muscles Activated: *contralateral* external oblique & transverso-spinalis, *ipsilateral* internal oblique

Tissue Stretched: *ipsilateral* external oblique & transverso-spinalis, *contralateral* internal oblique

Tissue Compressed: abdominal contents, ipsilateral intervertebral foramen

* T-spine & L-Spine are usually assessed together; to remove lower extremity influence consider performing in a seated position

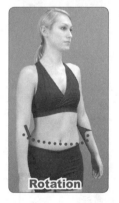

Rotation

Compare bilaterally; if possible palpate joint during PROM & use the shortest level possible; apply over pressure at end ROM; introduction statement:
"If any of the actions or movements are painful or uncomfortable please let me know."

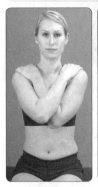 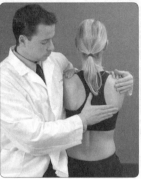 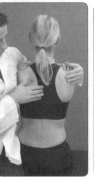 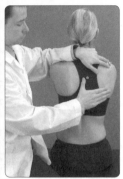

| Starting Position Patient's arms crossed | Thenar spinous contact to assess motion | Alternate finger-tip spinous contact | Alternate patient contact with forearm-shoulder stabilization |

Flexion (> 50°-70°)

Tissue Stretched: erector spinae, supraspinous & interspinous ligaments, posterior IVD, posterior facet joint capsule & intercostal muscles

Tissue Compressed: anterior thoracic structure, anterior longitudinal ligament, anterior IVD, lungs, heart, aorta

Extension (> 20°-30°)

Tissue Stretched: rectus abdominis, anterior longitudinal ligament, aorta, lungs, anterior intercostal muscles

Tissue Compressed: erector spinae, supraspinous & interspinous ligaments, posterior IVD & IVF, z-joint capsule & posterior intercostal muscles

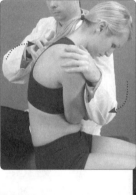

Lateral Flexion (> 25°-35°)

Tissue Stretched: *contralateral* erector spinae, transverso-spinalis, intercostal muscles, contralateral IVD & IVF, z-joints

Tissue Compressed: *ipsilateral:* erector spinae, transverso-spinalis, intercostal muscles, ipsilateral IVD & IVF, z-joints

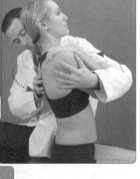

Rotation (> 40°-55°)

Tissue Stretched: *ipsilateral* external oblique & transverso-spinalis, *contralateral* internal oblique

Tissue Compressed: abdominal contents, ipsilateral IVF

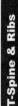

T-Spine & Ribs

Flexion (normal 20-45°)
- Patient standing
- Zero inclinometers over T1 & T12
- Ask patient to flex trunk, subtract T1 inclination from T12 inclination = ROM

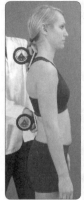

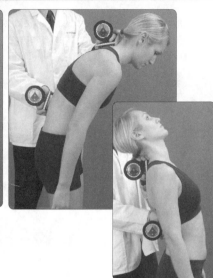

Extension (normal: 25-45°)
- Same as flexion except patient extends trunk

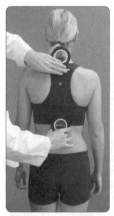

Lateral flexion (normal: 20-40°)
- Patient seated or standing
- Zero inclinometers over T1 & T12
- Ask patient to laterally flex trunk, subtract T1 inclination from T12 inclination = ROM
- Repeat on contralateral side

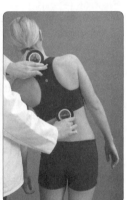

Rotation (normal: 35-50°)
- Patient standing with trunk flexed 90°
- Zero inclinometers over T1 & T12
- Ask patient to turn spine to one side, subtract T1 inclination from T12 inclination = ROM
- Repeat on contralateral side

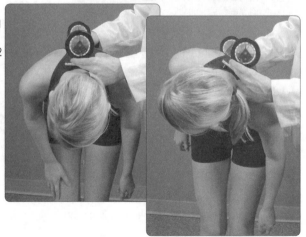

T-Spine & Ribs

Elevated 1st Rib

Indications: elevated anterior 1st rib

Position: patient supine; clinician at head of table

Contact: clinician's places finger tips, thumb or thenar eminence over patient's anterior portion of 1st rib (lateral to SCM)

Force: passively flex, laterally flex & rotate the patient's neck toward the contact hand & instruct patient take in a deep breath; with exhalation push 1st rib S-I; repeat & take up slack with each breath; repeat 3-5 times & reassess

Clinical notes: use a 'soft' contact

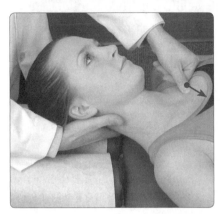

Elevated 2nd Rib

Indications: elevated anterior 2nd rib

Position: patient supine; clinician at head of table

Contact: clinician's places thumb or thenar eminence over patient's anterior portion of 2nd rib (just lateral to sternum)

Force: flex, laterally flex & rotate the patient's neck toward the contact hand & instruct patient take in a deep breath; with exhalation push 2nd S-I; repeat & take up slack with each breath; repeat 3-5 times & reassess

Clinical notes: use a 'soft' contact

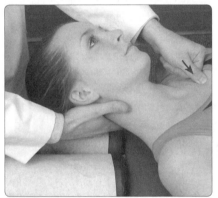

Anterior Rib Malposition

Indications: anterior rib #2-8 malposition

Position: patient supine; clinician in fencer stance

Contact: clinician places pincer grip or thenar eminence over patient's anterior portion of dysfunctional rib; abduct patient's shoulder ~90°

Force: have patient take in a deep breath; with exhalation apply gentle traction to the arm & mobilize rib P-A & M-L or L-M; repeat if necessary

Clinical notes: use a 'soft' contact

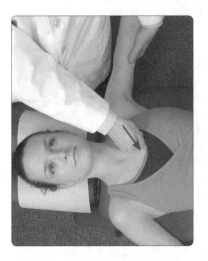

T-Spine & Ribs

Thumb Index Lamina Push

Indications: general ↓ thoracic segmental ROM

Position: patient prone; clinician in fencer or square stance

Contact: clinician's places thumb & index finger bilaterally over lamina (clinician may choose to reinforce contact hand with non-contact hand)

Force: develop tension by pushing through contact until tension is reached; then apply mobilization into direction of restriction (specific force varies depending on restriction)

   Extension restriction: tissue pull P-A, S-I

   Flexion restriction: tissue pull P-A, I-S

   Lateral Flexion & Rot: tissue pull P-A, L-M

Clinical notes: given common postural positions (slouching), most commonly the thoracic spine requires mobilizations that induce extension movements

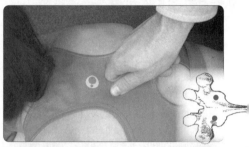

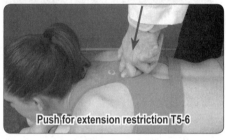

Push for extension restriction T5-6

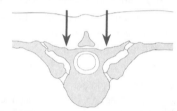

Thumb Spinous Push

Indications: general ↓ thoracic segmental rotational ROM

Position: patient prone; clinician in fencer or square stance

Contact: clinician's places thumbs bilaterally over the lateral side of patient's spinous process

Force: tissue pull L-M & slightly P-A; develop tension by pushing through contact until tension is reached; then apply mobilization (sustained glide or oscillations) into direction of restriction

Clinical notes: keep a 'soft' contact to ensure patient comfort

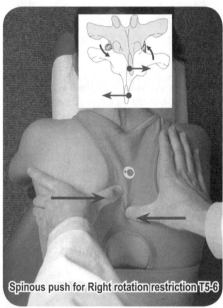

Spinous push for Right rotation restriction T5-6

S = stabilization (indifferent hand), ● = contact, ——▶ = examiner force, ·········▶ = patient motion

T-Spine & Ribs

Thumb Transverse Push

Indications: ↓ thoracic segmental rotation ROM

Position: patient prone; clinician in fencer or square stance

Contact: clinician's places reinforced thumb over patient's transverse process

Force: tissue pull P-A, M-L; develop tension by pushing through contact until tension is reached; then apply mobilization into direction of restriction

Clinical notes: remember breathing techniques may help patient further relax tissue, consider IASTM to save thumbs

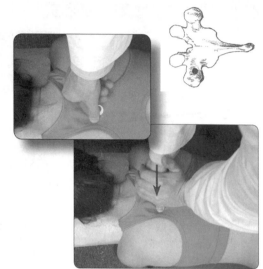

Diaphragm Release

1. Perform gently, slowly & with caution
2. Patient supine; place large pillow under knees
3. Place fingers of one or both hands flat on the anterior inferior margin of the rib cage
4. Ask patient to "*take a deep breath and slowly exhale*"
5. As patient exhales, curl fingertips under the rib cage, gently slide fingers along the interior surface of the ribs & costal cartilage
6. Note that palpation of the diaphragm is very difficult to perform even in the most flexible patient & only the anterior margin under the costal cartilage may be noted; it may be impossible to palpate in more muscular or obese patients
7. Treatment should also include costal mobilization & evaluation or QL and iliopsoas

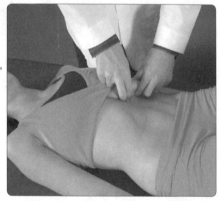

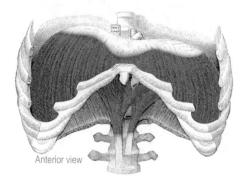

Anterior view

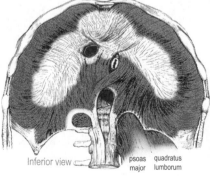

Inferior view

psoas major   quadratus lumborum

T-Spine & Ribs

S = stabilization (indifferent hand), ● = contact, ——► = examiner force, ·····► = patient motion

Bilateral Hypothenar Costal Push

Indications: general ↓ costal ROM

Position: patient prone; clinician in fencer or at head of table

Contact: clinician's bilaterally places hypothenar eminences over patient's costotransverse junctions (clinician may choose to interlock fingers)

Force: have patient take in a deep breath; with exhalation tissue pull M-L and P-A (I-S if clinician is facing superiorly, S-I if clinician is at head of table); develop tension by transferring body weight to contact until tension is reached; then apply mobilization

Clinical notes: this mobilization may be used as a manipulation with the addition of a HVLA thrust delivered at tissue tension

Also know as a 'Carver Bridge'

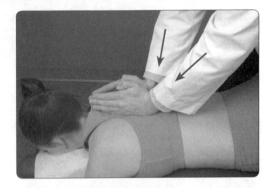

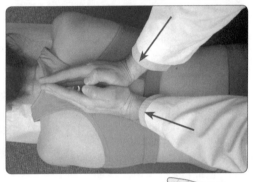

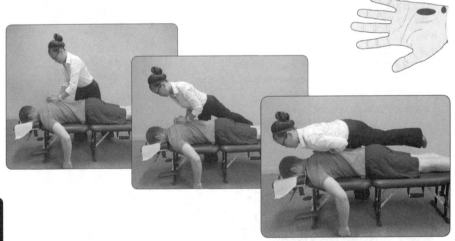

Chest hand drop variation - This variation allows smaller practitioners to generate more force by dropping their body weight on their hands (4'11" tall clinician in picture)

S = stabilization (indifferent hand), ● = contact, ⟶ = examiner force, ⌁⌁⌁▷ = patient motion

T-Spine & Ribs

Thenar Costal Push

Indications: general ↓ costal ROM

Position: patient prone; clinician at head of table

Contact: clinician's places reinforced thumb over patient's rib

Force: have patient take in a deep breath; with exhalation tissue pull I-S, M-L and P-A; develop tension by pushing through contact until tension is reached; then apply mobilization, repeat 2-3 times & reassess rib motion

Clinical notes: costal contacts can be sensitive, care must be taken to ensure a 'soft' contact

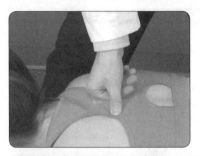

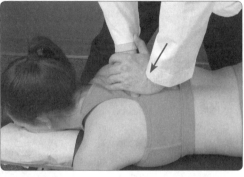

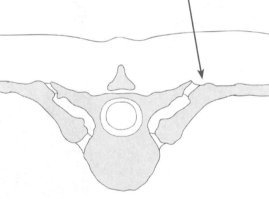

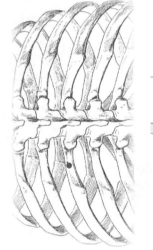

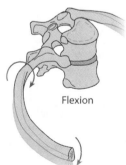

Flexion

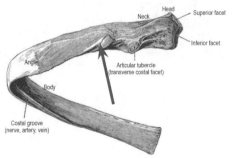

Head
Neck
Superior facet
Inferior facet
Articular tubercle
(transverse costal facet)
Angle
Body
Costal groove
(nerve, artery, vein)

S = stabilization (indifferent hand), ● = contact, ——▶ = examiner force, ·······▶ = patient motion

T-Spine & Ribs

prohealthsys

Active Bilateral Thenar TP Push

Indications: ↓ upper thoracic extension (T1-T4), reduce head forward posture

Position: patient prone with shoulders at edge of table & head hanging off table in a flexed position; clinician at head of table

Contact: clinician's bilaterally places thumbs over patient's laminar groove of specific segment

Force: have patient extend neck back to neutral position; as patient extends neck, clinician pushes laminar P-A & S-I direction; repeat until desired effect is reached (up to 10 x)

Clinical notes: the patient should be instructed to focus on elongating their neck as they extend their head back - can also be done as an IASTM technique to save clinicians hands

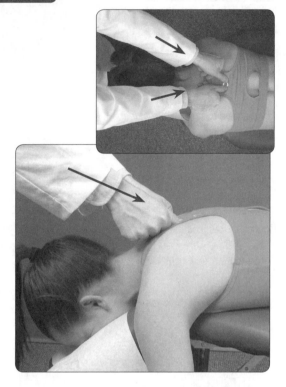

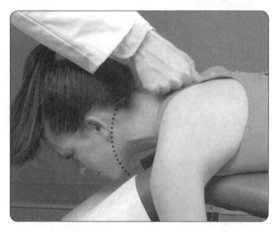

S = stabilization (indifferent hand),   ● = contact,   ⟶ = examiner force,   ┄┄┄▶ = patient motion

T-Spine & Ribs

Bilateral Thenar TP Pin & Stretch

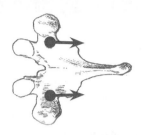

Indications: ↓ upper thoracic lower cervical myofascial tightness

Position: patient prone with shoulders at edge of table & head hanging off table in a flexed position; clinician at head of table

Contact: clinician's bilaterally places thumbs over patient's laminar groove of specific segment

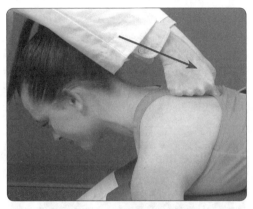

Force: have patient inhale & extend neck back to neutral position; as patient extends neck, clinician pushes laminar P-A & S-I direction; patient is then instructed to exhale & slowly flex neck while clinician maintains force over thoracic segment; repeat by taking up the slack & holding each time

Clinical notes: procedure may be repeated until desired effect is reached (usually 3-5x) - may also be done as an IASTM technique to take pressure off of the clinician's thumb

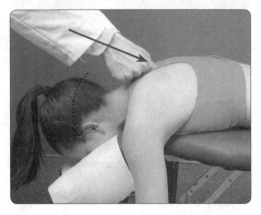

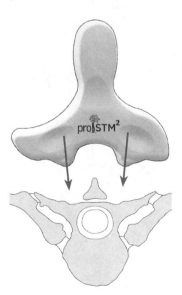

proISTM²

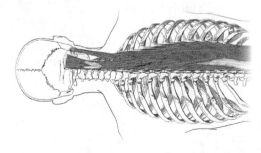

S = stabilization (indifferent hand), ● = contact, ⟶ = examiner force, ┈┈▶ = patient motion

T-Spine & Ribs

prohealthsys

Bilateral Thenar Transverse

Indication: extension, flexion, rotation, lateral flexion restrictions or malpositions

Position: patient prone; clinician in fencer or square stance

Contact: clinician's bilaterally places thenar eminences over transverse processes of the superior vertebrae (clinician may use a *bilateral hypothenar* contact - 'knife edge' contact)

Force: develop tension by transferring body weight to hand, thrust by dropping body & pushing through contact hands, breathing technique should be used

Extension restriction: tissue pull P-A, S-I   **Flexion restriction:** tissue pull P-A, I-S

Lateral Flexion: tissue pull P-A, M-L, I-S of main thrusting hand

Rotation: tissue pull P-A, M-L of main thrusting hand

Clinical notes: given common postural positions (slouching), most commonly the thoracic spine requires manipulations that induce extension movements

If rotational or lateral flexion restrictions are noted, when mobilization is applied more force may be directed through one hand to induce rotational or lateral flexion movement

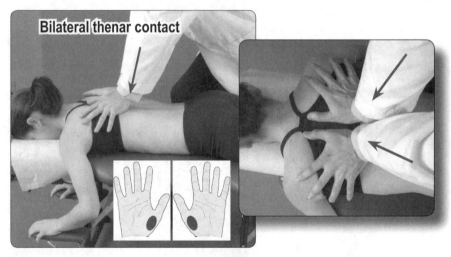

Bilateral thenar contact

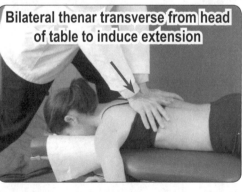

Bilateral thenar transverse from head of table to induce extension

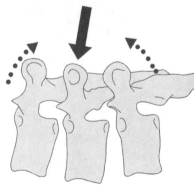

S = stabilization (indifferent hand), ● = contact, ———▶ = examiner force, ·········▶ = patient motion

T-Spine & Ribs

prohealthsys

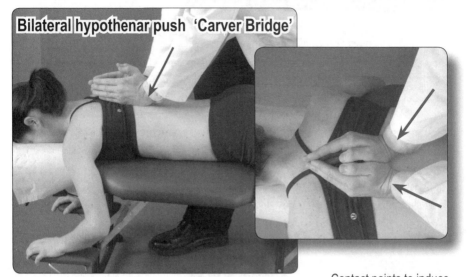

Bilateral hypothenar push 'Carver Bridge'

Contact points to induce **extension** with P-A thrust or mobilization

Contact to induce **lateral flexion** with rotational force

Contact points to induce **right rotation** of the inferior vertebra with P-A mobilization

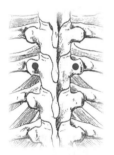

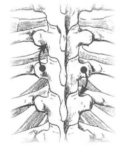

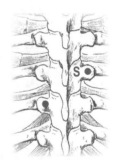

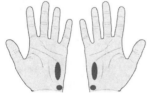

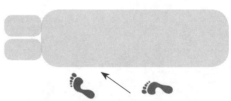

The treatments on these pages are among the best in office options to counteract the forces of gravity on the spine following prolonged sitting or smart phone use - by reversing the thoracic kyphosis and expanding the lung cavity - following these treatments **may patients express how they can breath better & stand taller**

Take a picture and measure the patients height pre and post treatment
(youtube: **prohealth**sys posture poster)

S = stabilization (indifferent hand), ● = contact, ⟶ = examiner force, ⋯⋯▶ = patient motion

T-Spine & Ribs

Crossed Bilateral Hypothenar Transverse

Indication: extension, flexion, rotation, lateral flexion restrictions or malpositions

Position: patient prone; clinician in fencer or square stance

Contact: clinician's bilaterally places hypothenar eminences over transverse processes of the superior vertebrae (clinician may use a *thenar* contact on the crossed hand)

Force: develop tension by transferring body weight to hand, thrust by dropping body & pushing through contact hands

Extension restriction: tissue pull P-A, S-I   **Flexion restriction:** tissue pull P-A, I-S

Lateral Flexion: tissue pull P-A, L-M of main thrusting hand

Rotation: tissue pull P-A, M-L of main thrusting hand

Clinical notes: given common postural positions (slouching), most commonly the thoracic spine requires manipulations that induce extension movements

If rotational or lateral flexion restrictions are noted, when the HVLA thrust is applied more force may be directed through one hand to induce rotational or lateral flexion movement

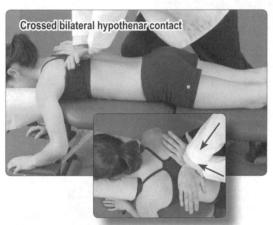

Crossed bilateral hypothenar contact

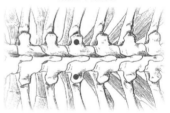

Contact points to induce **extension** with P-A thrust

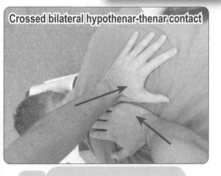

Crossed bilateral hypothenar-thenar contact

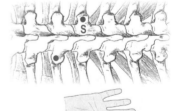

Contact points to induce **right rotation or right lateral flexion** of the superior vertebra

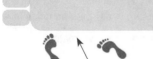

S = stabilization (indifferent hand),   ● = contact,   ➡ = examiner force,   ·······▷ = patient motion

T-Spine & Ribs

Unilateral Hypothenar Transverse Push

Indication: rotation or lateral flexion restrictions or malpositions (T2-T12)

Position: patient prone; clinician in fencer or square stance

Contact: clinician places thenar eminence over transverse processes (clinician's non-contact hand is used to reinforce contact hand by grasping wrist & stabilizing carpals/metacarpals)

Force: develop tension by transferring body weight to hand & tissue pull P-A, M-L & S-I or I-S depending on specific joint dysfunction; thrust by dropping body & pushing through contact

Clinical notes: use breathing technique to help relax patient muscles

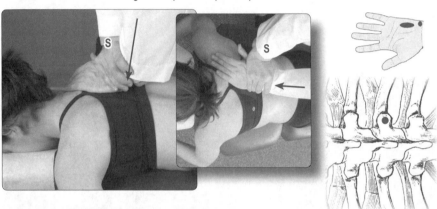

Unilateral Hypothenar Spinous Push

Indication: extension, flexion, rotation, lateral flexion restrictions or malpositions (T2-T12)

Position: patient prone; clinician in fencer or square stance

Contact: clinician's places hypothenar eminence over spinous processes (clinician's non-contact hand is used to reinforce contact hand by grasping wrist & stabilizing carpals/metacarpals)

Force: develop tension by transferring body weight to hand, thrust by dropping body & pushing through contact hand

Extension restriction: tissue pull P-A, S-I   **Flexion restriction:** tissue pull P-A, I-S

Lateral Flexion & Rotation: tissue pull P-A, L-M

Clinical notes: spinous process contacts can be very sensitive and care should be used to ensure patient comfort is maintained

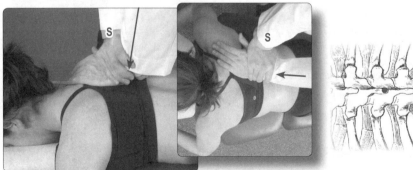

S = stabilization (indifferent hand),   ● = contact,   ➡ = examiner force,   ┈┈➤ = patient motion

T-Spine & Ribs

> Supine manipulation, while often difficult to learn, have the benefit of providing the clinician with the synergistic biomechanical advantage of using the patient's own body weight to help assist with the motion - resulting in a much more comfortable patient experience decreased stress on the clinicians body.

Contact: due to the nature of supine mobilizations & manipulation it is not possible to visualize the specific hand contacts, as such below are some optional contacts that may be used. Depending on the clinician's specific style and ability any option may be viable; also realize that by rolling the patient over more or applying more pressure with one side of the hand, rotational & lateral flexion forces may also be induced.

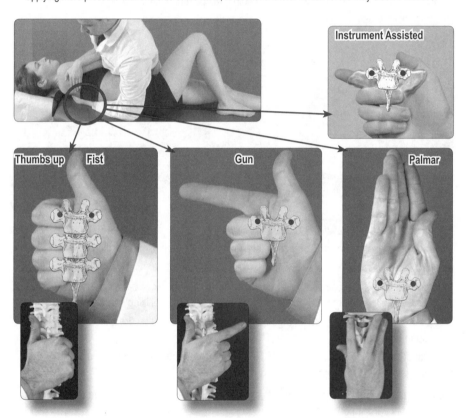

Instrument Assisted

Thumbs up   Fist

Gun

Palmar

Fist
- Thenar-2nd DIP contact
- Offers the largest fulcrum for mobilization
- May be uncomfortable on smaller, thinner patients
- Best used on patients with increased muscle or adipose mass

Gun
- Thenar-3rd DIP contact
- Slightly lower fulcrum than 'fist'
- Often more comfortable contact
- Excellent alternative to 'fist'

Palmar
- Thenar-hypothenar contact
- Offers the smallest fulcrum for mobilization
- Softest, most comfortable contact
- Best used on small thin patients
- Clinicians with smaller hand will find this contact difficult

Ultimately clinicians must develop or choose a style that works best for their individual ability and patient population

S = stabilization (indifferent hand), ● = contact, ⟶ = examiner force, ╌╌╌▶ = patient motion

T-Spine & Ribs

prohealthsys

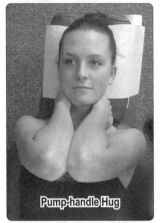

Pump-handle Hug

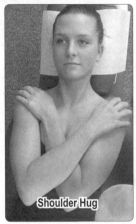

Shoulder Hug

Lat Hug

- Helps apply flexion distraction force to the upper spine
- Warning: lots of force on neck

- Makes patient very flat (may be useful for thicker pts)

- Best option - pulls scapulas apart to give maximum spine exposure, ribs & muscles

'Romantic Zone'

It is important the clinician avoid or spend as little time as possible with their face or chest directly over the patient's face or chest to avoid any misinterpretation of the therapeutic interaction - the 'V' on the patient show the region of the 'romantic zone' ☺

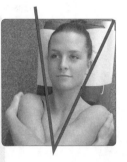

Patient elbows should contact ~2-5 cm below the clinicians xiphoid process (your abs are a 3rd hand).

Practitioners who are taller and have more upper body weight may also use a axillary or shoulder contact

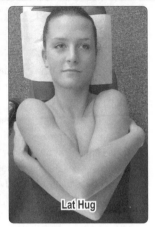

Elbows into Abs
work in your 'strike zone"

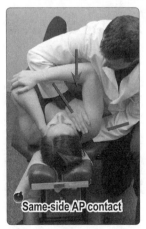

Same-side AP contact

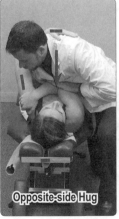

Opposite-side Hug

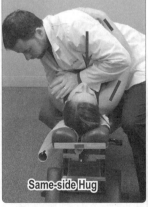

Same-side Hug

- Excellent method for specific anterior & posterior costal or sternal contacts

- Makes patient thinner (good for thick patients or smaller practitioners)

T-Spine & Ribs

Supine Crossed Arm Push

Indication: flexion, extension, rotation or lateral flexion restrictions vertibrae or ribs

Position: patient supine or seated with arms crossed over chest; clinician in fencer stance

Contact: clinician places the patient's elbows into their upper rectus abdominis & reaches behind patient for a posterior contact (bilateral or unilateral transverse process contact depending on joint dysfunction); clinician's 'non-contact hand' is used to support the patient's upper body (may use a same side or opposite side contact)

- If the patient starts supine, establish posterior contact then set the patient's elbows
- If the patient starts seated, set the patient's elbows then establish posterior contact

Force: varies depending on joint dysfunction and starting position of patient, develop tension by tractioning the patient body superiorly & transferring body weight; thrust by dropping body & pushing through abdominal muscles into the stationary posterior contact hand

Extension: bilateral contact on lower vertebra, traction superiorly tissue pull S-I

Flexion: bilateral contact on upper vertebra, patient supine but slightly flexed, traction superiorly tissue pull I-S

Rotation: unilateral thenar contact, tissue pull S-I & M-L

Lateral flexion: unilateral contact, patient supine but predisposed in lateral flexion, tissue pull S-I & L-M

Clinical notes: supine mobes require much less force as they **use the biomechanical advantage of the patient's body weight** to develop tension; techniques should be timed with patient full exhalation; the main disadvantage is the intimate nature of the procedure which can surprise patients the first time it is performed (good personal hygiene is a must ☺)

Starting position

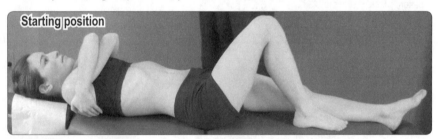

'Pick-up' Variation

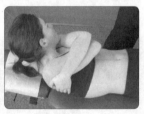

Instruct patient to perform a partial sit-up & look towards the wall (set-up may be started with patient seated then slowly lower them to table)

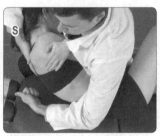

Stabilize patient's head & neck with forearm & hand, tuck patient's elbow into your abdominal muscles

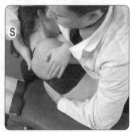

Tissue pull & find end-range to address specific restriction noted

S = stabilization (indifferent hand),   ● = contact,   ⟶ = examiner force,   ·········▷ = patient motion

T-Spine & Ribs

Same Side Variation

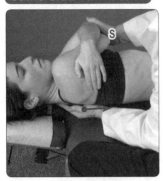

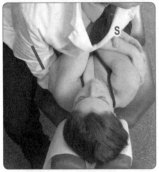

Clinician contact hand is on the
same side as stance

Place patient elbows into clinician's abdominal muscle (above umbilicus)
(A common error is to place the patients elbow too high into the clinician's sternum - this is very uncomfortable for both the patient and clinician)

Have patient take in a deep breath & as they breath out, apply I-S distraction with body; at end of breath apply a mobilization or HVT by bending legs & dropping body & contracting abdominal muscles

Image of vertebrae shows segmental force vectors developed

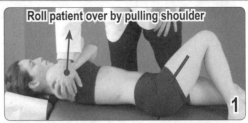

Roll patient over by pulling shoulder

1

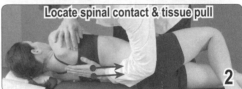

Locate spinal contact & tissue pull

2

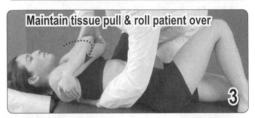

Maintain tissue pull & roll patient over

3

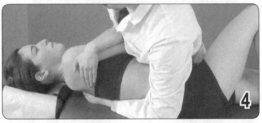

4

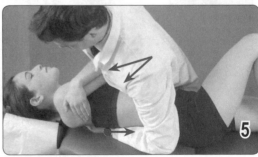

5

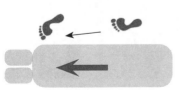

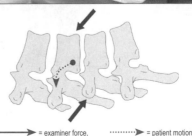

S = stabilization (indifferent hand), ● = contact, ⟶ = examiner force, ┈┈▶ = patient motion

T-Spine & Ribs

Indication: flexion, extension, rotation or lateral flexion restrictions or malpositions

Position: patient supine or seated with fingers interlaced behind their neck & elbows fully flexed; clinician in fencer stance

Contact: clinician places the patient's elbows into their upper rectus abdominis & reaches behind patient for a posterior contact (bilateral or unilateral transverse process contact depending on joint dysfunction); clinician's 'non-contact hand' is used to support the patient's upper body (can be a same side or opposite side contact)
- If the patient starts supine, establish posterior contact then set patient elbows
- If the patient starts seated, set patient's elbows then establish posterior contact

Force: varies depending on joint dysfunction and starting position of patient, develop tension by tractioning the patient body superiorly & transferring body weight;

thrust by dropping body & pushing through abdominal muscles into the stationary posterior contact hand

Extension: bilateral contact on lower vertebra, traction superiorly tissue pull S-I

Flexion: bilateral contact on upper vertebra, patient supine but slightly flexed, traction superiorly tissue pull I-S

Rotation: unilateral thenar contact, tissue pull S-I & M-L

Lateral flexion: unilateral contact, patient supine but predisposed in lateral flexion, tissue pull S-I & L-M

Clinical notes: supine manipulations have the advantage of requiring much less force as they use the biomechanical advantage of the patient's body weight to develop tension; the main disadvantage is the intimate nature of the procedure which can surprise patients the first time it is performed (good personal hygiene is a must) and the set-up may also put extra torque on the neck

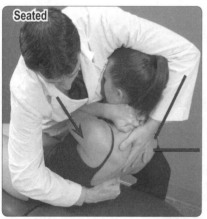

Seated

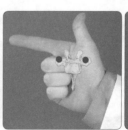

Supine

Contacts on spine

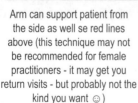

Arm can support patient from the side as well se red lines above (this technique may not be recommended for female practitioners - it may get you return visits - but probably not the kind you want ☺)

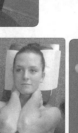

Pump-handle Hug

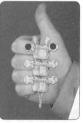

S = stabilization (indifferent hand), ● = contact, ——▶ = examiner force, ·········▶ = patient motion

Same Side Contact

Contact side is the same side as clinician stance. Useful for smaller clinicians treating larger patients, rather than having to reach across patient

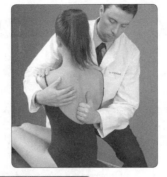
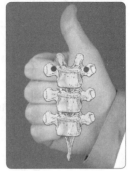

'Hug' Set-up with Reinforced Contact

Patient essentially hugs clinician. Useful for smaller clinicians treating larger patients, by making the patient effectively one arm width thinner. May be done as simple unilateral contact or reinforced contact. Can be a rather 'intimate' contact

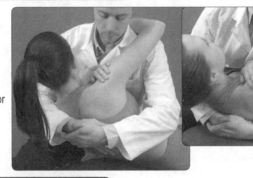

Head Rotation for Upper Thoracic

By rotating the cervical spine the upper thoracic spine may also be predisposed into rotation thus increasing the effectiveness of upper T-spine procedures that require rotation

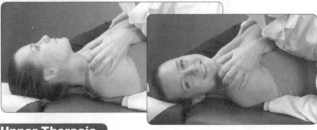

Pelvic Elevation for Upper Thoracic

Clinician sets-up contact and instructs patient to lift pelvis off table, increasing tension at the upper thoracic spine

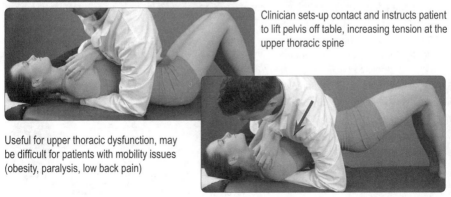

Useful for upper thoracic dysfunction, may be difficult for patients with mobility issues (obesity, paralysis, low back pain)

S = stabilization (indifferent hand),　● = contact,　——⟶ = examiner force,　⋯⋯▷ = patient motion

T-Spine & Ribs

Seated Thoracic or Costal

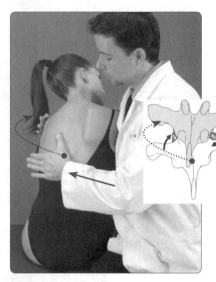

Indication: rotation or lateral flexion restrictions or malpositions (T3-T12)

Position: patient seated straddling table with arms crossed in front of chest; clinician seated or standing behind patient

Contact: clinician places thenar or hypothenar eminence over patient's TP or SP; clinician's 'non-contact hand' is used to support & tension the patient's upper body

Force: varies depending on joint dysfunction; tension is developed by rotating and/or laterally flexing the patient's upper body; thrust through contact hand

Rotation: tissue pull M-L & P-A

Lateral flexion: predispose the patient to lateral flexion & tissue pull M-L & I-S

Clinical notes: as clinical skill increases, seated adjustments may be done during spinal PROM assessment to improve clinical efficiency and patient management

Standing Thoracic or Costal

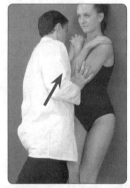

set-up is essentially the same as a supine thoracic manipulation except the patient is standing

Indication: flexion, extension, rotation or lateral flexion restrictions or malpositions

Position: patient standing with arms crossed over chest; clinician in fencer stance

Contact: clinician grips the patient's elbows & reaches behind patient for a posterior contact (bilateral or unilateral transverse process contact depending on joint dysfunction)

Force: varies depending on joint dysfunction and starting position of patient, develop tension by asking patient to lower body slightly; thrust by pushing through patient's elbows; specific forces & contacts are the same a supine crossed arm manipulations

Clinical notes: standing manipulations have the benefit of allowing the patients own body weight to be used as a distractive mechanism for the dysfunctional joint

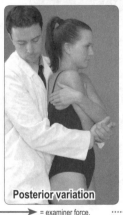

Posterior variation

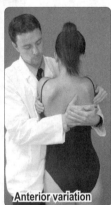

Anterior variation

S = stabilization (indifferent hand), ● = contact, ⟶ = examiner force, ┈┈▶ = patient motion

Indication: extension, rotation or lateral flexion restrictions or malpositions, spinal decompression

Position: patient seated with hands behind head

Contact: clinician slides hands through patient's arms& stabilizes the desired costal level with hands; clinician's knee contact is placed over desired spinal, costal or muscular contact

> The patient is instructed to take in a deep breath & as they breath out the clinician lifts & distracts over the fulcrum of the knee

Force: varies depending on joint dysfunction and starting position of patient, develop tension by tractioning the patient body superiorly & transferring body weight; Clinician can contract gastrosoleus to generate specific apical force

Clinical notes: This mobilization is very advanced and requires good clinician balance and skill; this maneuver is contraindicated in the presence of anterior glenohumeral instability

> Be sure to use the upper knee/lower thigh as your contact as a specific patellar contact it often to sharp and mobile

> Avoid excessive flexion force on the patients neck & injury to your own back by being sure to lean your body back with a straight spine

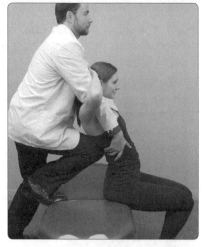

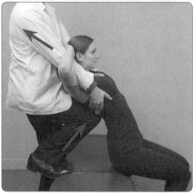

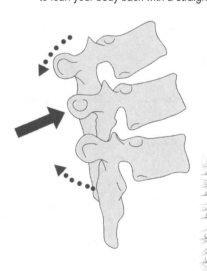

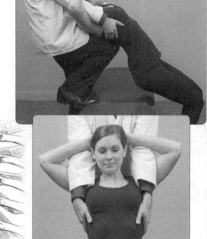

S = stabilization (indifferent hand),　● = contact,　——▶ = examiner force,　•••••••▶ = patient motion

T-Spine & Ribs

Indication: anterior rib dysfunction (rib 1-8)

Position: patient supine with affected side shoulder flexed 90°; clinician stands on patient affected side in lunge position

Contact: clinician places thenar or hypothenar eminence just lateral patient's costosternal junction of the affected segment; clinician's other contact hand is placed on the posterior aspect of the same rib segment

Force: tension is developed by tractioning and pulling the upper hand in the direction of restriction; tissue pull M-L & slightly A-P; mobilize through the upper contact hand

Clinical notes: depending on the specific dysfunction force vectors may also include I-S or S-I components

This is an excellent method to mobilize a specific rib segment from two points of contact

Another variation for anterior ribs is a bilateral hypothenar contact, where the clinician applies an A-P force while spreading the anterior costal-sternal junction (see image below)

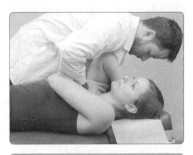

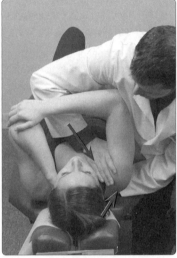

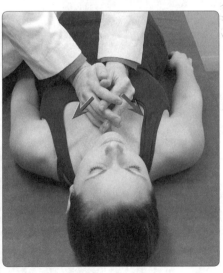

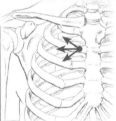

Anterior Contact

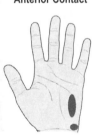

Posterior Contact

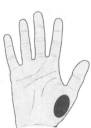

S = stabilization (indifferent hand), ● = contact, ——▶ = examiner force, ·········▶ = patient motion

Thenar Costal Push

Indication: rib dysfunction or malposition

Position: patient seated straddling table with arms crossed in front of chest; clinician seated or standing behind patient

Contact: clinician places thenar or hypothenar eminence just lateral to the patient's TP of the affected segment; clinician's 'non-contact hand' supports & tensions the patient's upper body

Force: tension is developed by rotating and/or laterally flexing the patient's upper body; tissue pull M-L & P-A; thrust through contact hand

Clinical notes: exact force vector (I-S, S-I) will depend on the specific lack of motion & corrective movement desired

As clinical skill increases seated adjustments may be done during spinal PROM assessment to improve clinical efficiency and patient management

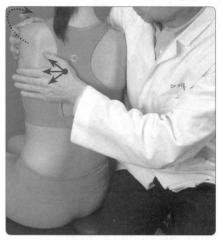

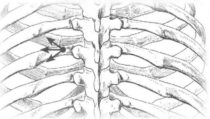

Thenar Sternocostal Pull

Indication: anterior rib dysfunction (rib 1-8)

Position: patient seated straddling table with arms relaxed at sides; clinician seated behind patient

Contact: clinician places thenar or hypothenar eminence just lateral patient's costosternal junction of the affected segment; clinician's 'non-contact hand' reinforces contact hand

Force: tension is developed by tractioning & rotating the patient's upper body; tissue pull M-L & slightly A-P; thrust through contact hand

Clinical notes: depending on the specific dysfunction force vectors may also include I-S or S-I components

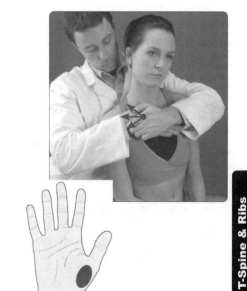

S = stabilization (indifferent hand), ● = contact, ➤ = examiner force, ┄┄┄➤ = patient motion

T-Spine & Ribs

Prone Costal Push

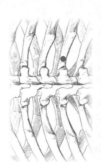

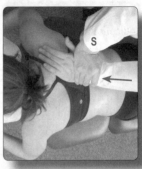

Indication: rib dysfunction (ribs 2-11)

Position: patient prone; clinician in fencer or square stance

Contact: clinician places thenar or hypothenar eminence just lateral to the patient's TP of the affected segment; 'non-contact' hand reinforces contact hand by grasping wrist

Force: tissue pull P-A & I-S for flexion restrictions or S-I for extension restrictions, develop tension by transferring body weight to hand, thrust by dropping body & pushing through contact hand

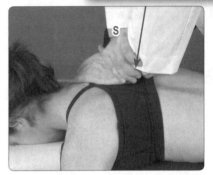

Clinical notes: this maneuver can be used as a mobilization if a HVLA is not applied

Side Posture Web Costal Push

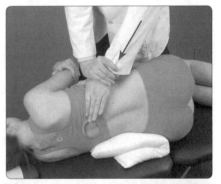

Indication: rib dysfunction (superior translation restriction, inferior malposition)

Position: patient side posture; clinician in fencer stance behind patient

Contact: clinician places web of thumb on inferior margin of the patient's affected rib; clinician's 'non-contact hand' reinforces the contact hand

Force: tissue pull I-S, develop tension by gently leaning into patient; thrust through contact hand

Clinical notes: this manipulation can be very uncomfortable if performed incorrectly, avoid excess lateral to medial to pressure on the rib cage. As with any manipulation, this maneuver can be used as a mobilization if a HVLA is not applied.

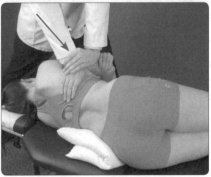

S = stabilization (indifferent hand), ● = contact, ⟶ = examiner force, ┈┈┈▷ = patient motion

T-Spine & Ribs

Bilateral Thenar or Crossed Costal Push

Indication: rib dysfunction (ribs 2-11)

Position: patient prone; clinician in fencer or square stance

Contact: clinician places thenar or hypothenar eminence just lateral to the patient's TP of the affected segment; stabilization hand is placed over the patient's contralateral thoracic TP

Force: tissue pull P-A, M-L & I-S for flexion restrictions or S-I for extension restrictions, develop tension by transferring body weight to hand, thrust by dropping body & pushing through contact hand

Clinical notes: this maneuver can be used as a mobilization if a HVLA is not applied

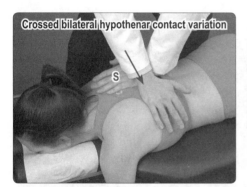
Crossed bilateral hypothenar contact variation

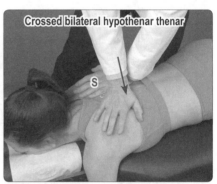
Crossed bilateral hypothenar thenar

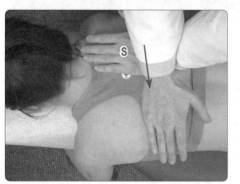

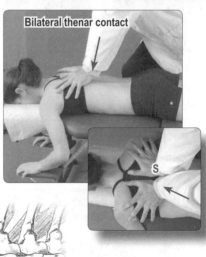
Bilateral thenar contact

Note that the rib contact is shown as multiple locations to indicate dispersion of contact hand force making the contact less sharp

S = stabilization (indifferent hand),　● = contact,　——▶ = examiner force,　⋯⋯▶ = patient motion

Covered Thumb

Indication: rib dysfunction (ribs 2-12)

Position: patient prone; clinician in fencer or square stance

Contact: clinician places thumb just lateral to the patient's TP (tubercle of rib) on the affected segment; 'non-contact' hand reinforces contact hand by grasping wrist

Force: tissue pull P-A, I-S & L-M, develop tension by transferring body weight to contact hand, thrust by dropping body & pushing through contact hand

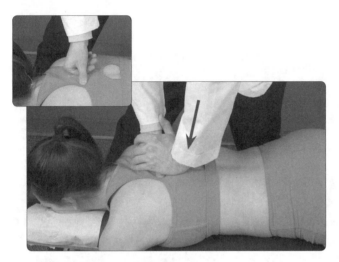
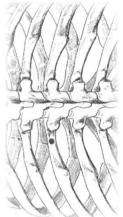

Ilial Costal Push-Pull

Indication: rib dysfunction (ribs 8-12)

Position: patient prone; clinician in fencer or square stance

Contact: clinician places thenar or hypothenar eminence just lateral to the patient's TP of the affected segment; pulling hand grasps the patient's ipsilateral ASIS

Force: tissue pull P-A, I-S & L-M, develop tension by transferring body weight to superior hand and pulling with lower hand, thrust by dropping body & pushing through contact hand

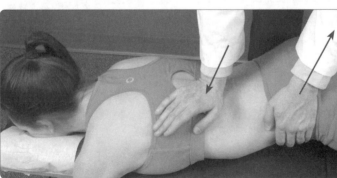

S = stabilization (indifferent hand), ● = contact, ——▶ = examiner force, ·········▶ = patient motion

Supine Thenar Costal Push

Indication: rib dysfunction (ribs 3-12)

Position: patient supine or seated with arms crossed over chest; clinician in fencer stance

Contact: clinician places the patient's elbows into their upper rectus abdominis & reaches behind patient for a posterior contact places **thenar eminence** just lateral to the patient's TP (tubercle of rib); clinician's 'non-contact hand' is used to support the patient's upper body (clinician may choose a same side or opposite side contact)
- If the patient starts supine, establish posterior contact then set the patient's elbows
- If the patient starts seated, set the patient's elbows then establish posterior contact

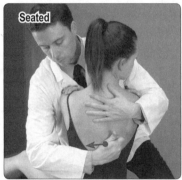
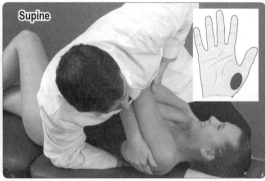

Force: tissue pull M-L & S-I for upper ribs & I-S for lower ribs, develop tension by transferring body weight; thrust by dropping body & pushing through abdominal muscles into the stationary posterior contact hand

Clinical notes: supine manipulations have the advantage of requiring much less force as they use the biomechanical advantage of the patient's body weight to develop tension; these techniques should be timed so the thrust occurs as the patient full exhales; the main disadvantage is the intimate nature of the procedure which can surprise patients the first time it is performed (good personal hygiene is a must)

Reinforced Variation

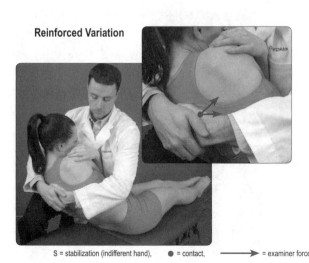

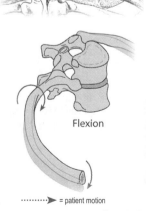

Flexion

S = stabilization (indifferent hand), ● = contact, ⟶ = examiner force, ┄┄▷ = patient motion

T-Spine & Ribs

Indication: rib dysfunction (ribs 1-3)

Position: clinician AP adjustment stance with superior leg at level of patient's head; patient supine with neck in neutral & ipsilateral shoulder & elbow flexed (instruct patient to wrap fingers behind neck)

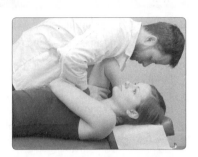

Contact: clinician places posterior hand **thenar eminence** over the angle of the patient's dysfunctional rib; clinician's anterior hand hypothenar eminence over desired rib, just lateral to sternum (thumb should be close to the axilla

Force: *posterior hand* tissue pull M-L & S-I ('J-hook'); *anterior hand* tissue pull M-L & A-P

thrust by dropping body & pushing through shoulder & hand to place maximal force over desired rib (consider using a breathing technique to avoid winding patient)

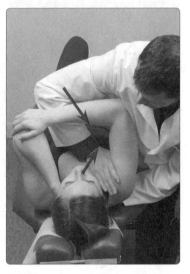

Clinical notes: take your time to ensure the appropriate end feel is felt prior to mobe/manip

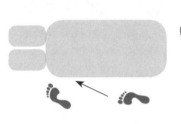

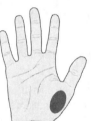

Pelvic Elevation for Upper Rib

Clinician sets-up contact and instructs patient to lift pelvis off table, increasing tension at the upper thoracic spine

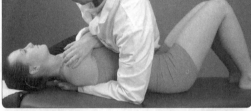

Useful for upper thoracic dysfunction, may be difficult for patients with mobility issues (obesity, paralysis, low back pain)

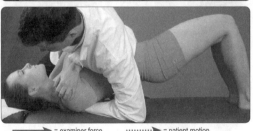

T-Spine & Ribs

S = stabilization (indifferent hand), ● = contact, ⟶ = examiner force, ┈┈┈▶ = patient motion

Hypothenar Costal Push

Indication: rib dysfunction (ribs 1-3)

Position: patient prone with neck in slight flexion & head slightly rotated; clinician in fencer stance with superior leg at level of patient's head

Contact: clinician places hypothenar eminence over the angle of the patient's dysfunctional rib; clinician's stabilization hand supports the patient's occipital bone & mastoid process (clinician may choose a same side or opposite side contact)

Force: tissue pull P-A & I-S or S-I, develop tension by stabilizing occipital bone & transferring body weight to lower hand; thrust by dropping body & pushing through contact hand

Clinical notes: avoid excessive force through the stabilization hand & patient's head

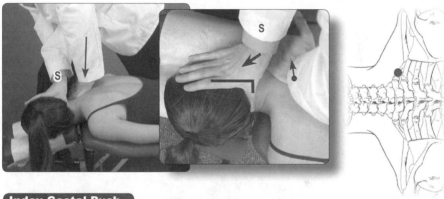

Index Costal Push

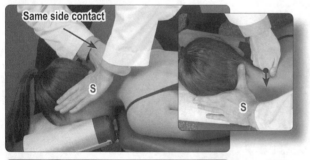

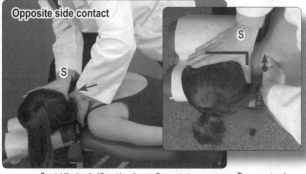

S = stabilization (indifferent hand), ● = contact, ➡ = examiner force, ┈┈➤ = patient motion

Thumb Spinous Push

Indication: lateral flexion or rotational joint dysfunction (C7-T3)

Position: patient prone with neck in slight flexion & head slightly rotated; clinician in fencer stance with superior leg at level of patient's head

Contact: clinician places thumb over the patient's dysfunctional SP; clinician's stabilization hand supports the patient's occipital bone & mastoid process (clinician may choose a same side or opposite side contact)

Force: tissue pull L-M & P-A (slight I-S or S-I if needed), develop tension by stabilizing occipital bone & transferring body weight to lower hand; thrust by dropping body & pushing through contact hand

Clinical notes: avoid excessive force through the stabilization hand

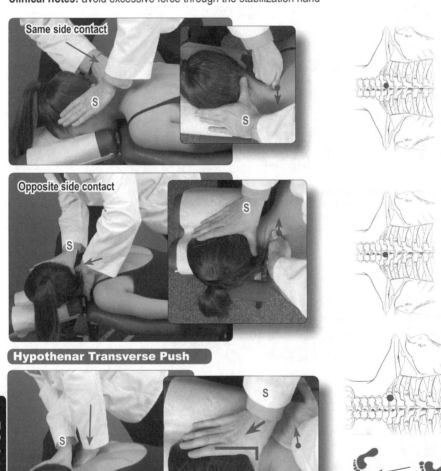

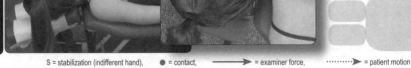

S = stabilization (indifferent hand), ● = contact, ——► = examiner force, ·········► = patient motion

Cephalad Spinous Push

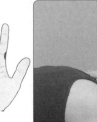

Indication: lateral flexion or rotational joint dysfunction (C7-T3)

Position: patient prone with neck in slight flexion & head slightly rotated; clinician in fencer stance standing at the head piece

Contact: clinician places hypothenar or MCP over the patient's ipsilateral SP; clinician's stabilization hand supports the patient's occipital bone & mastoid process

Force: tissue pull L-M & P-A (slight S-I), develop tension by stabilizing occipital bone & transferring body weight to lower contact hand; thrust/mobilize by dropping body & pushing through contact hand

Clinical notes: avoid excessive force through the stabilization hand

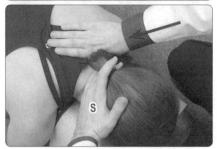

Supine Spinous Push

Indication: lateral flexion or rotational joint dysfunction (C7-T3)

Position: patient supine (or seated) with neck in slight flexion & head slightly rotated; clinician stands at ~45° to patient at head of table

Contact: clinician places anterolateral surface of index finger MCP joint on affected segment articular pillar or spinous process; clinician's stabilization hand supports the patient's contralateral occipital bone (very similar to regular cervical index pillar adjustment)

Force: tissue pull is L-M & P-A with a S-I component; develop tension by rotating the patient's head away & laterally flexing toward the segmental contact; thrust/mobilize by pushing through contact hand

Clinical notes: take your time to ensure the appropriate end feel is felt prior to mobilization - is take practice to sink through the soft tissue of the lower neck to a solid end feel

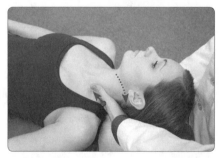

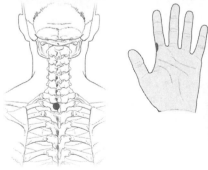

S = stabilization (indifferent hand), ● = contact, ➡ = examiner force, ┄┄➤ = patient motion

1. Vizniak, NA. Gross Anatomy Human Cadaver Dissections. 1999-2018.
2. Potter L, McCarthy C, Oldham J. Interexaminer Reliability of Identifying a Dysfunctional Segment in the Thoracic and Lumbar Spine. JMPT 29(3):203-207, 2006
3. McGee S. Evidence-Based Physical Diagnosis. Saunders. 2007.
4. Taylor MH, Monroe LG. Physical Rehabilitation: Evidence-Based Examination, Evaluation and Intervention. Saunders. 2007.
5. Warlow C, Hughes R, Uitehaag B, Liberati A. Evidence-Based Neurology. Blackwell Publishing Limited, BMJI Books. 2007.
6. Malanga GA & Nadler. Musculoskeletal Physical Exam, An Evidence-Based Approach. Mosby. 2006.
7. Hoppenfield S. Physical Examination of the Spine & Extremities. Lippincott Williams & Wilkins. 1976.
8. Hoppenfield S. Orthopaedic Neurology: A Diagnostic Guide to Neurologic Levels. Lippincott Williams & Wilkins. 1977.
9. Spencer JW, Jacobs JJ. Complementary and Alternative Medicine: An Evidence-Based Approach. Mosby. 2003.
10. Jewell D. Guide to Evidence-Based Physical Therapy Practice. Jones Barlett Publishers Inc. 2007.
11. Iesel SW. Operative Orthopaedics: An Illustrative Approach. Lippincott Williams & Wilkins. 2008.
12. Brismee JM, Gilbert K, Isom K, Hall R, Leathers B, Sheppard N, Sawyer S, Sizer P. Rate of false positive using the Cyriax Release test for thoracic outlet syndrome in an asymptomatic population. J Man Manipulative Ther. 2004;12:73-81.
13. Howard M, Lee C, Dellon AL. Documentation of brachial plexus compression (in the thoracic inlet) utilizing provocative neurosensory & muscular testing. J Reconstr Microsurg. 2003;1 9(5):303-31 2.
14. Lee AD, Agarwal S, Sadhu D. Doppler Adson's test: predictor of outcome of surgery in non-specific thoracic outlet syndrome. World J Surg.2006;30(3):291-292.
15. Lindgren KA, Leino E, Manninen H. Cervical rotation lateral flexion test in brachialgia. Arch Phys Med Rehabil. 1992;73(8):735-737.
16. Maitland GD. Maitland's Vertebral Manipulation. 6th ed. London; Butterworth-Heinemann: 2001.
17. Matsuyama T, Okuchi K, Coda K. Upper plexus thoracic outlet syndrome-case report. Neur Med Chir (Tokyo). 2002;42(5):237-241.
18. Plewa MC, Delinger M. The false-positive rate of thoracic outlet syndrome shoulder maneuvers in healthy patients. Acad Emerg Med. 1998;5(4):337-342.
19. Rayan CM, Jensen C. Thoracic outlet syndrome: provocative examination maneuvers in a typical population. J Shoulder Elbow Surg. 1995;4(2):113-117.
20. Smedmark V, Wallin M, Arvidsson I. Inter-examiner reliability in assessing passive intervertebral motion of the cervical spine. Man Ther. 2000;5:97-101.
21. Keene JS, Albert MJ, Springer SL, Drummond DS, Clancy WG Jr. Back injuries in college athletes. J Spinal Disord. Sep 1989;2(3):190-5.
22. Gourmelen J, Chastang JF, Ozguler A, et al. Frequency of low back pain among men and women aged 30 to 64 years in France. Results of two national surveys. Ann Readapt Med Phys. Nov 2007;50(8):640-4.
23. Louw QA, Morris LD, Grimmer-Somers K. The Prevalence of low back pain in Africa: a systematic review. BMC Musculoskelet Disord. Nov 1 2007;8(1):105.
24. Navar D, Zhou BH, Lu Y, Solomonow M. High-repetition cyclic loading is a risk factor for a lumbar disorder. Muscle Nerve. Nov 2006;34(5):614-22.
25. Radebold A, Cholewicki J, Panjabi MM, Patel TC. Muscle response pattern to sudden trunk loading in healthy individuals and in patients with chronic low back pain. Spine. Apr 15 2000;25(8):947-54.
26. Noonan TJ, Garrett WE Jr. Muscle strain injury: diagnosis and treatment. J Am Acad Orthop Surg. Jul-Aug 1999;7(4):262-9.
27. Panjabi MM. The stabilizing system of the spine. Part I. Function, dysfunction, adaptation, and enhancement. J Spinal Disord. Dec 1992;5(4):383-9; discussion 397.
28. Cholewicki J, Panjabi MM, Khachatryan A. Stabilizing function of trunk flexor-extensor muscles around a neutral spine posture. Spine. Oct 1 1997;22(19):2207-12.
29. Weksler N, Velan GJ, Semionov M, et al. The role of sacroiliac joint dysfunction in the genesis of low back pain: the obvious is not always right. Arch Orthop Trauma Surg. Dec 2007;127(10):885-8.
30. Taimela S, Kujala UM, Osterman K. Intrinsic risk factors and athletic injuries. Sports Med. Apr 1990;9(4):205-15.
31. Cholewicki J, Juluru K, Radebold A, Panjabi MM, McGill SM. Lumbar spine stability can be augmented with an abdominal belt and/or increased intra-abdominal pressure. Eur Spine J. 1999;8(5):388-95.
32. Almekinders LC. Anti-inflammatory treatment of muscular injuries in sport. An update of recent studies. Sports Med. Dec 1999;28(6):383-8.
33. Demoulin C, Distrée V, Tomasella M, Crielaard JM, Vanderthommen M. Lumbar functional instability: a critical appraisal of the literature. Ann Readapt Med Phys. Nov 2007;50(8):677-84.
34. Garrett WE Jr. Muscle strain injuries. Am J Sports Med. 1996;24(6 suppl):S2-8.
35. LeBlanc KE. Sacroiliac sprain: an overlooked cause of back pain. Am Fam Physician. Nov 1992;46(5):1459-63.
36. Panjabi MM. The stabilizing system of the spine. Part II. Neutral zone and instability hypothesis. J Spinal Disord. Dec 1992;5(4):390-6; discussion 397.
37. Tall RL, DeVault W. Spinal injury in sport: epidemiologic considerations. Clin Sports Med. Jul 1993;12(3):441-8.

Scoliosis

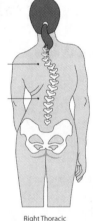

Right Thoracic Scoliosis

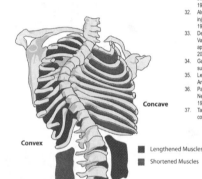

Convex

Concave

■ Lengthened Muscles
■ Shortened Muscles

Thoracic Quiz (answer page)

1. What are the joint type classifications for this region - z joint & disc? (160) _____

2. What is the orientation of the facet joints? (160)

   _____

3. What is the normal ROM for _____? (160)
   • Flexion/Ext.: _____, _____
   • Lateral flexion: _____
   • Rotation _____

4. What is the joint resting position? _____

5. What is the joint tight packed position? (160)

   _____

6. What ligaments resist extension? (159)

   _____

7. What muscles cause flexion to occur? (160)

   _____

8. Flexion of thoracic vertebrae is associated with what rib motion? (161)

   _____

9. What motions increase tensile (pulling load on intervertebral discs? (160)

   _____

10. Can you palpate _____ ? (152)

S = stabilization (indifferent hand),   ● = contact,   ⟶ = examiner force,   ·········▶ = patient motion

Learning Objectives

After completing this chapter, students will be able to:

1. Perform a regional exam and recognize common pathologies of the region

2. Identify and palpate body region bony landmarks, ligaments and muscles

3. Evaluate & identify risk factors of cervical mobilization (**5Ds And 3Ns**)

   - **Dizziness, vertigo, giddiness**
   - **D-LOC** (decreased level of consciousness)
   - **Diplopia** (or other visual disturbances)
   - **Dysarthria** (difficulty speaking)
   - **Dysphagia** (difficulty swallowing)
   - **Ataxia** (loss of motor control or gait)
   - **Nausea & vomiting**
   - **Numbness** (unilateral over face)
   - **Nystagmus** (lateral beating of the eyes)

4. Discuss regional kinematics and joint organ biomechanics

5. Demonstrate regional AROM, PROM & inclinometry, stretch and strengthen protocols

6. Recognize and execute the steps of effective mobilization and joint-play including indications, position, contact, force and relevant clinical notes

7. Perform supine, prone, seated assessment and mobilizations of

   - Rotation, flexion, lateral flexion restrictions
   - Extension restrictions
   - Lateral glides, P-A & A-P glides
   - Muscle Energy Technique
   - TMJ motion restrictions

Head & Neck

Cluster for patients with neck pain that will benefit from C-spine / T-spine osseous mobilization, exercise & patient education

- Symptoms <30 days
- No symptoms distal to the shoulder
- Looking up does not aggravate symptoms
- Diminished upper thoracic spine kyphosis
- Cervical extension ROM <30 degrees
- FABQ Physical Activity Score <12
- 3 positive: +LR: 5.5
- 4 positive: +LR: 12 - 5-6 positive: +LR: >12

1. Cleland JA, Childs JD, Fritz JM, Whitman JM, Eberhart SL. "Development of a clinical prediction rule for guiding treatment of a subgroup of patients with neck pain: use of thoracic spine manipulation, exercise, and patient education." Phys Ther. 2007 Jan. Web. 08/18/2014.
2. Cleland JA, Flynn TW, Whitman JM. User's Guide to the Musculoskeletal Examination Fundamentals for the Evidence-Based Clinician: Evidence in Motion; 2015.
3. Wainner RS, Fritz JM, Irrgang JJ, Boninger ML, Delitto A, Allison S. "Reliability and diagnostic accuracy of the clinical examination and patient self-report measures for cervical radiculopathy." Spine (Phila Pa 1976) 2003 Jan 1. Web. 08/18/2014.

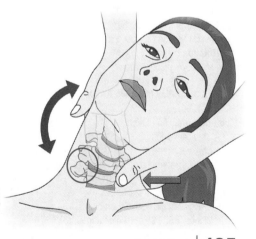

Head & Neck

History considerations
- Patient age? (OA after 60)
- Specific mechanism of injury & forces involved?
- Any impact trauma? Loss of consciousness?
- Associated headache? Dizziness? Nausea? trouble speaking? Double vision?
- Any numbness, tingling or weakness?
- Type of work, typical posture, sleeping posture?

Inspection
- Inspection of head & neck, skin, general appearance
- Posture of head, neck & thoracic spine, shoulder

Auscultate heart & carotid arteries

Palpation (may be done after ROM assessment)

Mandible	Articular pillars
Masseter/Parotids	Facet joints
Submandibular gland	Spinous processes
Submental gland	Upper trapezius
Thyroid gland	Levator scapulae
Trachea	Splenius cerv./cap.
Lymph nodes	Semispinalis capitis
SCM	Suboccipitals
Doorbell Sign	Upper rib motion
Mastoid processes	Supraclavicular fossa
Carotid artery	Clavicle

Functional assessment (ADLs)
- Breathing, swallowing, shoulder check, looking up at ceiling & down at floor

AROM
Flexion........................60°
Extension...................60°
Lateral flexion (x2).....45°
Rotation (x2)..............80°
TMJ ROM (pain, clicking?)

PROM & Joint Play (if lacking AROM in any motion)

Myotomes (may be done prone)
- Cervical flexion (C1-C2)
- Cervical extension (C2, C3, XI)
- Cervical lateral flexion (C3)
- Shoulder elevation (C4, XI)
- Deltoid (**C5**, C6 - axillary)
- Brachioradialis (C5, C6 - radial)
- Biceps (C5, **C6** - musculocutaneous)

- Triceps (C6, **C7**, C8, T1 - radial)
- Wrist extensors (**C6**, C7, C8 - radial)
- Wrist flexors (C6, **C7** - median/ulnar)
- Finger flexors (C7, **C8**, T1 - ulnar/median)
- Interossei (C7, C8, **T1** - ulnar)

Cranial nerve exam (if indicated)

EENT (if indicated)
Ophthalmic exam, Otoscope exam
Rhinoscopic & pharyngeal exam

Neurovascular screen
Sensory:
- Cranial nerve exam (if indicated)
- Corneal reflex (V, VII)
- Light touch (face/arms)
- Sharp/dull or pinwheel (face/arms)
- Vibration (DIP, 3rd digit)

DTR: Biceps (C5), brachioradialis (C6), triceps (C7), patella (L4), hamstring (L5), Achilles (S1)
- Hoffman (or dynamic Hoffman)
- Dynamometer (grip strength)
- Girth measurement (arm, forearm)
- Radial & brachial pulse, blanching, temperature

Orthopedic tests (as indicated)
VBI (may be done before AROM)
- Vertebral basilar artery function test
- Dekleyn's test

Instability
- Alar ligament stress test
- Lateral shear test
- Sharp-Purser test
- Transverse ligament stress test
- Rust's Sign

Radiculopathy/Nerve tension
- Cervical compression/distraction
- Brachial plexus compression test
- Soto-Hall Test
- Upper limb tension test
- Valsalva maneuver

Sprain/Strain
- Cervical distraction
- Cervical AROM/PROM & Muscle Tests
- O'Donoghue maneuver
- Scalene cramp test

Thoracic spine & shoulder screen

Diagnostic imaging (if indicated)

▶ youtube: Wrist/hand Exam Brief Vizniak

prohealthsys.com

Condition	Clinical notes
Radiculopathy	*Hx:* numbness, tingling, weakness or shooting electrical pain down arm *SSx:* ↓ pain when supine; (+) neurologic signs (↓ DTR, muscle weakness, ↓ sensation); (+) cervical compression for arm pain *DDx:* disc herniation, IVF encroachment, space occupying lesion, TOS
Osteoarthritis	*Hx:* patient > 50 yrs; gradual onset; crepitus; morning stiffness; dull achy pain *SSx:* ↓ pain with movement, worse at rest; limited AROM; confirm on x-ray (decreased joint space, osteophyte formation) *DDx:* rheumatoid, IVF encroachment, ankylosing spondylitis
Cervical strain	*Hx:* trauma or overuse; muscle pain/soreness *SSx:* tender to palpation; AROM limited by pain; pain with muscle testing *DDx:* cervical sprain, facet syndrome, meniscoid entrapment
Cervical joint dysfunction	*Hx:* insidious onset of local pain or discomfort *SSx:* tender to palpation; limited joint play; local myospasm; bone out of place *DDx:* cervical sprain, facet syndrome, meniscoid entrapment
Facet syndrome	*Hx:* well localized unilateral pain that may radiate to shoulder, antalgic posture *SSx:* ↑ pain w/ extension (loading facets); (+) cervical compression (local pain) *DDx:* cervical sprain, meniscoid entrapment, torticollis
Instability	*Hx:* recurrent neck pain or 'clicking or clunking' sensation *SSx:* ↑ PROM w/ over pressure; x-ray flexion/extension views will show ↑ ROM *DDx:* cervical sprain, osteoarthritis
Headache — **Cervico-genic**	*Hx:* ipsilateral head pain localized to the neck & occiput (may refer over eye) *SSx:* ↓ ROM due to pain; neck tenderness or symptoms reproduction with palp. *DDx:* rule out other causes of headache
Migraine	*Hx:* possible prodrome (visual changes) triggers (stress, rapid hormonal change, rapid blood sugar changes, vasoactive foods, Seasonal allergies, meds) *SSx:* unilateral mod/severe throbbing pulsating or photophobia nausea *DDx:* rule out other causes of headache
Cluster	*Hx:* <u>**severe**</u> ipsilateral head pain, "feels like a red hot poker in eye", men>women *SSx:* <u>lacrimation & rhinorrhea</u>, with restlessness, 15 min – 3 hour, can's sit still *DDx:* rule out other causes of headache
Pathologic	*Hx:* Recent head trauma? LOC? Abrupt severe headache for the first time? Patient's age (worrisome for over 50 or a child with persistent headache)? *Red Flags:* abrupt onset, very severe "worst headache I have ever had", nuchal rigidity – high diastolic pressure (>115), persistent/severe HA in child, drug/alcohol abuse, known cancer, papilledema (swollen optic disk) Fever
TMJ syndrome	*Hx:* jaw/facial pain worse with eating; locking/catching of jaw; chronic headaches *SSx:* ↓ ROM due to pain; crepitus; tenderness to palpation *DDx:* Bell's palsy, trigeminal neuralgia, dental infection
Vertebral basilar ischemia (VBI)	*Hx:* atherosclerosis, hypertension, diabetes, smoking, ligamentous hypermobility *SSx:* vertigo, dizziness, unsteadiness, visual changes, nystagmus; (+) VBI tests *DDx:* stroke, transient ischemic attack, positional vertigo

↑ = increased, ↓ = decreased, Hx = history, SSx = signs & symptoms, DDx = differential diagnosis

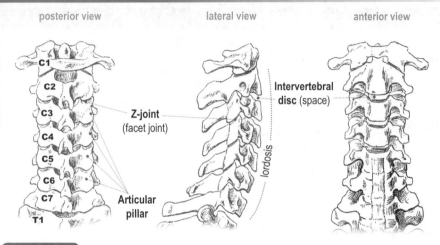

posterior view   lateral view   anterior view

C1
C2
C3
C4
C5
C6
C7
T1

Z-joint (facet joint)

Articular pillar

Intervertebral disc (space)

lordosis

C1 - Atlas

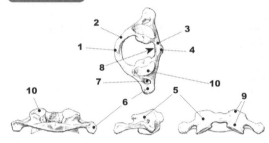

1. Posterior tubercle (no spinous process)
2. Posterior arch
3. Anterior arch
4. Anterior tubercle
5. Lateral mass (no vertebral body)
6. Transverse process
7. Transverse foramen
8. Articular facet for dens
9. Articular process (superior & inferior)
10. Superior articular facet

C2 - Axis

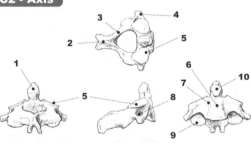

1. Dens (odontoid process)
2. Spinous process (bifid)
3. Lamina
4. Transverse process
5. Superior articular facet
6. Body
7. Pedicle
8. Transverse foramen
9. Inferior articular facet
10. Facet for anterior arch of C1

Typical Cervical Vertebra

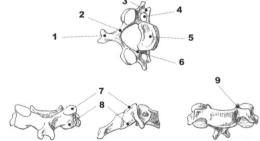

1. Spinous process (bifid)
2. Lamina
3. Transverse process
4. Transverse foramen
5. Body
6. Pedicle
7. Superior articular facet
8. Inferior articular process
9. Uncinate process (uncus)

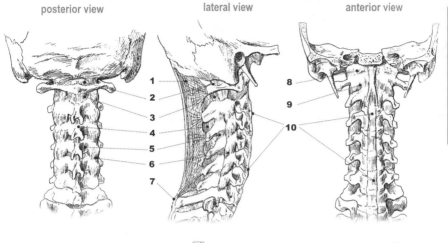

posterior view

lateral view

anterior view

1.
2.
3.
4.
5.
6.
7.
8.
9.
10.

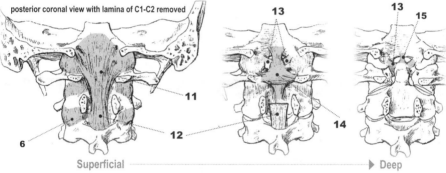

posterior coronal view with lamina of C1-C2 removed

13

13 15

11

6

12

14

Superficial ▷ Deep

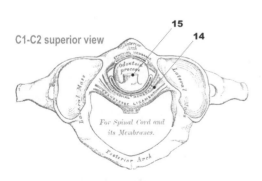

C1-C2 superior view

15 14

1. Nuchal ligament
2. Posterior atlanto-occipital membrane
3. Posterior atlantoaxial membrane
4. Interspinous Ligament
5. Ligamentum flavum
6. Capsular ligaments (zygapophyseal)
7. Supraspinous ligament
8. Anterior atlanto-occipital membrane
9. Anterior atlantoaxial membrane
10. Anterior longitudinal ligament
11. Tectorial membrane
12. Posterior longitudinal ligament
13. Alar ligaments (off dens)
14. Cruciform ligament (transverse ligament of dens)
15. Apical ligament (off dens)

- Cervical Instability - Atlantodental interval - standard cervical x-rays with flexion & extension views (normal child: 1-5 mm, adult: 1-3 mm) - see ortho conditions manual for more

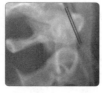

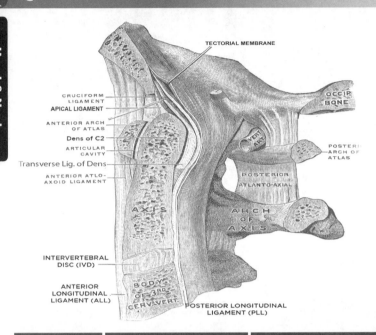

Ligament	Attaches (origin/insertion)	Function
Anterior longitudinal	Anterior vertebral body & disc to next vertebrae	Resists neck extension
Annulus fibrosus	Vertebral bodies from C3-S1	Shock absorption, resists all spinal motions
Posterior longitudinal	Posterior vertebral body & disc to next vertebrae	Resists neck flexion
Z-joint capsule	Facet to facet	Resist flexion & lateral flexion of neck
Ligamentum flavum	Laminae to laminae	Resists flexion of trunk, elasticity assists extension of trunk
Interspinous	Spinous process to spinous process	Resists flexion of trunk, & shear forces on vertebrae
Supraspinous	Spinous process to SP above	Resists trunk flexion & forward shear force on spine
Nuchal	EOP to C7-T1 Sps	Resists flexion, attachment point for muscles
Alar	Apex of dens to medial occipital	Resists lateral flexion & rotation of head; holds dens into atlas
Apical	Apex of dens to front foramen magnum	Holds dens into atlas & skull
Cruciform	Odontoid bone to arch of atlas (C1-2 stability) **Transverse Ligament of Dens** connects lateral masses	Stabilizes C1-C2, resists anterior translation of C1 relative to C2 (prevents brainstem compression)

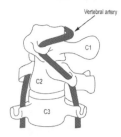

Vertebral artery

C1

C2

C3

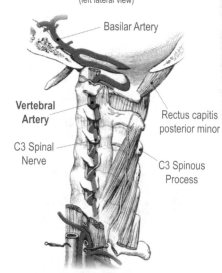

Vertebral Arteries & Basilar Artery
(left lateral view)

Basilar Artery

Vertebral Artery

Rectus capitis posterior minor

C3 Spinal Nerve

C3 Spinous Process

Cervical osseous mobilization is contraindicated if vertebral basilar artery issues or instability are suspected - literature review suggests that extreme *cervical rotation with extension* may be the primary causative motion causing injury following treatment; however evidence suggests that there may be no greater risk of following treatment than many common activities of daily living

- Remember there are alternate treatments available (mild mobilization, stretching, ROM exercises, soft tissue therapies, heat, massage, electrotherapy)
- Arterial issues been documented to occur with chiropractic doctors, medical doctors, osteopathic doctors & physical therapists as well as non-healthcare professions (MVAs, hair dresser, yoga, tai chi, wrestling, football)

Warning signs

5Ds And 3Ns vertebral basilar ischemia VBI

Dizziness, vertigo, giddiness

D-LOC (decreased level of consciousness)

Diplopia (or other visual disturbances)

Dysarthria (difficulty speaking)

Dysphagia (difficulty swallowing)

Ataxia (loss of motor control or gait)

Nausea & vomiting

Numbness (unilateral over face)

Nystagmus (lateral beating of the eyes)

Medical Legal

- Failure to recognize neurovascular signs of VBA may result in malpractice litigation
- 'VBA stroke is a very rare event in the population. The increased risks of VBA stroke associated with health visits is likely due to patients with headache and neck pain from VBA dissection seeking care **before** their stroke. We found no evidence of excess risk of VBA stroke associated chiropractic care compared to primary care'

Other Risk Factors - Neck Rotary Mobes

Long thin neck (longer levers = more force, less muscle support)

Hyper flexible (connective tissue variation)

Birth control medication (increase risk)

History of smoking or headaches

- (Cassidy JD, Boyle E, Côté P, et al. Risk of vertebrobasilar stroke and chiropractic care: results of a population-based case-control and case-crossover study. Spine 2008: 33(suppl 4):S176-S83)
1. H.A. Kranenburg. Et. al. Adverse events associated with the use of cervical spine manipulation or mobilization and patient characteristics: A systematic review. Musculoskeletal Science and Practice. Volume 28, April 2017, Pages 32–38.
2. Puentedura EJ, March J, Anders J, et al. Safety of cervical spine manipulation: are adverse events preventable and are manipulations being performed appropriately? A review of 134 case reports. The Journal of Manual & Manipulative Therapy. 2012;20(2):66-74. doi:10.1179/2042618611Y.0000000022.
3. Ernst E. Adverse effects of spinal manipulation: a systematic review. Journal of the Royal Society of Medicine. 2007;100(7):330-338.
4. Cassidy JD, Boyle E, Côté P, et al. Risk of vertebrobasilar stroke and chiropractic care: results of a population-based case-control and case-crossover study. Spine 2008; 33(suppl 4):S176-S83
5. Dvorak J, Orelli F. How dangerous is manipulation to the cervical spine? Manual Medicine 1985; 2: 1-4.
6. Jaskoviak P. Complications arising from manipulation of the cervical spine. J Manip Physiol Ther 1980; 3: 213-19.
7. Henderson DJ, Cassidy JD. Vertebral Artery syndrome. In: Vernon H. Upper cervical syndrome: chiropractic diagnosis and treatment. Baltimore: Williams and Wilkins, 1988: 195-222.
8. Eder M, Tilscher H. Chiropractic therapy: diagnosis and treatment (English translation). Rockville, Md: Aspen Publishers, 1990: 61.
9. Haldeman S, Chapman-Smith D, Petersen DM. Guidelines for chiropractic quality assurance and practice parameters. Gaithersburg, Md: Aspen Publishers, 1993: 170-2.
10. Coulter ID, Hurwitz EL, Adams AH, et al. The appropriateness of manipulation and mobilization of the cervical spine. Santa Monica, CA: RAND Corporation 1996: xiv. (RAND Home page: http://www.rand.org).
11. Patijn J. Complications in Manual Medicine: A Review of the Literature. J Manual Medicine 1991; 6: 89-92.
12. Lee KP, Carlini WG, McCormick GF, Albers GW. Neurologic complications following chiropractic manipulation: A survey of California neurologists. Neurology 1995; 45: 1213-5.
13. Guttman G: Injuries to the vertebral artery caused by manual therapy (English abstract), Manuelle Medizin 1983; 21: 2-14.
14. Plamondon RL. Summary of 1992 ACA annual statistical survey. ACA J Chiropractic 1993; 30 (Feb): 36-42.
15. Curtis P, Bove G. Family physicians, chiropractors, and back pain. J Family Practice 1992; 35 (5): 551-5.
16. Carey PF. A report on the occurrence of cervical cerebral vascular accidents in chiropractic practice. J of Canadian Chiropractic Assoc 1993; 37 (2): 104-6.
17. Klougart N, Leboeuf-Yde C, Rasmussen LR. Safety in chiropractic practice. Part I: The occurrence of cerebrovascular accidents after manipulation to the neck in Denmark from 1978-1988. J Manipulative Physiol Ther 1996; 19: 371-7.
18. Terrett AG. Vascular accidents from cervical spine manipulation: Report of 107 cases. J Aust Chiro Assoc 1987; 17: 15-24.
19. Terrett AG, Kleynhans AM. Cerebrovascular complications of manipulation. In: Haldeman S., ed. Principals and Practice of Chiropractic. Norwalk, Ct.: Appleton & Lange, 1992: 579-98.
20. Fries, JF. Assessing and understanding patient risk. Scand J Rheumatol 1992; Suppl. 92: 21

Head & Neck

Superficial

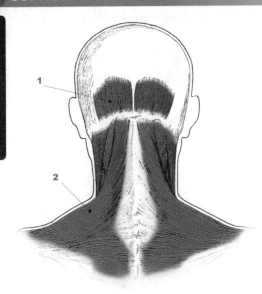

1. Occipitalis
2. Trapezius (upper fibers)
3. Splenius capitis
4. Splenius cervicis
5. Levator scapulae
6. Rhomboid minor
7. Spinalis capitis
8. Semispinalis capitis
9. Longissimus capitis

Deep

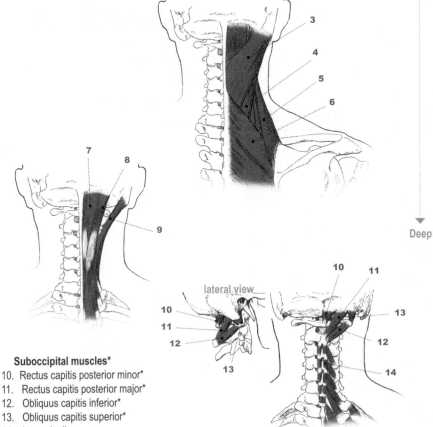

lateral view

Suboccipital muscles*
10. Rectus capitis posterior minor*
11. Rectus capitis posterior major*
12. Obliquus capitis inferior*
13. Obliquus capitis superior*
14. Interspinalis

prohealthsys

Superficial

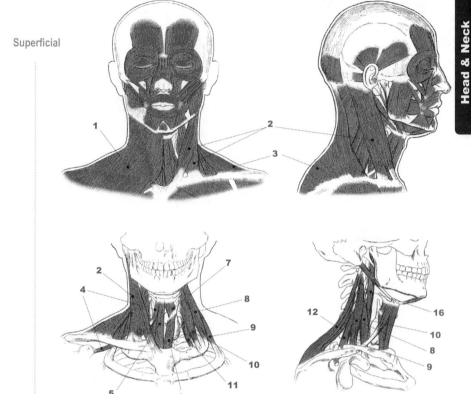

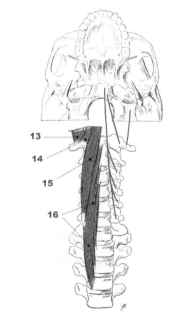

Deep

1. Platysma
2. Sternocleidomastoid
3. Trapezius
4. Omohyoid
5. Sternohyoid
6. Sternothyroid
7. Thyrohyoid
8. Middle scalene
9. Posterior scalene
10. Anterior scalene
11. Scalenus minimus
12. Levator scapulae
13. Rectus capitis lateralis
14. Rectus capitis anterior
15. Longus capitis
16. Longus cervicis (coli)

Lines indicate muscle attachments to the
base of the skull

prohealthsys

Flexion-Extension

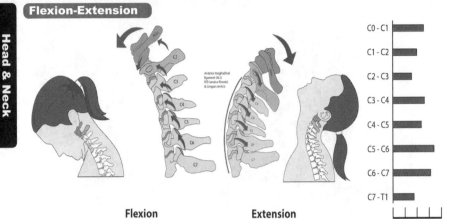

Anterior longitudinal ligament (ALL) IVD (anulus fibrosis) & Longus cervicis

Flexion   **Extension**

C0 - C1	
C1 - C2	
C2 - C3	
C3 - C4	
C4 - C5	
C5 - C6	
C6 - C7	
C7 - T1	

0 5 10 15 20°

Lateral Flexion

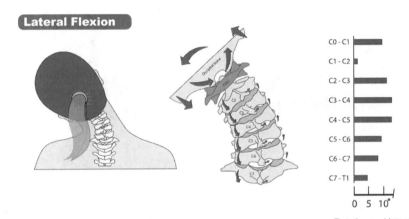

Occipital bone

C0 - C1	
C1 - C2	
C2 - C3	
C3 - C4	
C4 - C5	
C5 - C6	
C6 - C7	
C7 - T1	

0 5 10°

Rotation and lateral flexion are coupled motions in the same direction - C2-C7 - left rotation also induces left lateral flexion

Rotation

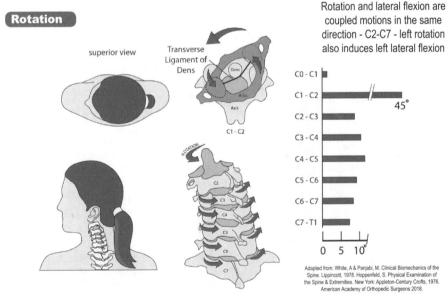

superior view

Transverse Ligament of Dens

Dens

Atlas

Axis

C1 - C2

ROTATION

C0 - C1	
C1 - C2	45°
C2 - C3	
C3 - C4	
C4 - C5	
C5 - C6	
C6 - C7	
C7 - T1	

0 5 10°

Adapted from: White, A & Panjabi, M. Clinical Biomechanics of the Spine. Lippincott, 1978. Hoppenfeld, S. Physical Examination of the Spine & Extremities. New York: Appleton-Century Crofts, 1976. American Academy of Orthopedic Surgeons 2018.

Cervical sprain/strain 'whiplash'

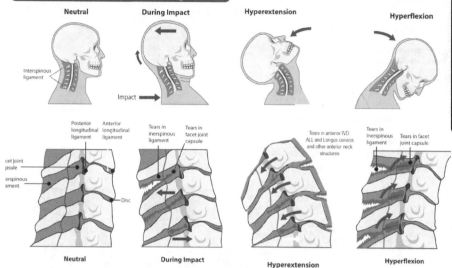

In whiplash injuries be aware that clinical presentation & perceived severity of injury do not correlate! - lower speed impacts often result in more significant & potentially chronic injuries. Damage or tearing of soft tissue around the cervical spine and resulting inflammation

- Tearing of muscles/ligaments (ALL, nuchal, longus cervicis, SCM, scalenes)
- Cervical facet capsular ligaments (z-joints) and disc injury
- Muscles attached to periosteum contract causing myofascial pain
- Can involve reversal or straightening of cervical lordosis (protective myospasm of deep neck flexors)

C-spine xray

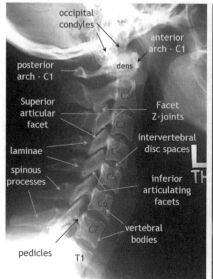
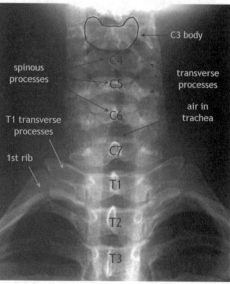

All palpation methods involve tactile movement of soft tissues & osseous structures to evaluate **variations in elasticity, tone, motion from side to side, pain and/or discomfort.** - clinical style & preference will determine which specific methods clinicians use (use what works best for you)

'Neck Walk'

Procedure
Patient supine, examiner starts superficially to introduce touch & assess integrity of superficial tissues; examiner then proceeds to palpate deeper soft tissue & osseous structures (walk over neck with hands and give your self an anatomy review!)

Interpretation
(+) Nonuniform motion, muscle spasm, hypertonicity, pain → joint dysfunction (subluxation), trigger point, muscle tightness, sprain/strain, local joint irritation (possible degeneration)

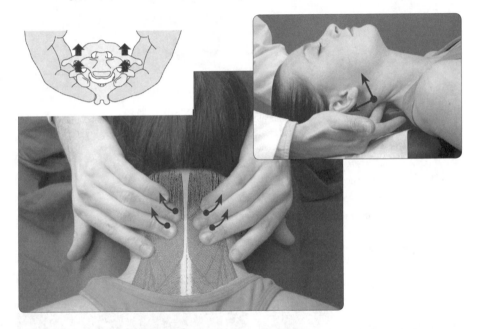

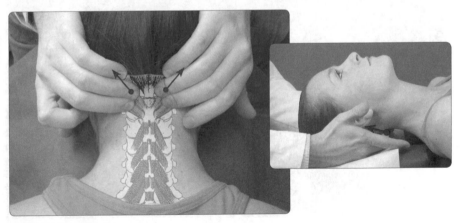

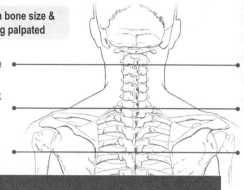

Realize that normal anatomical variation in bone size & shape may alter exact spinal levels being palpated

- **C2** - first palpable SP below the occipital bone

- **C7 or T1** - most prominent SP at base of neck (C7 will usually move from a palpating finger with cervical flexion/extension)

- **T4** - level with the root of the spine of scapula or apex of axillary fold

Structure	Location
EOP	midline of occipital base
C1 TP	~1 cm (½" inch) anterior & inferior to mastoid process (under ear lobe)
C2 SP	1st prominent SP below EOP
C4 SP	hyoid bone
C5 SP	thyroid cartilage
C7 SP	usually second most prominent SP, slides anterior during cervical extension
T1 SP	most prominent SP (usually)

TP = transverse process, SP = spinous process

Segmental Assessment

Procedure: Patient supine, examiner palpates through musculature to articular pillars; flexes, laterally flexes & finally rotates patient head/neck - (lateral flex one direction/rotate opposite direction) **'walk' hands up & down the c-spine - observe end feels at each individual segment**

Interpretation: (+) Nonuniform motion → joint dysfunction (subluxation), malposition or restriction of motion, soft tissue contracture

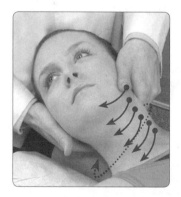

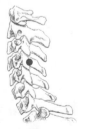 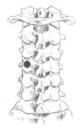

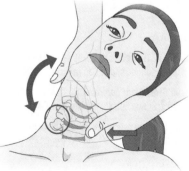

Use a **soft or gentle end range pressure to reduce guarding and discomfort**. When learning do NOT hold people in a hard end-ROM - relax your hands/body for more effective application.

Introduction statement: "Try and move as far as possible, if any of the actions or movements are painful please let me know, do not do any action you feel will cause you further injury."

Flexion (50°-70°)

Muscles Activated: sternocleidomastoid (SCM), longus cervicis, longus capitis, rectus capitis anterior; *eccentric* contraction of upper trapezius, splenius, semispinalis, longissimus capitis

Tissue Stretched: trapezius, splenius cervicis & capitis, longissimus capitis, suboccipitals, nuchal ligament, interspinous ligament, posterior IVD, posterior facet joint capsule

Tissue Compressed: anterior neck muscles, trachea, esophagus, carotid arteries

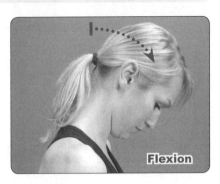

Flexion

Extension (50°-70°)

Muscles Activated: trapezius (upper), splenius cervicis & capitis, longissimus capitis, suboccipitals

Tissue Stretched: anterior neck muscles, anterior longitudinal ligament, anterior IVD, trachea, esophagus, carotid arteries

Tissue Compressed: posterior neck muscles, posterior intervertebral discs, facet (z-joints) joints, vertebral arteries

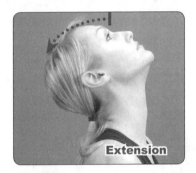

Extension

Lateral Flexion (45°-60°)

Muscles Activated: *ipsilateral:* trapezius (upper), splenius cervicis & capitis, longissimus capitis, levator scapulae, suboccipitals

Tissue Stretched: *contralateral:* trapezius (upper), longissimus capitis, SCM, lateral IVD, carotid artery, z-joints

Tissue Compressed: *ipsilateral:* trapezius (upper), longissimus capitis, SCM, lateral IVD, carotid artery, z-joints

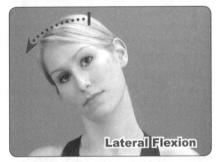

Lateral Flexion

Rotation (80°-90°)

Muscles Activated: *ipsilateral:* splenius cervicis & capitis, suboccipitals; *contralateral:* SCM

Tissue Stretched: *contralateral:* splenius cervicis & capitis, suboccipitals; *ipsilateral:* SCM

Tissue Compressed: *ipsilateral:* splenius cervicis & capitis, suboccipitals; *contralateral:* SCM

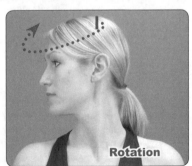

Rotation

Compare bilaterally; if possible palpate joint during PROM & use the shortest level possible, apply over pressure at end ROM; introduction statement:
"If any of the actions or movements are painful or uncomfortable please let me know."

PROM may be performed with the patient seated or supine

 Seated **Supine**

Flexion (> 50°-70°)
Tissue Stretched: upper trapezius, splenius cervicis & capitis, longissimus capitis, suboccipitals, nuchal ligament, interspinous ligament, posterior IVD, posterior facet joint capsule
Tissue Compressed: anterior neck muscles, trachea, esophagus, carotid arteries

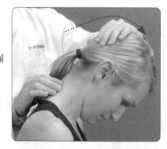

Extension (> 50°-70°)
Tissue Stretched: anterior neck muscles, anterior longitudinal ligament, anterior IVD, trachea, esophagus, carotid arteries
Tissue Compressed: posterior neck muscles, posterior intervertebral discs, facet (z-joints) joints, vertebral artery

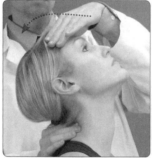
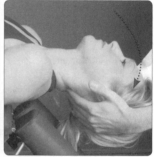

Lateral Flexion (> 45°-60°)
Tissue Stretched:
contralateral: trapezius (upper), longissimus capitis, SCM, lateral IVD, carotid artery, z-joints
Tissue Compressed:
ipsilateral: trapezius (upper), longissimus capitis, SCM, lateral IVD, carotid artery, z-joints

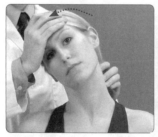
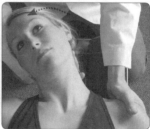

Rotation (> 80°-90°)
Tissue Stretched:
contralateral: splenius cervicis & capitis, suboccipitals; *ipsilateral:* SCM
Tissue Compressed:
ipsilateral: splenius cervicis & capitis, suboccipitals

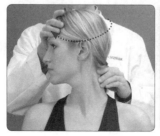
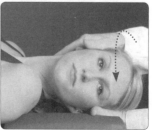

Flexion (normal 50°-70°)

- Patient seated, neutral c-spine
- Zero inclinometers over T1 & skull
- Ask patient to flex neck, **subtract T1 inclination from skull inclination = ROM**

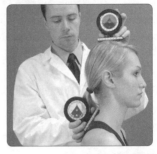

Extension (normal: 50°-70°)

- Same as flexion except patient extends neck

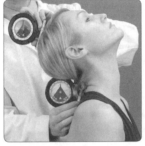

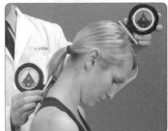

Lateral flexion (normal: 45°-60°)

- Patient seated, neutral c-spine
- Zero inclinometers over T1 & skull
- Ask patient to flex neck, subtract T1 inclination from skull inclination = ROM
- Repeat on contralateral side

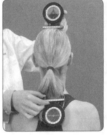

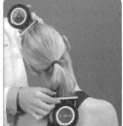

Rotation (normal: 80°-90°)

- Patient prone, neutral c-spine
- Zero inclinometer over forehead
- Ask patient to turn neck to one side
- Repeat on contralateral side

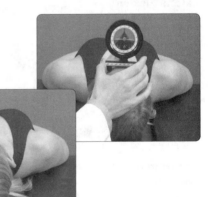

Joint types:
Gliding (zygapophyseal joints)
Pivot (atlantoaxial joint)
Fibrocartilaginous (intervertebral joints)
Hinge & gliding (TMJ)

Articular surfaces
Atlanto-occipital joint: *convex* (occipital condyles of occiput) on *concave* (superior articular facets of atlas)
Atlantoaxial: *concave* (articular facet for dens on atlas) *on convex* (anterior facet of dens on axis)
Zygapophyseal: facets are oriented 45°
Intervertebral discs: horizontal plane
TMJ: *convex* (mandibular condyle & disc) *on concave* (mandibular fossa of temporal bone)

Main muscle actions
Flexion: sternocleidomastoid (SCM), longus cervicis, longus capitis, rectus capitis anterior
Extension: trapezius, splenius cervicis & capitis, longis. capitis, levator scapulae, suboccipitals
Lateral flexion: scalenes, levator scapula, longissimus capitis, splenius capitis & cervicis, rectus capitis lateralis
Rotation: SCM, longus capitis & coli, rotatores, splenius, suboccipitals

Resting position
C-spine: slight extension
TMJ: mouth closed with teeth not in contact

Close packed position
C-spine: full extension
TMJ: teeth clenched

Capsular pattern of restriction
C-spine: lateral flexion = rotation, extension
TMJ: limitation of mouth opening

Normal end feel: tissue stretch (for all actions)

Abnormal end feel
Early myospasm → muscle/ligament tear
Late myospasm → instability
Empty → ligament rupture
Hard → bone approximation (osteophyte)

Coupled motions (C2-C7 vertebral segments)
Left lateral flexion coupled with left rotation
Right lateral flexion coupled with right rotation

Cervical Facet Angles

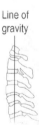

Line of gravity

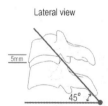

Lateral view

5mm

45°

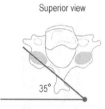

Superior view

35°

'Text Neck' - force to cervical spine with neck flexion

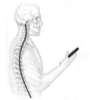 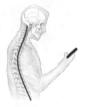   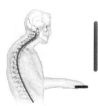

Neutral - 0°	15°	30°	60°	45°
~10 lbs	~27 lbs	~40 lbs	~60 lbs	~49 lbs
4.5 kg	12 kg	18 kg	27 kg	22 kg

Indications: hypertonic suboccipitals, muscle tension headaches, upper cervical hyperlordosis

Position: patient supine with head in slight extension; clinician at head of table

Contact: clinician bilaterally places finger tips just superior to the C2 spinous process

Force: tissue force is P-A, I-S & M-L; push into space superior to C2 until tissue tension is reached then pull fingers laterally & superiorly depending on the tissue restriction encountered, hold tension until muscle relaxation is noted

Clinical notes: use a soft finger pad contact, verbally check patient tolerance to pressure (more pressure is better, within patient tolerance)

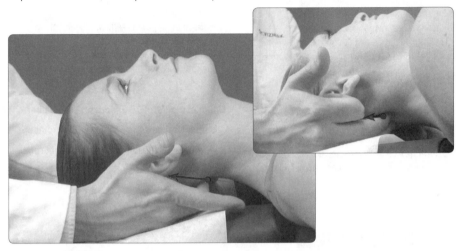

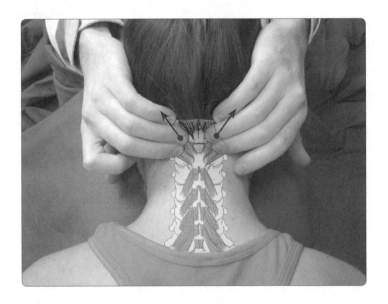

S = stabilization (indifferent hand), ● = contact, ➤ = examiner force, ┈┈┈➤ = patient motion   **prohealthsys.com**

Indications: muscle tension headaches, cervical hyperlordosis, neck stiffness

Position: patient supine with head in slight extension; clinician at head of table

Contact: clinician bilaterally places finger tips just lateral to cervical spinous processes

Force: tissue force is P-A, I-S & M-L; push into tissue until tension is reached then pull fingers laterally & superiorly depending on the tissue restriction encountered, hold tension until muscle relaxation is noted

Clinical notes: use a soft finger pad contact, verbally check patient tolerance to pressure (more pressure is better, within patient tolerance)

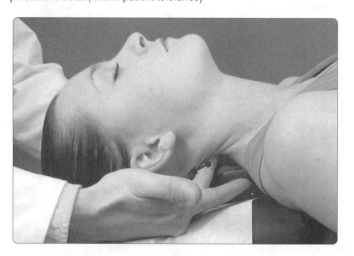

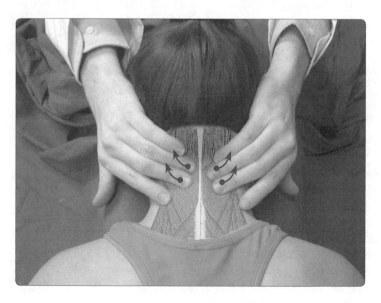

Anterior Scalene Stretch

Indications: muscle hypertonicity, ↓ 1st rib mobility

Position: patient supine; clinician at head of table

Contact: clinician places thumb on insertion at 1st rib & supports patient's head with other hand

Force: laterally flex away and rotate toward the side to be stretched; have patient take a deep breath, on exhalation as the rib cage depresses apply more lateral flexion pressure, hold tension until muscle relaxation is noted, repeat as necessary

Clinical notes: verbally check patient tolerance to pressure; discontinue if the patient feels light headed or experiences numbness and tingling into the upper extremity

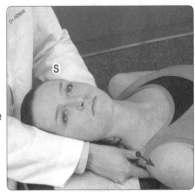

Middle Scalene Stretch

Indications: muscle hypertonicity, ↓ 1st rib mobility

Position: patient supine; clinician at head of table

Contact: clinician places thumb or thenar eminence on insertion at 1st rib & supports patient's head

Force: laterally flex away from side to be stretched; have patient take a deep breath, on exhalation as the rib cage depresses apply more lateral flexion pressure, hold tension until muscle relaxation is noted, repeat as necessary

Clinical notes: verbally check patient tolerance to pressure; discontinue if the patient feels light headed or experiences numbness and tingling into the upper extremity

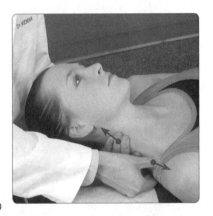

Posterior Scalene Stretch

Indications: muscle hypertonicity, ↓ 2nd rib mobility

Position: patient supine; clinician at head of table

Contact: clinician places thenar eminence on insertion at 2nd rib, stabilizes the shoulder & supports patient's head with the other hand

Force: flex and laterally flex away from side to be stretched; have patient take a deep breath, on exhalation as the rib cage depresses apply more lateral flexion pressure, hold tension until muscle relaxation is noted, repeat as necessary

Clinical notes: same as above, note that superior hand is also tractioning on scalene attachment

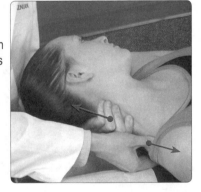

Posterior & Lateral Neck Stretches

Indications: muscle hypertonicity, ↓ mobility

Position: patient supine; clinician at head of table

Contact: clinician bilaterally supports patient's occiput

Force: flex or laterally flex the patient's neck to the point of tension; have patient take a deep breath, on exhalation as the rib cage depresses apply more flexion pressure, hold tension until muscle relaxation is noted, repeat as necessary

Clinical notes: verbally check patient tolerance to pressure; discontinue if the patient feels light headed or experiences numbness and tingling into the upper extremity

By changing the rotation of the head & neck with lateral flexion pressure different myofascial fibers may be selectively stretched

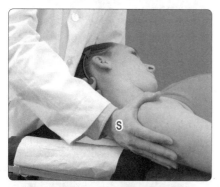
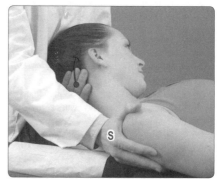

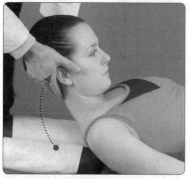
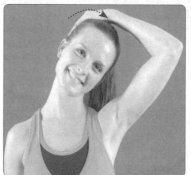

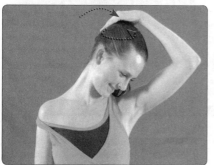
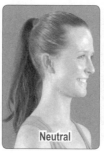
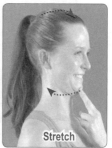

Neutral

Stretch

Head & Neck

Altered head/neck flexion
- Weak agonist: deep neck flexors
- Overactive antagonist: suboccipitals
- Overactive synergist: SCM

Symptoms related to altered neck flexion
- Headache, neck & shoulder blade pain
- TMJ dysfunction/pain

Evaluation
- Patient is supine & is instructed to bring chin to chest
- Overpressure may be added at end point
- More sensitive test (fewer false (-)'s if patient's neck is pre-positioned in chin tuck & raised 2 cm off table - hold for 4 seconds

Note: fail
- If chin juts forward or if there is shaking
- If there is chin jutting or shaking with mild overpressure added
- If head elevates from 2 cm position (this indicates a change in the center of mass of the head)
- If chin juts forward during movement or shaking before 4 seconds

Rationale
- To identify if neck flexor weakness or in-coordination is present
- In particular to identify if deep neck flexors are weak & the SCM is tight or overactive

Postural analysis
- Head forward posture
- Prominence of SCM

Myofascial trigger points
- SCM, suboccipitals
- Mid traps, masticatory muscles
- Mastoid process

Mobility (joint dysfunction)
- C0-C1, lower cervicals, cervical-thoracic junction
- TMJ

Treatment
- Mobilize/adjust C0-C1 & cervical-thoracic junction
- Relax/stretch SCM & suboccipitals
- Facilitate/strengthen deep neck flexors
- Correct poor sitting posture
- Lumbo-pelvic stabilization exercises (neutral pelvis)

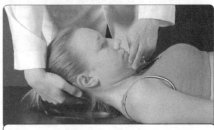

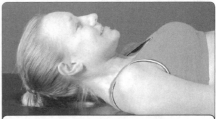

1. Instruct patient to bend neck
2. Examiner may pre-position patient with neck retracted (~2cm off table)

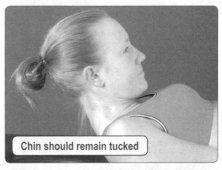

Patient should be able to hold without losing chin tuck or shaking for more than 4 seconds (synonym: Jull test)

Chin should remain tucked

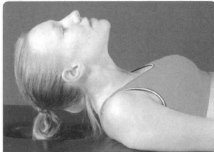

If the patient leads with their chin "jutting" or "poking" this suggests overactive SCM recruitment &/or weak deep neck flexors

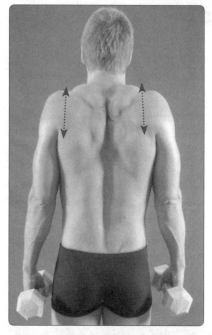

Exercises demonstrated in this text may be performed at home with weights, therapy bands, soup cans, pots or any other device that can provide muscle resistance.

KIS - Keep it simple. Exercises & stretches should be easy to do & easy to remember (**show patients how to do it, have them demonstrate it & give handouts with pictures to use at home**)

Keep it short. Time is precious, so keep the home routine to under 15 minutes.

Keep it pain-free. The patient should not work in painful areas; the amount of stretch, weight & reps should be started at below what the practitioner believes the patient's ability is & progress slowly

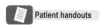
Patient handouts

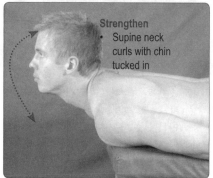

Strengthen
• Supine neck curls with chin tucked in

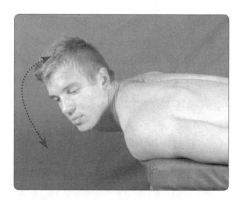

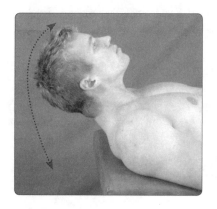

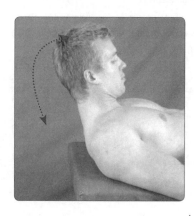

Head & Neck

Atlanto-occipital Flexion Restriction

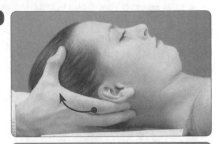

Indications: hypertonic suboccipitals, muscle tension headaches, ↓ head flexion

Position: patient supine with head in flexion; clinician at head of table

Contact: clinician supports occiput with inferior hand & frontal bone with other hand

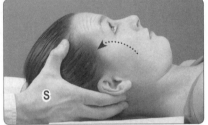

Force: flex patient's head; ask patient to look upwards & attempt to extend head against resistance; hold for ~5 seconds; ask patient to relax and take up the slack by further flexing the head & hold for ~10 seconds; repeat procedure 2-5 times & reassess ROM

Clinical notes: verbally check patient tolerance to pressure (more pressure is better, within patient tolerance)

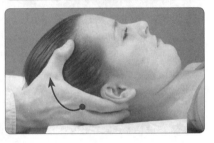

Atlanto-axial Rotation Restriction

Indications: hypertonic suboccipitals, muscle tension headaches, ↓ neck rotation

Position: patient supine with neck in mild flexion; clinician at head of table

Contact: clinician supports occiput with inferior hand & frontal bone with other hand

Force: flex & rotate the patient's head until the restriction is reached; ask patient to attempt to extend & rotate head against resistance; hold for ~5 seconds; ask patient to relax and take up the slack by further rotating the head & hold for ~10 seconds; repeat procedure 2-5 times & reassess ROM

Clinical notes: breathing technique may be applied (stretch during deep exhalation), some clinicians suggest that the C-spine should be in full flexion to help limit lower cervical spine motion

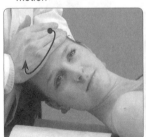

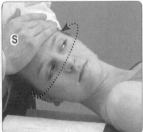

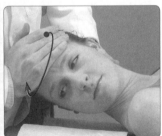

S = stabilization (indifferent hand), ● = contact, ⟶ = examiner force, ┈┈┈▶ = patient motion

prohealthsys.com

Flexion Rotation & Lateral Translation

Indications: ↓ neck rotation, joint dysfunction, neck stiffness, reduce posteriolateral restrictions

Position: patient supine; clinician at head of table

Contact: clinician supports patient's head with both hands & uses finger tips to palpate involved segment

Force: flex the patient's head to tension, then laterally flex to tension and finally rotate to tension; ask patient to push towards neutral against resistance; hold for ~5 seconds; ask patient to relax and take up the slack by further flexing, laterally flexing & rotating the head (micromovements) & hold for ~10 seconds; repeat procedure 2-5 times & reassess ROM

Clinical notes: verbally check patient tolerance to pressure

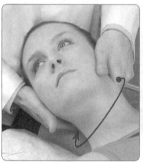
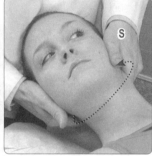
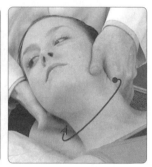

Extension Rotation & Lateral Translation

Indications: ↓ neck rotation, joint dysfunction, neck stiffness, reduce anterolateral restrictions

Position: patient supine; clinician at head of table

Contact: clinician supports patient's head with both hands

Force: extend the patient's head to tension, then laterally flex to tension and finally rotate to tension; ask patient to push towards neutral against resistance; hold for ~5 seconds; ask patient to relax and take up the slack by further extending, laterally flexing & rotating the head (micromovements) & hold for ~10 seconds; repeat procedure 2-5 times & reassess ROM

Clinical notes: verbally check patient tolerance to pressure, note that extremes of rotation & extension are contraindicated when performed in combination

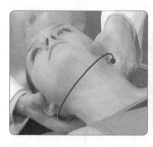
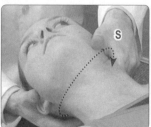
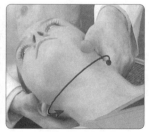

Head & Neck

Vertebral Lateral Translation

Indications: restricted lateral flexion, neck stiffness (C1-C7)

Position: patient supine (or seated) with neck in slight flexion; clinician at head of table

Contact: clinician places index finger or finger tips on affected segment articular pillar/lamina; clinician's stabilization hand supports the patient's contralateral occipital bone & palpates translation

Force: tissue force is L-M; develop tension by gently pushing the affected segment medially

Clinical notes: this maneuver can be uncomfortable, a 'soft' contact is required. Lateral translation may also be performed with an index pillar contact or combined with passive lateral flexion

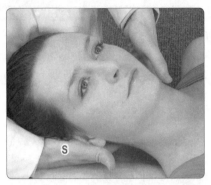

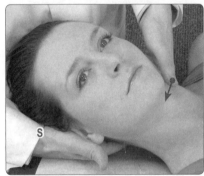

Vertebral Anterior Translation

Indications: restricted extension, neck stiffness, reduce cervical hypolordosis (C1-C7)

Position: patient supine (or seated); clinician at head of table

Contact: clinician places finger tips on affected segment's articular pillar/lamina; clinician stabilizes & supports the patient's occipital bone

Force: tissue force is P-A

Clinical notes: this maneuver may be combined with simultaneous soft tissue massage therapies and/or cervical distraction

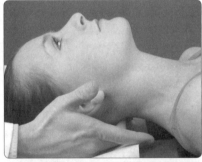

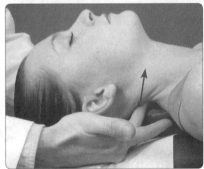

prohealthsys

Head & Neck

Atlantoaxial Rotation

Indications: restricted atlantoaxial rotation, neck stiffness (C1-C2)

Position: patient supine (or seated) with neck in slight flexion; clinician at head of table

Contact: clinician places thumb on the posterior lateral mass/transverse process; clinician's stabilization hand supports the patient's contralateral occipital bone

Force: tissue force is M-L & rotational; develop tension by rotating head & neck away from contact; apply over pressure at end range

Clinical notes: a 'soft' contact is required. May also be performed with an index pillar contact or IASTM

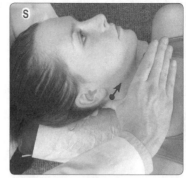

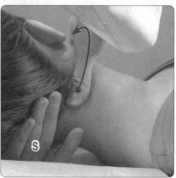

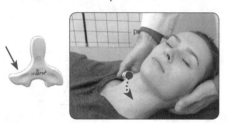

Mid-Cervical Rotation

Indications: restricted mid cervical rotation, neck stiffness (C3-C7)

Position: patient supine (or seated) with neck in slight flexion; clinician at head of table

Contact: clinician places thumb on the posterior articular pillar; clinician's stabilization hand supports the patient's contralateral occipital bone

Force: tissue force is M-L & rotational; develop tension by rotating head & neck away from contact; apply over pressure at end range

Clinical notes: a 'soft' contact is required. May also be performed with an index pillar contact or IASTM

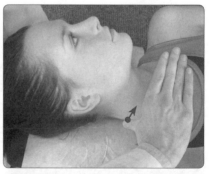

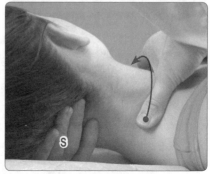

Head & Neck

Indications: spinal decompression, neck stiffness, IVF encroachment (C1-T1)

Position: patient supine (or seated) with head in slight extension; clinician at head of table

Contact: clinician bilaterally grasps the patient's occiput

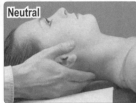

Neutral

Force: tissue force is I-S; have patient take a deep breath, as they exhale gently pull superiorly on the occiput

Clinical notes: this technique may also be performed with a reinforcing towel or strap

Note that increased cervical flexion causes more distraction further down the cervical spine (more flexion to distract lower segments, less flexion for upper segments)

Use IASTM or mobilization belts to take pressure off of your hands

Most patients love cervical distraction

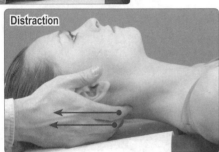

Distraction

Variation for cervical distraction (chin pull)

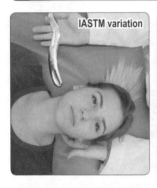

IASTM variation

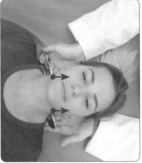

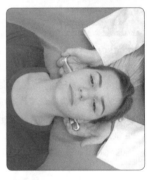

Unilateral Distraction

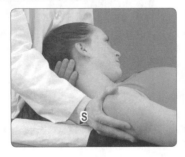

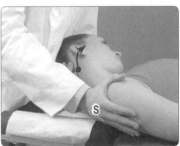

prohealthsys

Indications: spinal decompression, neck stiffness, IVF encroachment (C1-T1)

Position: patient supine (or seated) with head in slight flexion; clinician at head of table

Contact: clinician bilaterally grasps the patient's occiput

Force: tissue force is I-S; have patient take a deep breath, as they exhale gently pull superiorly

Clinical notes: this technique may also be performed with a reinforcing towel or strap. Note that increased cervical flexion causes more distraction further down on the cervical spine (more flexion to distract lower segments, less flexion for upper segments)

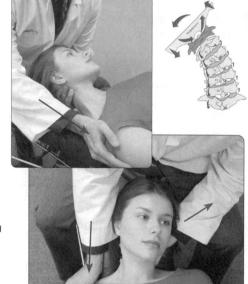

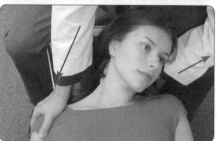

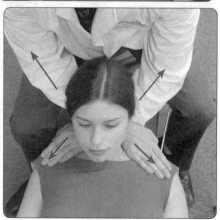

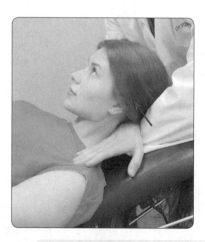

The method above has the advantage of distraction with external shoulder rotation at the same time - use a breathing technique, increase pressure on the exhale

Indication: rotation, lateral flexion & extension restrictions or malpositions (C1-C7)

Position: patient supine (or seated) with neck in slight flexion & head slightly rotated; clinician stands at ~45°-90° to patient at head of table

Contact: clinician places anterolateral surface of index finger on affected segment articular pillar; clinician's stabilization hand supports the patient's contralateral occipital bone

Force: tissue pull is M-L-M & P-A with a slight I-S component (more P-A induces extension, more M-L-M to induce lateral flexion); develop tension by rotating the patient's head away & laterally flexing toward the segmental contact; mobilize by pushing through contact hand (consider using grade 4 mobilizations at end ROM before a grade 5 to help with muscle relaxation/patient guarding)

Clinical notes: Avoid extreme rotation & extension forces in the cervical spine. *Variation:* thumb pillar push where a thumb contact is used instead of an index contact; also consider instrument assisted mobilization (see images)

Clinician's Contact for Index Push
Variations in patient & clinician size will alter exact contact point

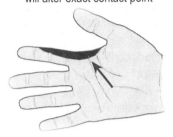

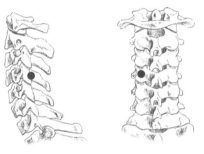

- Sternum over contact
- Knees & hips bent
- Forearm low to direct force vector
- Wrist neutral or slightly extended to soften contact
- Toes point in direction of force

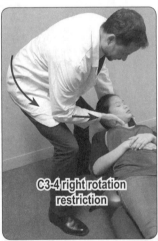

C3-4 right rotation restriction

Arrow indicates clinician hip motion to help improve force/ speed

Foot direction dictates the direction of the joint mobilization forces you will generate

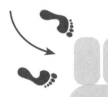

force is developed from the hips and refined with the upper limb/ hands

Index Pillar Push

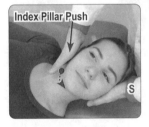

S

Instrument assisted variation

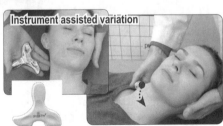

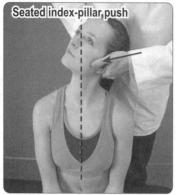

Seated index-pillar push

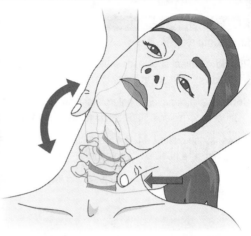

For most cervical set-ups (spine & seated)
keep nose in alignment with sternum

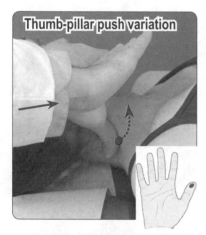

Thumb-pillar push variation

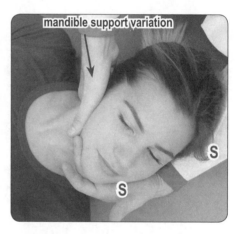

mandible support variation

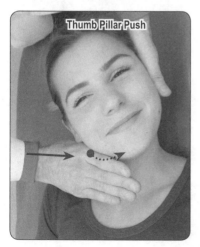

Thumb Pillar Push

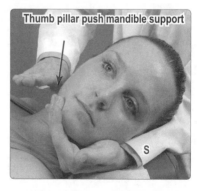

Thumb pillar push mandible support

Use a **soft or gentle end range pressure to
reduce guarding and discomfort**. When learning
do NOT hold people in a hard end-ROM - relax
your hands/body for more effective application.

prohealthsys

Head & Neck

Index Spinous Push

Indication: rotation, lateral flexion & extension restrictions or malpositions (C2-T2)

Position: patient supine (or seated) with neck in slight flexion & head slightly rotated; clinician stands at ~45°-90° to patient at head of table

Contact: clinician places anterolateral surface of index finger on the lateral side of the spinous process; clinician's stabilization hand supports the patient's contralateral occipital bone

Force: tissue pull is L-M, P-A & slightly S-I; develop tension by laterally flexing toward & rotating the patient's head away from the segmental contact; thrust by pushing through contact hand

Clinical notes: spinous contacts can be very sensitive, care must be taken to ensure a soft contact

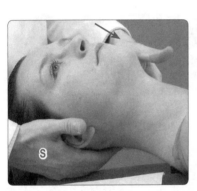

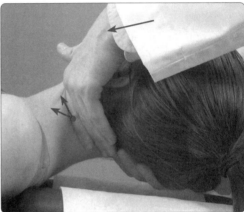

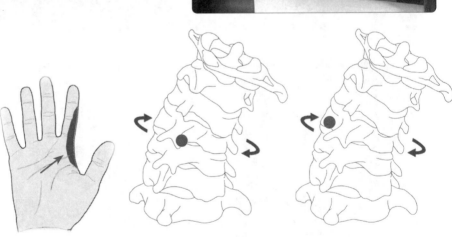

index spinous push   index pillar push

S = stabilization (indifferent hand),   ● = contact,   ——▶ = examiner force,   ·······▶ = patient motion   **prohealthsys.com**

Head & Neck

Thumb Anterior Pillar Pull

Indication: rotation and/or lateral flexion restrictions or malpositions (C2-C7)

Position: patient supine (or seated) with neck in slight flexion & head slightly rotated; clinician stands at ~45º-90º to patient at head of table

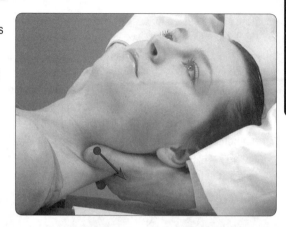

Contact: clinician places contact thumb on anterior lateral side of the articular pillar and fingers supporting the neck; stabilization hand supports the patient's contralateral occipital bone

Force: tissue pull is A-P & slightly I-S; develop tension by laterally flexing away & rotating toward the segmental contact; thrust by pulling through contact hand

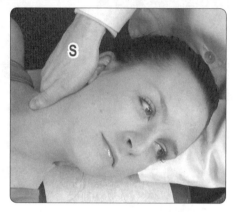

Clinical notes: This maneuver may be combined with a contralateral index pillar push to aid in the motion or an index spinous push to create a local counter resistive force. Anterior cervical contacts can be very sensitive and care should be taken to avoid compression of key anatomical structures (carotid arteries)

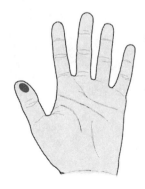
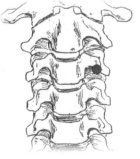
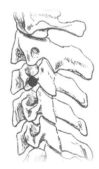

Head & Neck

Digital Pillar Pull

Indication: rotation, lateral flexion & extension restrictions or malpositions (C2-C7)

Position: patient seated (or supine) and relaxed in chair with back support; clinician stands at ~45°-90° to patient on the opposite side of the contact hand

Contact: clinician places anterior surface of middle finger on affected segment articular pillar; clinician's stabilization hand supports the patient's contralateral C-spine & occipital bone

Force: tissue pull is P-A with a slight I-S component (more P-A induces extension, L-M to induce lateral flexion); develop tension by rotating the patient's head away & laterally flexing toward the segmental contact; thrust by pulling through contact hand

Clinical notes: This maneuver may be used as a mobilization if a HVLA thrust is not delivered (grade 1-4 mobilizations). Avoid excessive extension forces in the cervical spine

Variation: thumb pillar push where a thumb contact is used instead of an index contact

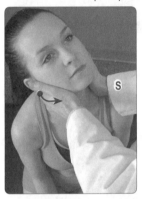
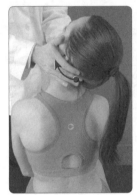
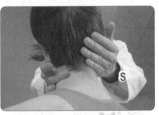
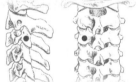

Hypothenar Anterior Pillar Push

Indication: rotation and/or lateral flexion restrictions or malpositions (C2-C7)

Position: patient seated (or supine) with neck in slight flexion & head slightly rotated; clinician stands in front of patient

Contact: clinician places contact hypothenar eminence on anterior lateral side of the articular pillar and fingers supporting the neck; stabilization hand supports the patient's contralateral occipital bone & C-spine

Force: tissue pull is A-P & slightly I-S; develop tension by laterally flexing away & rotating toward the segmental contact; thrust by pushing through contact hand

Clinical notes: This maneuver may be combined with a contralateral digital pillar pull to aid in the motion Anterior cervical contacts can be very sensitive and care should be taken to avoid key anatomical structures (arteries)

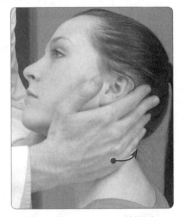

S = stabilization (indifferent hand), ● = contact, ⟶ = examiner force, ┈┈┈▷ = patient motion   prohealthsys.com

Thenar Pillar Push

Indication: flexion, extension, rotation and/or lateral flexion restrictions or malpositions (C2-C7)

Position: patient prone with neck in slight flexion; clinician in fencer stance on either side of patient

Contact: clinician places thumbs on posterolateral side of the articular pillars

Force: tissue pull is P-A & I-S; develop tension by traction in the desired direction; thrust through contacts

Clinical notes: mild distractive forces maintained during tension may increase manipulation success

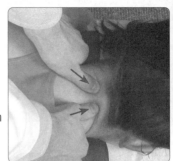

Hypothenar Spinous

Indication: flexion or extension restrictions or malpositions (C2-C7)

Position: patient prone with neck in slight flexion & head slightly rotated; clinician in fencer stance on either side of patient

Contact: clinician places hypothenar eminence on patient's spinous process; clinician's non-contact hand reinforces contact hand

Force: tissue pull P-A & I-S for flexion and purely P-A for extension; develop tension by transferring body weight & mildly dropping body, thrust by pushing through contact hand

Clinical notes: spinous-hypothenar contacts can be very uncomfortable and great care should be taken to avoid painful mobilizations

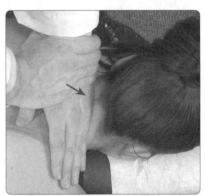

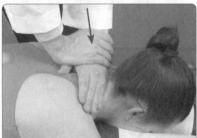

Bilateral Index Pillar Push

Indication: same as above

Position: same as above

Contact: clinician bilaterally places index fingers (proximal phalynx) of both hands on posterolateral side of the articular pillars

Force: tissue pull P-A & slightly I-S for flexion (P-A only for extension restrictions); develop tension by transferring body weight & dropping body, thrust by pushing through contact hand

Clinical notes: mild distractive forces maintained during tension may increase manipulation success

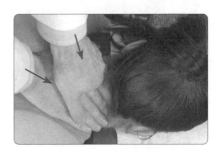

C1 is often difficult to assess, one easier method is to place your fingers just anterior & inferior to the mastoid process, **palpate the C1 TPs bilaterally**, then palpate for local tenderness, asymmetrical lateral displacement, muscle hypertonicity, or asymmetrical motion as the patient is taken through cervical ROM (flex, lat flex, rot.)

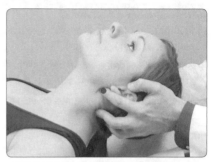

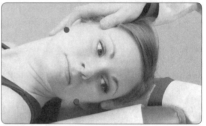

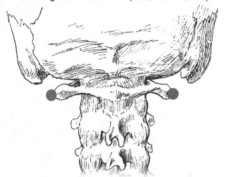

The Egg in the Spoon: many clinicians find it useful to assess C0-C1 motion in multiplanar arching actions - try and visualize an egg (C0) sitting in a spoon (C1) and then move into multiple directions looking for asymmetry or restriction of motion

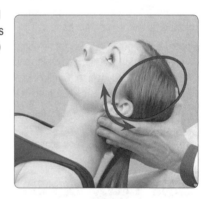

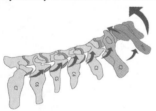

By fully flexing the lower cervical spine many of the posterior ligaments & joint capsules may be stretched and tightened allowing for a more isolated assessment of C0-C1

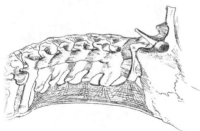

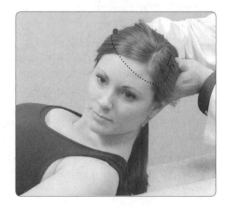

Mastoid Push/Occipital Lift

Indication: rotation, lateral flexion & extension restrictions or malpositions (C0-C1), long axis distraction

Position: patient supine (or seated) with neck in slight flexion & head rotated away from clinician; clinician in low fencer stance

Contact: clinician places anterolateral surface of index finger, hypothenar eminence or thumb on patient's medial aspect of mastoid process, occipital bone or C1; clinician's stabilization hand supports the patient's contralateral occipital bone, zygomatic process & mandible

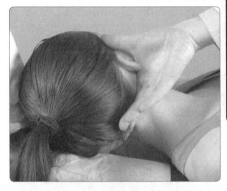

Force: tissue pull is I-S (L-M to induce lateral flexion & P-A to induce rotation); develop tension by applying long axis distraction; thrust by pushing through contact hand

Clinical notes: Avoid cupping of the patient's ear & excessive extension forces in the cervical spine

Remember you can move C1 in relation to C0 or move C0 in relation to C1

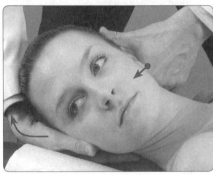

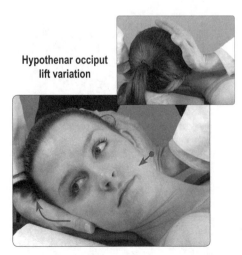

Hypothenar occiput lift variation

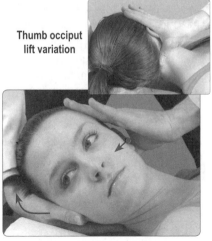

Thumb occiput lift variation

Head & Neck

Bilateral Occiput Push

Indication: flexion, extension restrictions or malpositions (C0-C1), long axis distraction

Position: patient prone with neck in slight flexion or extension depending on joint dysfunction; clinician in low fencer stance

Contact: clinician bilaterally places thenar or hypothenar eminences over patient's inferior-medial aspect of mastoid process

Force: tissue pull is I-S & P-A for flexion restriction (just P-A for extension restriction); develop tension by applying long axis distraction; thrust by pushing through contact hands

Clinical notes: Avoid cupping of the patient's ears & excessive extension forces in the cervical spine

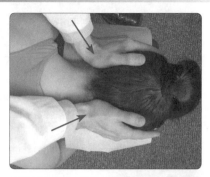

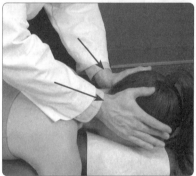

Hypothenar Zygomatic

Indication: lateral flexion restrictions or malpositions (C0-C1), long axis distraction

Position: patient supine (or seated) with neck in slight flexion & head rotated away from clinician; clinician in low fencer stance

Contact: clinician places hypothenar eminence over patient's zygomatic arch; clinician's stabilization hand supports the patient's contralateral occipital bone, zygomatic process & mandible

Force: tissue pull L-M & I-S; develop tension by applying long axis distraction; thrust by pushing through contact hand

Clinical notes: Avoid cupping of the patient's ear & excessive extension forces in the cervical spine

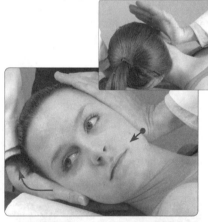

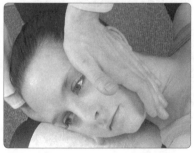

S = stabilization (indifferent hand), ● = contact, ⟶ = examiner force, ·····▷ = patient motion **prohealthsys.com**

Indication: rotation, lateral flexion & extension restriction or malposition (C0-C1)

Position: patient seated (or supine) and relaxed in chair with back support; clinician stands at ~45°-90° to patient on the opposite side of the contact hand

Contact: clinician places hypothenar eminence onto occipital bone/ posterior mastoid process; clinician reinforces with the other hand and uses their body to help direct lateral flexion forces

Force: tissue pull is L-M with a slight I-S component (more P-A induces extension, A-P to induce flexion); develop tension by laterally flexing the patient's head away from the clinician's body; mobilize by pulling through contact hand

Clinical notes: great care and skill are required to deliver a controlled mobilization; female clinician's must be aware of their body position and may choose to use a pillow for separation over their chest

Variation: thenar contact may also be used

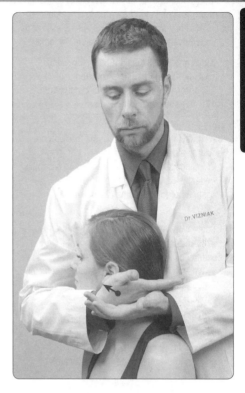

Contact & vector for right rotation restriction of C0

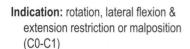

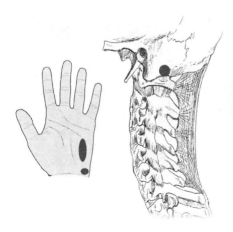

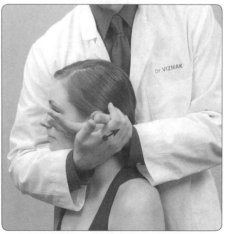

Contact & vector for left rotation, left lateral flexion restriction of C0

Head & Neck

Definition: pain & tenderness due to a dysfunction of the TMJ or surrounding musculature & soft tissue
- an often overlooked cause for patient discomfort

- Divided into 3 subtypes (that often co-exist):
  1. **Myofascial pain dysfunction**
  2. **Internal derangement** (disc/cartilage)
  3. **Degenerative joint disease**

History
- Jaw or facial pain - increased with mastication
- Locking or catching with motion
  - Limited ROM, TMJ clicking, grinding & popping
- Headache, earache & neck pain
- Past head or facial trauma (whiplash)

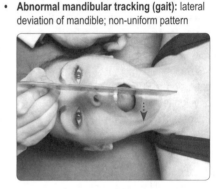
Measurement of TMJ ROM (32 mm)

Physical
- Observation: asymmetry, muscle hypertrophy
  - Malocclusion of jaw, abnormal dental wear
- Tenderness to palpation over mastication muscles
  - Myospasm in muscles of mastication & facial muscles (masseter, pterygoids), TMJ via the external auditory meatus

- Check ROM - decreased jaw opening (normal 40 mm minimum or ~ 3 knuckles inserted between upper & lower incisors); protrusion, lateral deviation (movement is normally ~10 mm)

- **Abnormal mandibular tracking (gait):** lateral deviation of mandible; non-uniform pattern

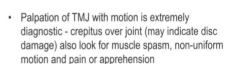

Temporomandibular Joint

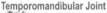

- Palpation of TMJ with motion is extremely diagnostic - crepitus over joint (may indicate disc damage) also look for muscle spasm, non-uniform motion and pain or apprehension

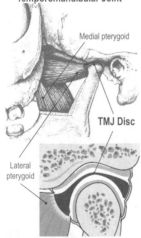
Medial pterygoid

TMJ Disc

Lateral pterygoid

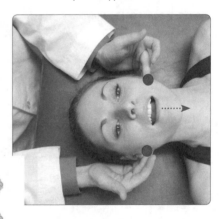

Normal   Locking   Clicking

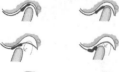

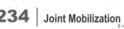

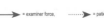

prohealthsys

External Mandibular Traction

Indications: hypertonic masseter/temporalis / medial pterygoid, joint capsule contracture

Position: patient supine; clinician at head of table

Contact: clinician supports patient's head & uses thenar, hypothenar or thumb

Force: gently load into mandible & apply S-I force to distract the mandible - verbally check patient tolerance

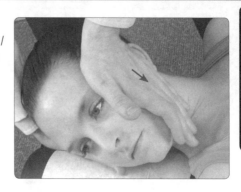

Bilateral Mandibular Traction

Indications: hypertonic masseter/temporalis / medial pterygoid, joint capsule contracture

Position: patient supine; clinician at side of table

Contact: clinician places gloved hands inside patient's mouth with distal thumb on lower molars & IP joint of thumb on upper molars

Force: gently load or flex thumbs to create a traction force of the most noted restriction of motion (may be used as a mobilization or contract relax technique)

Note - similar index finger digital contacts may be used to release the pterygoids - warn the patient ahead of time these may be mildly uncomfortable

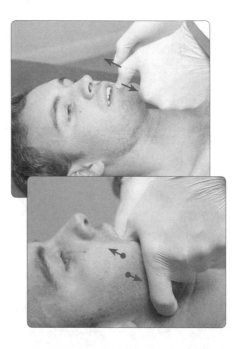

IASTM of Masseter

Indications: hypertonic masseter, joint capsule contracture

Position: patient supine; clinician at side of table

Contact: clinician places gloved hand inside patient's mouth to lift masseter and instrument is used to release soft tissue

Force: gently load & stroke through soft tissue and restriction - note that excessive force over the very large parotid gland may have undesired damaging effects to the tissue

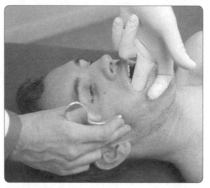

1. Vizniak, NA. Gross Anatomy Human Cadaver Dissections. 1999-2018.
2. Cassidy JD, Boyle E, Côté P, et al. Risk of vertebrobasilar stroke and chiropractic care: results of a population-based case-control and case-crossover study. Spine 2008; 33(suppl 4):S176-S83
3. H.A. Kranenburg. Et. al. Adverse events associated with the use of cervical spine manipulation or mobilization and patient characteristics: A systematic review. Musculoskeletal Science and Practice. Volume 28, April 2017, Pages 32–38.
4. Puentedura EJ, March J, Anders J, et al. Safety of cervical spine manipulation: are adverse events preventable and are manipulations being performed appropriately? A review of 134 case reports. The Journal of Manual & Manipulative Therapy. 2012;20(2):66-74. doi:10.1179/2042618611Y.0000000022.
5. Ernst E. Adverse effects of spinal manipulation: a systematic review. Journal of the Royal Society of Medicine. 2007;100(7):330-338.
6. Cassidy JD, Boyle E, Côté P, et al. Risk of vertebrobasilar stroke and chiropractic care: results of a population-based case-control and case-crossover study. Spine 2008; 33(suppl 4):S176-S83
7. Dvorak J, Orelli F. How dangerous is manipulation to the cervical spine? Manual Medicine 1985; 2: 1-4.
8. Jaskoviak P. Complications arising from manipulation of the cervical spine. J Manip Physiol Ther 1980; 3: 213-19.
9. Henderson DJ, Cassidy JD. Vertebral Artery syndrome. In: Vernon H. Upper cervical syndrome: chiropractic diagnosis and treatment. Baltimore: Williams and Wilkins, 1988: 195-222.
10. Eder M, Tilscher H. Chiropractic therapy: diagnosis and treatment (English translation). Rockville, Md: Aspen Publishers, 1990: 61.
11. Haldeman S, Chapman-Smith D, Petersen DM. Guidelines for chiropractic quality assurance and practice parameters. Gaithersburg, Md: Aspen Publishers, 1993: 170-2.
12. Coulter ID, Hurwitz EL, Adams AH, et al. The appropriateness of manipulation and mobilization of the cervical spine. Santa Monica, Ca: RAND Corporation 1996: xiv. (RAND Home page: http://www.rand.org).
13. Patijn J. Complications in Manual Medicine: A Review of the Literature. J Manual Medicine 1991; 6: 89-92.
14. Lee KP, Carlini WG, McCormick GF, Albers GW. Neurologic complications following chiropractic manipulation: A survey of California neurologists. Neurology 1995; 45: 1213-5.
15. Guttman G: Injuries to the vertebral artery caused by manual therapy (English abstract). Manuelle Medizin 1983; 21: 2-14.
16. Plamandon RL. Summary of 1992 ACA annual statistical survey. ACA J Chiropractic 1993; 30 (Feb): 36-42.
17. Curtis P, Bove G. Family physicians, chiropractors, and back pain. J Family Practice 1992; 35 (5): 551-5.
18. Carey PF. A report on the occurrence of cervical cerebral vascular accidents in chiropractic practice. J of Canadian Chiropractic Assoc 1993; 37 (2): 104-6.
19. Klougart N, Leboeuf-Yde C, Rasmussen LR. Safety in chiropractic practice. Part I: The occurrence of cerebrovascular accidents after manipulation to the neck in Denmark from 1978-1988. J Manipulative Physiol Ther 1996; 19: 371-7.
20. Terrett AG. Vascular accidents from cervical spine manipulation: Report of 107 cases. J Aust Chiro Assoc 1987; 17: 15-24.
21. Terrett AG, Kleynhans AM. Cerebrovascular complications of manipulation. In: Haldeman S., ed. Principals and Practice of Chiropractic. Norwalk, Ct.: Appleton & Lang, 1992: 579-98.
22. Fries, JF. Assessing and understanding patient risk. Scand J Rheumatol 1992; Suppl. 92: 21
23. Haraldsson BG, Gross AR, Myers CD, et al. Massage for mechanical neck disorders. Cochrane Database Syst Rev. Jul 19 2006;3:CD004871.
24. Taylor MH, Monroe LG. Physical Rehabilitation: Evidence-Based Examination, Evaluation and Intervention. Saunders. 2007.
25. Warlow C, Hughes R, Uitehaag B, Liberati A. Evidence-Based Neurology. Blackwell Publishing Limited, BMJI Books. 2007.
26. Malanga GA & Nadler. Musculoskeletal Physical Exam, An Evidence-Based Approach. Mosby. 2006.
27. Hoppenfield S. Physical Examination of the Spine & Extremities. Lippincott Williams & Wilkins. 1976.
28. Hoppenfield S. Orthopaedic Neurology: A Diagnostic Guide to Neurologic Levels. Lippincott Williams & Wilkins. 1977.
29. Spencer JW, Jacobs JJ. Complementary and Alternative Medicine: An Evidence-Based Approach. Mosby. 2003.
30. Jewell D. Guide to Evidence-Based Physical Therapy Practice. Jones Barlett Publishers Inc. 2007.
31. Tall RL, DeVault W. Spinal injury in sport: epidemiologic considerations. Clin Sports Med. Jul 1993;12(3):441-8.
32. Tsao B. The electrodiagnosis of cervical and lumbosacral radiculopathy. Neurol Clin. May 2007;25(2):473-94.
33. Dishman JD, Cunningham BM, Burke J. Comparison of Tibial Nerve H-Reflex Excitability After Cervical and Lumbar Manipulation. JMPT 25(5):318-325, 2002.
34. Bandiera G, Stiell IG, Wells GA, Clement C, DeMaio V. Vandemheen KL, Greenberg GH, Lesiuk H, Brison R, Cass D, Dreyer J, Eisenhauer MA, Macphail I, McKnight RD, Morrison L, Reardon M, Schull M, Worthington J; Canadian C-Spine & CT Head Study Group. The Canadian C-spine rule performs better than unstructured physician judgment. Ann Emerg Med. 2003;42(3):395-402.
35. Bertilsson B, Grunnesjo M, Strender LE. Reliability of clinical tests in the assessment of patient with neck/shoulder problems-impact of history. Spine. 2003;19:2222-2231.
36. Catttysse E, Swinkels RA, Oostendorp RA, Duquet W. Upper cervical instability: are clinical tests reliable? Man Ther. 1997;2(2):91-97.
37. Davidson R, Dunn E, Metzmaker J. The shoulder abduction test in the diagnosis of radicular pain in cervical extradural compression monoradiculopathies. Spine. 1981 ;6.441 -445.
38. Dickinson G, Stiell IG, Schull M, Brison R, Clement CM, Vandemheen KL, Cass D, McKnight D, Greenberg G, Worthington JR, Reardon M, Morrison L, Eisenhauer MA, Dreyer J, Wells GA. Retrospective application of the NEXUS low-risk criteria for cervical spine radiography in Canadian emergency departments.Ann Emerg Med. 2004;43(4):507-5 14.
39. Dobbs A. Manual therapy assessment of cervical instability. Orthopaedic Physical Therapy Clinics of North America. 2001;10:431-454.
40. Hall I, Robinson K. The flexion-rotation test & active cervical mobility-a comparative measurement study in cervicogenic headache. Man Ther. 2004;9(4):1 97-202.
41. Harris KD, Heer DM, Roy IC, Santos DM, Whitman JM, Wainner RS. Reliability of a measurement of neck flexor muscle endurance. Phys Ther. 2005;85(1 2):1 349-1 355.
42. Hoffman jR, Mower WR, Wolfson AB, Todd KH, Zucker MI. Validity of a set of clinical criteria to rule out injury to the cervical spine in patients with blunt trauma. National Emergency X-Radiography Utilization Study Group. N Eng J Med. 2000;343(2):94-99.
43. Hum phreys BK, Delahaye M, Peterson CK. An investigation into the validity of cervical spine motion palpation using patients with congenital block vertebrae as a "gold standard". BMC Musculoskelet Disord. 2004;5:1 9.
44. Jull G, Bogduk N, Marsland A. The accuracy of manual diagnosis for cervical zygapophysial joint pain syndromes. Med JAust. 1988;148(5):23 3-236.
45. Olsen L, Millar L, Dunker j, Hicks J, Glanz D. Reliability of a clinical test for deep cervical flexor endurance. j Manipulative Physiol Therapeutics. 2006;29:1 34-1 38.
46. Sandmark H, Nisell R. Validity of five common manual neck pain provoking tests. Scand Rehabil Med. 1 995;27(3):1 31-1 36.
47. Shah KC, Rajshekhar V. Reliability of diagnosis of soft cervical disc prolapse using Spurling's test. Br J Neurosurg. 2004;1 8(5):480-483.
48. Sharp J, Purser DW, Lawrence is. Rheumatoid arthritis of the cervical spine in the adult. Ann Rheum Dis. 1958;1 7(3):303-1 3.
49. Smedmark V, Wallin M, Arvidsson I. Inter-examiner reliability in assessing passive intervertebral motion of the cervical spine. Man Ther. 2000;5(2):97-101.
50. Spurting RG, Scoville WB. Lateral rupture of the cervical intervertebral disc. Surg Gynecol Obstet. 1944; 78:350-358.
51. Stiell IG, Clement CM, McKnight RD, Brison R, Schull MJ, Rowe BH, Worthington JR, Eisenhauer MA, Cass D, Greenberg G, MacPhail I, Dreyer J, Lee JS, Bandiera G, Reardon M, Holroyd B, Lesiuk H, Wells GA. The Canadian C-spine rule versus the NEXUS low-risk criteria in patients with trauma. N Engi I Med. 2003; 349(26):251 0-2518.
52. Stiell IC, Wells GA, Vandemheen KL, Clement CM, Lesiuk H, De Maio VJ, Laupacis A, Schull M, McKnight RD, Verbeek R, Brison R, Cass D, Dreyer j, Eisenhauer MA, Greenberg GH, MacPhail I, Morrison L, Reardon M, Worthington I. The Canadian C-spine rule for radiography in alert & stable trauma patients. JAMA. 2001 ;286(1 5):1 841-1848.
53. Tong HC, Haig AJ, Yamakawa K. The Spurting test & cervical radiculopathy. Spine. 2002;27(2):1 56-159.
54. Uchihara T, Furukawa T, Tsukagoshi H. Compression of brachial plexus as a diagnostic test of cervical cord lesion. Spine. 1994;1 9(1 9):21 70-21 73.
55. Uitvlugt G, Indenbaum S. Clinical assessment of atlantoaxial instability using the Sharp-Purser test. Arthritis Rheum. 1988;31(7):91 8-922.
56. Van Suijlekom HA, De Vet HC, Van Den Berg SG, Weber WE. Interobserver reliability in physical examination of the cervical spine in patients with headache. Headache. 2000;40(7):581 -586.
57. Viikari-juntura E, Porras M, Laasonen EM. Validity of clinical tests in the diagnosis of rootcompression in cervical disc disease. Spine. 1989;14(3):253-257.
58. Viikari-Juntura E, Takala E, Riihimaki H, Martikainen R, Jappinen P. Predictive validity of symptoms & signs in the neck & shoulders. J Clin Epidemiol. 2000;53(8):800-808.
59. Wainner RS, Fritz JM, trrgang JJ, Boninger ML, Delitto A, Allison S. Reliability & diagnostic accuracy of the clinical examination & patient self-report measures for cervical radiculopathy. Spine. 2003;28(1):52-62.
60. Richter RR, Reinking MF: How does evidence on the diagnostic accuracy of the vertebral artery test influence teaching of the test in a professional physical therapist education program? PHYS THER Vol. 85, No. 6, June 2005, pp. 589-599
61. Anderssen GBJ: The epidemiology of spinal disorders. In Frymoyer JW, ed. The Adult Spine: Principles & Practice. New York: Raven Press; 1997: 93-141.
62. Argoff CA, Wheeler AH: Spinal & radicular pain disorders. . Neurol Clin 1998 Nov; 23: 1662-7.
63. Bats-Baril WL, Frymoyer JW: The economics of spinal disorders. In: Frymoyer JW, ed. The Adult Spine: Principles & Practice. New York: Raven Press; 1991: 85-105.
64. Rachlin ES, ed. Myofascial pain & fibromyalgia: trigger point management. St. Louis: Mosby, 1994:3-29.
65. Rachlin ES. History & physical examination for regional myofascial pain syndrome. In: Rachlin ES, ed. Myofascial pain & fibromyalgia: trigger point management. St. Louis: Mosby, 1994:159-72.
66. Rachlin ES. Trigger points. In: Rachlin ES, ed. Myofascial pain & fibromyalgia: trigger point management. St. Louis: Mosby, 1994:145-57.

Head & Neck Quiz (answer page)

1. What are the joint type classifications for this region? (211) _____

2. What is the orientation of the facet joints? (211)

    _____

3. What is the normal ROM for _____? (196)
    - Flexion/Ext.: _____, _____
    - Lateral flexion: _____
    - Rotation _____

4. What is the resting position? (211) _____

5. What is the joint tight packed position? (211)

    _____

6. What motions are coupled in the c-spine? (211)

    _____

7. What muscles cause flexion to occur? (211)

    _____

8. Articular surfaces shape for the c-spine? (211)

    _____

9. What are the 5D And 3Ns of vertebral basilar ischemia? (201)

    _____

10. Can you palpate _____ ? (196)

Learning Objectives

After completing this chapter, students will be able to:

1. Perform a regional exam and differentiate common pathologies of the region

2. Identify and palpate body region bony landmarks, ligaments and muscles

3. Discuss regional kinematics and joint organ biomechanics including scapulohumeral rhythm and throwing mechanics

4. Demonstrate regional AROM, PROM & goniometry, stretch and strengthen protocols

5. Recognize and execute steps of effective mobilization and joint-play including indications, position, contact, force and relevant clinical notes

6. Perform supine, prone, seated assessment and mobilizations including

   - Shoulder pin & stretch & MET
   - GH joint (glides, rotation, flex/extension, long axis distraction, abduction, adduction)
   - AC Joint (glides)
   - SC joint (glides)
   - Scapulocostal (distraction, upward & downward rotation)

Shoulder & Arm

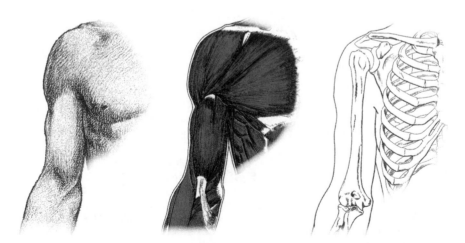

Realize that any mobilization (grade 1-4) can be made into a manipulation (grade 5) with the addition of a high velocity low amplitude (HVLA) thrust & vise versa with the lack of a HVLA thrust

Conversely any technique can be adapted to use IASTM where indicated to save your hands...

Follow **HIP-MNRS** (see Yellow "Physical Assessment" text for specific details or review)
History, Inspection, Palpation - Motion, Neurovascular screen, Referred pain, Special tests

Special history questions
- Specific mechanism of injury & forces involved?
  - Did you fall on outstretched hand?
- Any numbness, tingling or weakness?
- Type of work, typical posture, sleeping posture?
  - Overuse/overhead work? (Impingement)
- Prior injuries?

Inspection
- Asymmetry, bruising, bumps, color, swelling, height, head tilt, winging of scapula
- Posture of head, neck & thoracic spine, shoulder

Palpation (may be done after ROM assessment)

Middle trapezius	Rotator cuff superior
Lower trapezius	Rotator cuff anterior
Rhomboids	Teres major
Thoracic spine	Latissimus dorsi
Ribs 1-9 posterior	Subscapularis
Levator scapulae	Serratus anterior
Upper trapezius	Triceps brachii
Scalenes	Deltoid
Thoracic outlet	Deltoid tuberosity
Cervical spine	Pectoralis minor
Supraspinatus	Coracoid process
AC joint	Coracobrachialis
Infraspinatus	Biceps brachii
Teres minor	Bicipital groove
AC step defect	Pectoralis major
Rotator cuff posterior	SC joint

Functional assessment (ADLs)
- Apley's superior & inferior

AROM
Flexion .... 180°
Extension .... 50°
Int./ext. rotation .... 90°/80°
Abduction .... 180°
Adduction .... 35°
Horizontal Add./Abd. 130°/30°
Scapulocostal rhythm

PROM & Joint Play (if lacking AROM in any motion)

Myotomes (resisted isometric movements)
- Shoulder elevation (C4, XI)
- Deltoid (**C5**, C6 - axillary)
- Brachioradialis (C5, C6 - radial)
- Biceps (C5, **C6** - musculocutaneous)
- Triceps (C6, **C7**, C8, T1 - radial)
- Wrist extensors (**C6**, C7, C8 - radial)
- Wrist flexors (C6, **C7** - median/ulnar)
- Finger flexors (C7, **C8**, T1 - ulnar/median)
- Interossei (C7, C8, **T1** - ulnar)

Neurovascular screen
- **Sensory:** light touch, two point discrimination, Vibration (3rd digit), Tinel's
- **DTR's:**
  - Biceps (C5), Brachioradialis (C6), Triceps (C7)
- Girth measurements
- Grip strength (Dynamometer)
- Radial & brachial pulse, blanching, temperature

Orthopedic tests (as indicated)
Screening
- Apley's scratch
- Codman's arm drop
- Mouth Wrap-around Test

Impingement
- Hawkins-Kennedy
- Impingement sign
- Painful arc

Biceps tendinitis
- Hyperextension
- Speed's, Yergason's
- Modified Yergason's

Rotator cuff
- Empty can
- Lift-off test

Labral tear (SLAP lesion)
- Hyperabduction
- Clunk, Crank, O'brien's test
- Biceps Load Test II

Glenohumeral joint stability
- Ant/post drawer
- Ant/post apprehension
- Load & shift

Elbow & Spinal Screen

Diagnostic imaging (if indicated)

 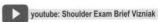

Condition	Clinical notes
AC separation	*Hx:* prior trauma - fall onto shoulder or impact over shoulder *SSx:* possible step defect; tenderness to palpation over AC joint; (+) AC shear, cross-body test, O'Brien's *DDx:* supraspinatus rupture, impingement syndrome, rotator cuff tear
Adhesive capsulitis **(Frozen shoulder)**	*Hx:* patient age 40-60, usually female, weeks of shoulder pain & restriction *SSx:* restricted AROM in clear capsular pattern (external rotation > abduction > internal rotation); extremely painful & limited PROM *DDx:* cervical pathology, impingement syndrome, rotator cuff tear
Bicipital tendonitis	*Hx:* pain over anterior shoulder, history of repetitive elbow flexion (weight lifter) *SSx:* exquisite pain with direct palpation of biceps long head tendon; pain with resisted horizontal adduction *DDx:* cervical pathology, rotator cuff strain
Bursitis (subacromial)	*Hx:* pain over superior or lateral GH joint, pain at night difficulty sleeping *SSx:* tender palpation over acromion/deltoid; ↓ shoulder ROM in abduction & flexion; pain may be relieved by GH inferior distraction *DDx:* cervical pathology, rotator cuff strain, impingement syndrome
Glenoid Labral Tear	*Hx:* usually repetitive shoulder motion, throwing athletes or weight-lifters *SSx:* ↓ shoulder ROM in abduction & flexion; pain may be relieved by GH inferior distraction (+) O'Brien's, clunk or crank test *DDx:* Bicipital Tendonitis, Impingement Syndrome, Rotator Cuff Injury
Glenohumeral osteoarthrosis	*Hx:* insidious onset of pain, morning stiffness, worse with excessive activity *SSx:* crepitus & pain w/ ROM; (+) Ellman compression test (GH scour test) *DDx:* AC osteoarthrosis, GH instability, impingement syndrome
Impingement	*Hx:* pain with overhead movements, may refer pain down lateral arm *SSx:* pain with ROM; (+) painful arc, Hawkin's-Kennedy, Neer's *DDx:* cervical pathology, GH instability, poor posture
Instability	*Hx:* prior trauma; patient may be able to demonstrate ↑ motion; patient may have impingement type symptoms due to excess GH movement *SSx:* observation of sulcus sign; (+) load & shift test *DDx:* rotator cuff strain, impingement syndrome, congenital ligament laxity
Rotator cuff tear	*Hx:* prior trauma - lifting or throwing injury; degeneration of rotator cuff? (elderly) *SSx:* weakness in specific rotator cuff movements, abnormal scapulohumeral rhythm; (+) Codman's arm drop, impingement signs, painful arc *DDx:* supraspinatus rupture, impingement syndrome, congenital ligament laxity
Supraspinatus tendonitis	*Hx:* pain with overhead movements or hand placed behind back *SSx:* exquisite pain with resisted supraspinatus movements; (+) empty can test, impingement, pain with direct palpation *DDx:* cervical pathology, GH instability, complete supraspinatus rupture
Thoracic outlet syndrome	*Hx:* pain & paresthesia, possible muscle weakness into shoulder, arm &/or hand *SSx:* myospasm of cervical musculature (depending on cause); (+) TOS tests *DDx:* cervical radiculopathy, cervical disc herniation, carpal tunnel syndrome

↑ = increase, ↓ = decrease, Hx = history, SSx = signs & symptoms, DDx = differential diagnosis
see blue 'Orthopedic Conditions' text for more details

Shoulder & Arm

prohealthsys

anterior view

posterior view

lateral view

Clavicle

1. Acromial end
2. Conoid tubercle
3. Costal tubercle
4. Sternal end

Scapula

5. Superior angle
6. Superior border
7. Medial (vertebral) border
8. Medial angle
9. Inferior angle
10. Lateral (axillary) border
11. Acromion
12. Coracoid process
13. Supraglenoid tubercle

14. Infraglenoid tubercle
15. Suprascapular notch
16. Spinoglenoid notch
17. Supraspinous fossa
18. Infraspinous fossa
19. Subscapular fossa
20. Glenoid fossa
21. Spine of the scapula

Humerus

22. Head
23. Anatomical neck
24. Surgical neck
25. Greater tubercle
26. Crest of greater tubercle

27. Intertubercular sulcus (bicipital groove)
28. Lesser tubercle
29. Crest of lesser tubercle
30. Radial/spiral groove
31. Deltoid tuberosity
32. Lateral supracondylar ridge
33. Lateral epicondyle
34. Medial supracondylar ridge
35. Medial epicondyle
36. Coronoid fossa
37. Trochlea
38. Capitulum
39. Notch for the ulnar nerve
40. Olecranon

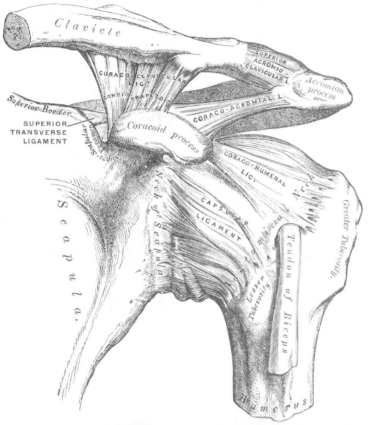

Shoulder & Arm

Ligament	Attaches (origin/insertion)	Function
Acromioclavicular	Acromion process to clavicle	Resists AC joint separation
Coracoacromial	Corocoid process to acromion process	Forms arch over shoulder
Coracoclavicular Trapezoid Conoid	Coracoid process to clavicle	Resists anterior and posterior scapula movements & upward/downward movements of clavicle on scapula
Coracohumeral	Coracoid process to greater and lesser tuberosity on humerus	Resists upward humeral head movement & external rotation Supports weight of arm
Costoclavicular	Clavicle to 1st rib	Resists clavicle elevation, anterior, posterior, and lateral movement Supports weight of arm
Glenohumeral Superior Middle Inferior	Upper, anterior edge of glenoid to over, in front, and below humeral head	Tight with external rotation & abduction past 100° Prevents anterior dislocation of humerus; resists clavicular motion, supports weight of arm
Interclavicular	Clavicle to clavicle	Checks motion of clavicle, supports arm weight

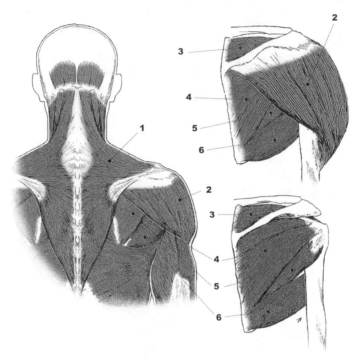

1. Trapezius
2. Deltoid
3. Supraspinatus
4. Infraspinatus
5. Teres minor
6. Teres major
7. Subscapularis
8. Serratus anterior
9. Pectoralis major
10. Latissimus dorsi

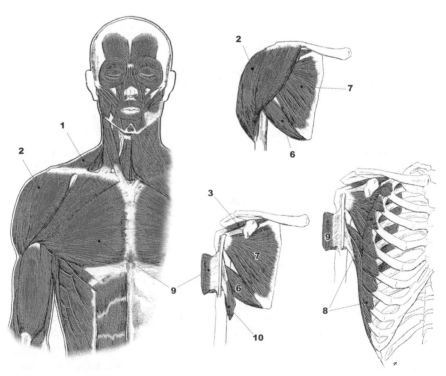

Joint type: synovial
Ball & socket (glenohumeral)
Gliding (scapulothoracic)

Articular surfaces
Glenohumeral: *convex* (head of humerus) on *concave* (glenoid fossa)
Scapulothoracic: *concave* (subscapular fossa) *on convex* (posterior ribs)

Active range of motion (shoulder)
Flexion ....180°
Extension ....60°
Int./ext. rotation ....90°/80°
Abduction ....180°
Adduction ....35°
Horizontal Add./Abd. ..130°/45°
Scapulohumeral (humerus: scapula)
120°:60° (2:1)

Main muscle actions
Flexion: anterior deltoid, biceps brachii, coracobrachialis, pectoralis major
Extension: posterior deltoid, latissimus dorsi, triceps brachii, teres major
Abduction: middle deltoid, supraspinatus
Adduction: latissimus dorsi, teres major, pectoralis major
Horizontal adduction: pectoralis major, coracobrachialis, anterior deltoid
Horizontal abduction: posterior deltoid, teres major
Internal rotation: subscapularis, pectoralis major, latissimus dorsi
External rotation: infraspinatus, teres minor

Resting position
GH: 55°-70° abduction, 30° horizontal abduction
Acromioclavicular: arm at side
Sternoclavicular: arm at side

Close packed position
Glenohumeral: maximal abduction & lateral rotation
Acromioclavicular: 90° abduction
Sternoclavicular: full elevation

Normal end feel
Flexion: elastic, firm-bony contact
Abduction: elastic
Extension: firm
Internal/External : elastic / firm
Horizontal adduction: soft tissue
Horizontal abduction: firm/elastic

Abnormal end feel
Empty → subacromial bursitis
Hard capsular → frozen shoulder
Late myospasm → instability

Capsular pattern of restriction
Glenohumeral: external rotation > abduction > internal rotation

Capsular pattern restrictions (detailed)
Posterior capsule: ↓ horizontal adduction, internal rotation & end range flexion, ↓ posterior glide
Posterior inferior capsule: ↓ elevation, internal rotation & horizontal adduction
Posterior superior capsule: ↓ internal rotation
Anterior superior capsule: ↓ end range flexion & extension, ↓ external rotation & horizontal abduction
Anterior capsule: ↓ abduction, extension, external rotation & horizontal adduction

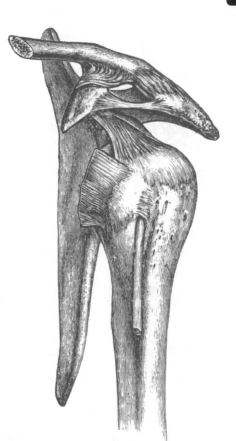

Shoulder & Arm

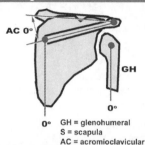

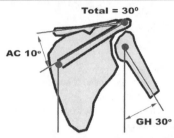

AC 0°

GH

0°

0°   GH = glenohumeral
     S = scapula
     AC = acromioclavicular

Total = 30°

AC 10°

GH 30°

Resting phase (neutral)	Phase 1 (0°-30°)
Shoulder ROM is measured from standard anatomical position	Important abductors
	Deltoid (60%-70%)
Shoulder hiking (elevation) in phase 1 may indicate shoulder pathology	Supraspinatus (30%-40%)
	When arm is externally rotated, long head of biceps will help in abduction (coracobrachialis & biceps short head help with GH flexion when the arm is externally rotated)
Clavicle follows the humerus	
The inferior capsule folds like an accordion, & unfolds for abduction, loss of this motion = *"frozen shoulder"* or *adhesive capsulitis*	
	Rotator cuff as a group
Most important shoulder girdle stabilizer is serratus anterior	Depresses humerus*, cancels superior translation by deltoid
Rotator cuff = SITS muscles	**GH:** 15°-20°, superior roll with inferior slide
Supraspinatus	**Scapula:** 10°-15°, external rotation
Infraspinatus	Serratus anterior is the major stabilizer, at this point, of the shoulder girdle
Teres minor	Upper & lower trapezius are minor stabilizers at this point
Subscapularis	

Shoulder Stability

Muscles provide a full 50% of the GH joint stability (bone shape, glenoid labrum, synovial fluid surface tension & ligaments provide the other 50%)

SC: Distal end elevates 10°-15°
Superior roll with inferior glide (same as GH)
Upper trapezius is not very active

GH = glenohumeral joint, AC = acromioclavicular joint, SC = sternoclavicular joint

*note that the action of supraspinatus is not to directly depress the humerus, rather the space occupied by the muscle helps keep the humerus inferior, following a full supraspinatus rupture it is possible to observe the humerus in an elevated position relative to the glenoid fossa on MRI or X-ray

Scapulohumeral rhythm serves at least two purposes:

1. Preserves length-tension relationships of glenohumeral muscles; the muscles do not shorten as much as they would without the scapula's upward rotation, so they can sustain their force production through a larger range of motion

2. Prevents impingement between humerus & acromion. Because of the difference in size between the glenoid fossa & the humeral head, subacromial impingement can occur unless relative movement between the humerus & scapula is limited. Simultaneous movement of the humerus & scapula during shoulder elevation limits relative (arthrokinematic) movement between the two bones

Total Motion = 180°, 2:1 (GH : Scapula)

GH: 120°   **Shoulder Girdle** (Scap./SC/AC): 60°

prohealthsys

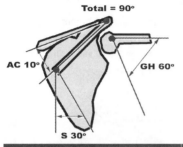

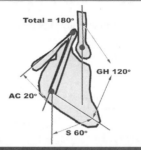

Total = 90°

AC 10°   GH 60°

S 30°

Total = 180°

GH 120°

AC 20°

S 60°

Phase 2 (30°-90°)

GH: 40°-45° (55°-65° total)
Superior roll with inferior slide
Deltoid & supraspinatus - abduction
Rotator cuff - depress & externally rotate
Greatest impingement: 70°-120°

Scapula: 15°-20° (30° total)
Externally rotates
Serratus anterior prevents winging
Upper & lower trapezius - forces couple
& cancel each other out

SC: 15°-20° (30° total)
Elevation of distal clavicle
At end of 1st 30° the coracoclavicular
ligaments become taut & stop the
superior roll & inferior slide that make
up the hinge action, this will cause
rotation in the 3rd phase

AC: twisting/rotation: 0°-5° (10°-15° total)
AC: 5°-10° scapula rotation

Phase 3 (90°-180°)

GH: 60° (120° total)
Deltoid & supraspinatus active, biceps joins in after 90°;
above 90° rotator cuff & ligaments act to depress, externally
rotate & stabilize GH joint
Biceps, Pec major & Lats also help depress the humerus
Triceps long head tendon resists inferior translation
Pec major & subscap. reinforce anterior capsule & resists
anterior translation & dislocation
Structures resisting abduction: inferior capsule, latissimus
dorsi, pec. major, teres major, subscapularis, inferior GH
ligament, long head of triceps (resist inferior translation)

Scapula: 30° (60° total) upper trapezius, serratus anterior
upward rotates scapula
Structures that limit upward rotation; rhomboids, lower trap.

SC: rotates externally & points upwards
Crank-shaped clavicle allows elevation at distal end, while
proximal rotates; this causes a 30° elevation at the distal
clavicle due to taut coracoclavicular ligaments, which stop
the hinge & cause rotation. Resisted by costoclavicular ligs
from the 1st rib & eccentric contraction of subclavius

AC: 10° (20° total) final 10° rotation during phase 1-2, AC
rotation is due to scapular rotation

Throwing

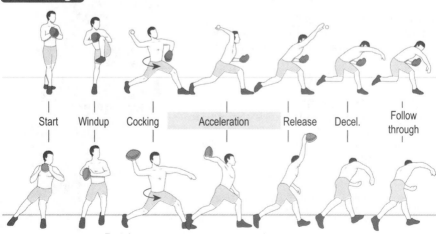

| Start | Windup | Cocking | Acceleration | Release | Decel. | Follow through |

Foot down   Max external rotation &
weight transfer forward

Compare bilaterally, examiner should make an introduction statement:
"Try and move as far as possible, if any of the actions or movements are painful or uncomfortable please let me know, do not do any action you feel will cause you further injury."

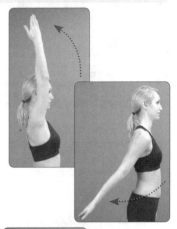

Flexion (160°-180°)
Muscles Activated: deltoid (anterior fibers), biceps brachii, pectoralis major & coracobrachialis (1st 60° only)
Tissue Stretched: latissimus dorsi, teres major, pectoralis major (lower fibers), triceps brachii (long head), inferior GH capsule, conoid ligament
Tissue Compressed: supraspinatus tendon, subdeltoid bursa, upper GH joint capsule

Extension (40°-60°)
Muscles Activated: deltoid (posterior fibers), latissimus dorsi, teres major/minor, infraspinatus, triceps brachii
Tissue Stretched: deltoid (anterior fibers), biceps brachii, pectoralis major, anterior GH capsule
Tissue Compressed: posterior GH capsule

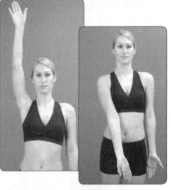

Abduction (160°-180°)
Muscles Activated: supraspinatus, deltoid (middle fibers), trapezius, serratus anterior
Tissue Stretched: latissimus dorsi, teres major, pectoralis major (lower fibers), triceps brachii (long head), inferior GH capsule, conoid ligament
Tissue Compressed: supraspinatus tendon, subdeltoid bursa, upper GH joint capsule

Adduction (30°-40°)*
Muscles Activated: deltoid (anterior fibers), pectoralis major, latissimus dorsi, teres major, coracobrachialis, trapezius
Tissue Stretched: deltoid (middle fibers), posterior GH capsule
Tissue Compressed: pectoralis major, AC & SC joint, anterior GH capsule

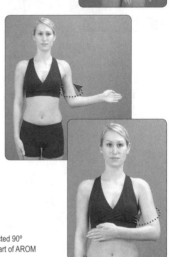

Lateral Rotation (80°-100°)**
Muscles Activated: infraspinatus, teres minor, posterior deltoid
Tissue Stretched: pectoralis major, subscapularis, anterior GH capsule
Tissue Compressed: posterior GH capsule

Medial Rotation (70°-90°)**
Muscles Activated: pec major, subscapularis, anterior deltoid, teres major, latissimus dorsi
Tissue Stretched: infraspinatus, teres minor, posterior deltoid posterior GH capsule
Tissue Compressed: anterior GH capsule

*Adduction may also be assessed with the patient moving the arm behind their back
**Medial & lateral rotation should be tested with the shoulder in neutral & again abducted 90°
Horizontal adduction & abduction & scapular movements may also be assessed as part of AROM

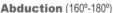

prohealthsys

Compare bilaterally; if possible palpate joint during PROM & use the shortest lever possible, start with unaffected; apply over pressure at end ROM; introduction statement: "If any of the actions or movements are painful or uncomfortable please let me know."

Flexion (> 160°-180°)
Tissue Stretched: latissimus dorsi, teres major, pectoralis major (lower fibers), triceps brachii (long head), inferior GH capsule, conoid ligament
Tissue Compressed: supraspinatus tendon, subdeltoid bursa, upper GH joint capsule

Extension (> 40°-60°)
Tissue Stretched: deltoid (anterior fibers), biceps brachii, pectoralis major, anterior GH capsule
Tissue Compressed: posterior GH capsule

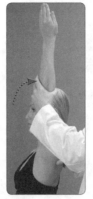
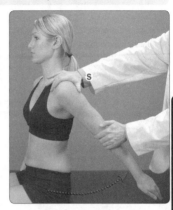

Shoulder & Arm

Abduction (> 160°-180°)
Tissue Stretched: latissimus dorsi, teres major, pectoralis major (lower fibers), triceps brachii (long head), inferior GH capsule, conoid ligament
Tissue Compressed: supraspinatus tendon, subdeltoid bursa, upper GH joint capsule

Adduction (> 30°-40°)
Tissue Stretched: deltoid (middle fibers), posterior GH capsule
Tissue Compressed: pectoralis major, AC & SC joint, anterior GH capsule

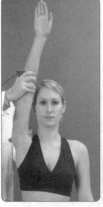
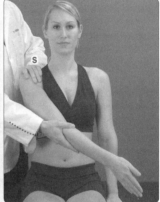

Medial Rotation (> 70°-90°)
Tissue Stretched: infraspinatus, teres minor, posterior deltoid posterior GH capsule
Tissue Compressed: anterior GH capsule

Lateral Rotation (> 80°-100°)
Tissue Stretched: pectoralis major, subscapularis, anterior GH capsule
Tissue Compressed: posterior GH capsule

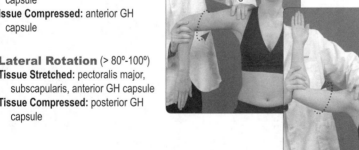

*shoulder PROM may also be assessed with the patient supine

Patient instructions for assessing general muscle strength testing:
"I am going to try and move you in _____ direction, don't let me do it" or "resist my force"

Flexion
Muscles Activated: deltoid (anterior fibers), biceps brachii, pectoralis major & coracobrachialis

Extension
Muscles Activated: deltoid (posterior fibers), latissimus dorsi, teres major/minor, infraspinatus, triceps brachii

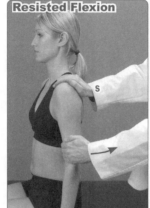
Resisted Flexion

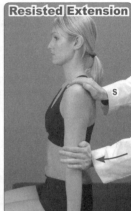
Resisted Extension

Adduction
Muscles Activated: deltoid (anterior fibers), pectoralis major, latissimus dorsi, teres major, coracobrachialis, trapezius

Abduction
Muscles Activated: supraspinatus, deltoid (middle fibers), trapezius, serratus anterior

Resisted Adduction   **Resisted Abduction**

Lateral Rotation
Muscles Activated: infraspinatus, teres minor, posterior deltoid

Medial Rotation
Muscles Activated: pectoralis major, subscapularis, anterior deltoid, teres major, latissimus dorsi

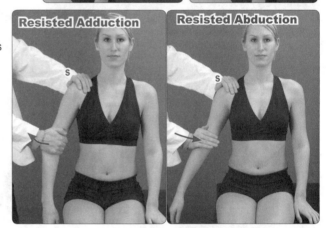

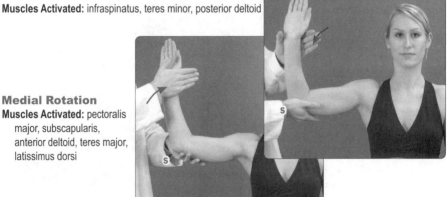

Flexion (normal 160°-180°)

- Patient prone
- Fulcrum aligned with the acromion
- Stationary & moving arm are aligned to the lateral epicondyle & midline of humerus
- Ask patient to flex shoulder

Extension (normal: 40°-60°)

- Patient prone
- Goniometer position the same as flexion
- Ask patient to extend shoulder

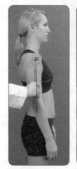
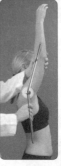
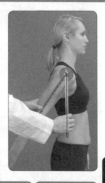

Abduction (normal: 160°-180°)

- Patient seated with arm relaxed at side
- Fulcrum aligned with the acromion
- Stationary & moving arm are aligned to the anterior midline of humerus
- Ask patient to abduct shoulder

Adduction (normal: 30°-40°)

- Same as abduction except patient is instructed to adduct shoulder

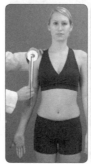
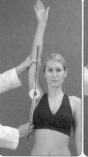
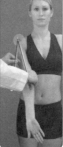

Medial rotation (normal: 70°-90°)

- Patient supine with shoulder & elbow flexed 90°
- Fulcrum aligned with the olecranon process
- Stationary arm aligned perpendicular to floor; moving arm aligned with styloid process of ulna
- Ask patient to move medially rotate shoulder

Lateral rotation (80°-100°)

- Same as medial rotation, except patient is instructed to laterally rotate shoulder

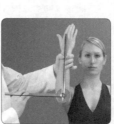
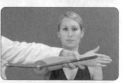
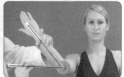

Horizontal abd. (normal: 120°-130°)

- Patient supine with shoulder abducted 90°
- Fulcrum aligned with the acromion
- Stationary & moving arm are aligned to the midline of humerus
- Ask patient to horizontally adduct shoulder

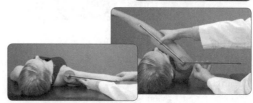

Horizontal add. (normal: 30°-45°)

- Patient prone with shoulder abducted 90°
- Fulcrum aligned with the acromion
- Stationary & moving arm are aligned to the midline of humerus
- Ask patient to horizontally abduct shoulder

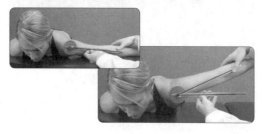

Shoulder & Arm

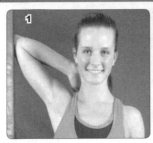
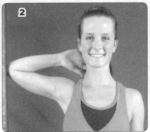
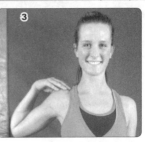

1. **Pec Lower fibers:** elbow flexed, shoulder abduct 150° & extended against door or wall

2. **Pec Middle fibers:** elbow flexed, shoulder abduct 100° & extended against door or wall

3. **Pec Upper fibers:** elbow flexed, shoulder abduct 60° & extended against door or wall

By flexing the elbow the stretches are more specific to pectoralis major; may also be done with the arm straight but will also stretch anterior arm muscles. Stretches may be done bilaterally through a door.

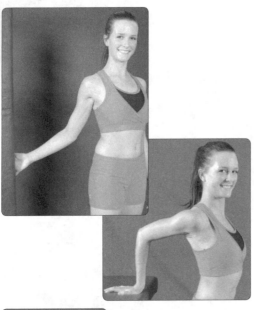
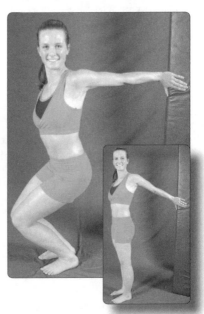
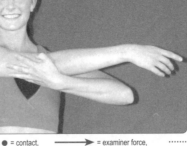
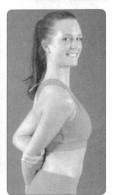

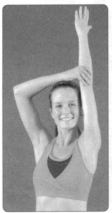
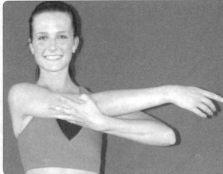

S = stabilization (indifferent hand), ● = contact, ⟶ = examiner force, ┈┈┈▶ = patient motion

Stretch: deliberate lengthening of muscles & fascia, in order to increase muscle flexibility and/or joint range of motion (stretches develop passive tension); **it is crucial to ask patients to demonstrate the stretches they are performing to ensure proper technique & injury avoidance**
Stretches should be held for 15-30 seconds & performed after a mild warm up

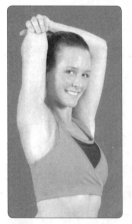

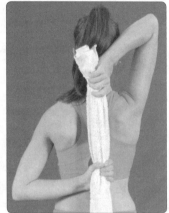

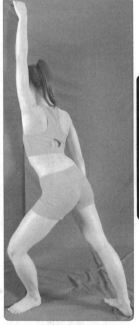

Shoulder

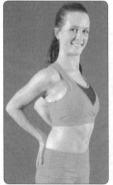

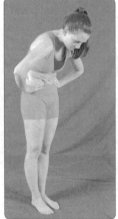

 Patient handouts on prohealthsys

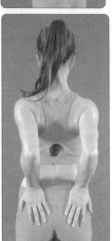

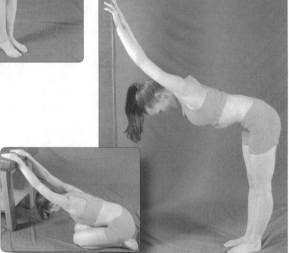

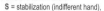 **S** = stabilization (indifferent hand), ● = contact, ⟶ = examiner force, ┈┈┈▶ = patient motion

Exercises demonstrated in this text may be performed at home with weights, therapy bands, soup cans, pots or any other device that can provide muscle resistance.

KIS - Keep it simple. Exercises & stretches should be easy to do & easy to remember **(show patients how to do it, have them demonstrate it & give handouts with pictures to use at home)**

Keep it short. Time is precious, so keep the home routine to under 15 minutes.

Keep it pain-free. The patient should not work in painful areas; the amount of stretch, weight & reps should be started at below what the practitioner believes the patient's ability is & progress slowly

Shoulder

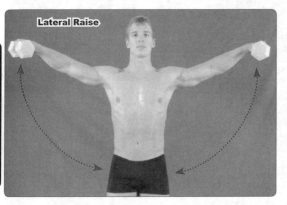

Lateral Raise

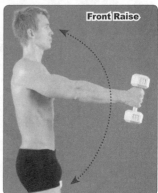

Front Raise

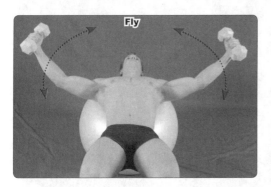

Fly

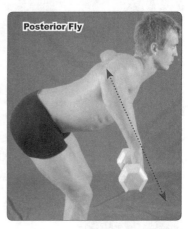

Posterior Fly

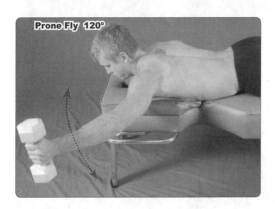

Prone Fly 120°

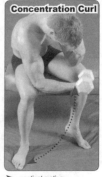

Concentration Curl

S = stabilization (indifferent hand), ● = contact, ➞ = examiner force, ·······▶ = patient motion

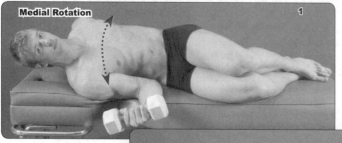

Medial Rotation 1

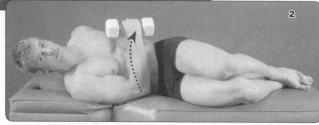

2

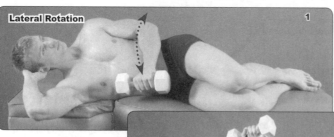

Lateral Rotation 1

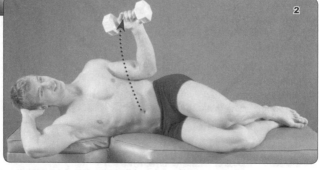

2

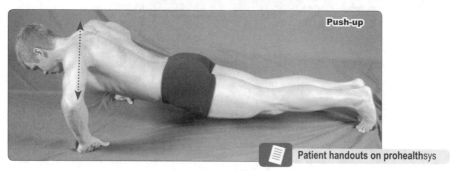

Push-up

Patient handouts on prohealthsys

S = stabilization (indifferent hand), ● = contact, ——▶ = examiner force, ⋯⋯▶ = patient motion

> **Pin & Stretch treatments can be adapted & applied to any myofascial structure if the clinician has a detailed understanding of basic anatomy & biomechanics**
> 1. Clinician places muscle in shortened position & pins specific myofascial fibers with other hand
> 2. Patient is then <u>passively</u> moved to lengthen muscle while pinning force is maintained
> 3. Hold at tension for ~10 seconds or until myofascial release is felt; repeat & reassess as needed

Middle Deltoid Example

1. Clinician places muscle in shortened position (shoulder abducted - origin & insertion approximated) & pins specific myofascial fibers with other hand
2. Patient is then passively moved to lengthen muscle (shoulder adduction - move insertion away from origin) while pinning force is maintained
3. Hold at tension for ~10 sec or until release is felt; repeat as needed

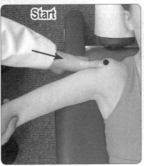
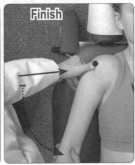

Pectoralis Major Example

1. Clinician places muscle in shortened position (origin & insertion approximated) & pins specific myofascial fibers with other hand
2. Patient is then passively moved to lengthen muscle (shoulder abduction - move insertion away from origin) while pinning force is maintained
3. Hold at tension for ~10 sec or until release is felt; repeat as needed

Note: any region of pectoralis major may be stretched by altering the specific pinning contact

This is an especially useful method to apply to patients with rounded shoulders secondary to poor posture or tight pectoralis muscles

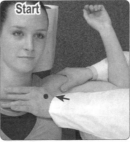
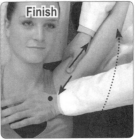

Teres Major Example

1. Clinician places muscle in shortened position (shoulder adducted - origin & insertion approximated) & pins specific myofascial fibers with other hand
2. Patient is then passively moved to lengthen muscle (shoulder abduction - move insertion away from origin) while pinning force is maintained
3. Hold at tension for ~10 sec or until release is felt sec; repeat as needed

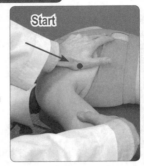
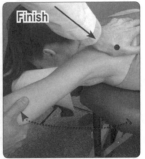

S = stabilization (indifferent hand), ● = contact, ⟶ = examiner force, ┈┈┈▶ = patient motion

prohealthsys

Shoulder External Rotation Restriction

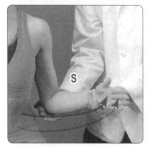
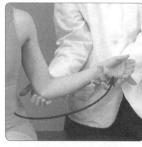

External rotation tissue resistance | Patient contracts ~10% in internal rot. | Clinician finds new end range

Shoulder Abduction Restriction

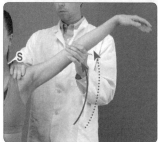
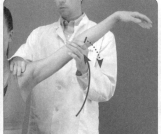
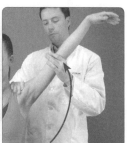

Abduction tissue resistance | Patient contracts ~10% in adduction | Clinician finds new end range

Shoulder Flexion Restriction

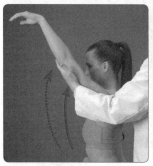
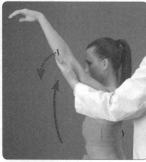
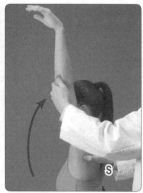

Flexion tissue resistance | Patient contracts ~10% in extension

Clinician finds new end range

S = stabilization (indifferent hand), ● = contact, ——→ = examiner force, ·······▶ = patient motion

Shoulder

Long Axis Distraction

Indications: ↓ GH inferior glide, adhesions, contracture, joint dysfunction

Position: patient supine, seated or standing

Contact: clinician stabilizes patient's scapula & clavicle while contacting distal humerus

Force: S-I pulling force at distal humerus

Clinical notes: maneuver can be performed as a mobilization or manipulation - maneuver is contraindicated in cases of GH instability

Verbally check patient tolerance to pressure

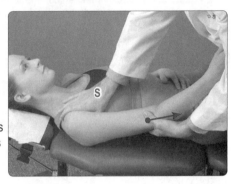

Inferior Glide 90° Flexion

Indications: ↓ GH inferior glide, adhesions, contracture, joint dysfunction

Position: patient supine with shoulder flexed 90° & elbow fully flexed

Contact: clinician contacts proximal humerus

Force: S-I pulling force at proximal humerus

Clinical notes: maneuver can be performed as a mobilization or manipulation - maneuver is contraindicated in cases of GH instability

Verbally check patient tolerance to pressure

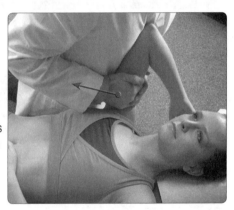

Lateral Distraction

Indications: ↓ GH lateral glide, adhesions, contracture, joint dysfunction

Position: patient supine, seated or standing

Contact: clinician stabilizes patient's elbow while contacting proximal medial humerus

Force: M-L force at proximal humerus

Clinical notes: maneuver can be performed as a mobilization or manipulation - maneuver is contraindicated in cases of GH instability

Verbally check patient tolerance to pressure

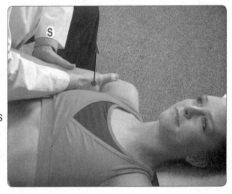

S = stabilization (indifferent hand),　　● = contact,　　——▶ = examiner force,　　·········▶ = patient motion

Lateral Long-axis Glide

Indications: ↓ GH lateral glide, adhesions, contracture, joint dysfunction

Position: patient supine, seated with shoulder abducted 90º

Contact: clinician stabilizes patient's proximal humerus

Force: S-I pulling force down long axis of humerus

Clinical notes: maneuver can be performed as a mobilization or manipulation - maneuver is contraindicated in cases of GH instability

Verbally check patient tolerance to pressure

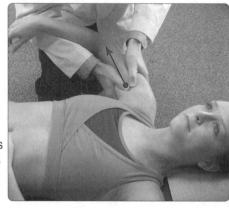

Shoulder

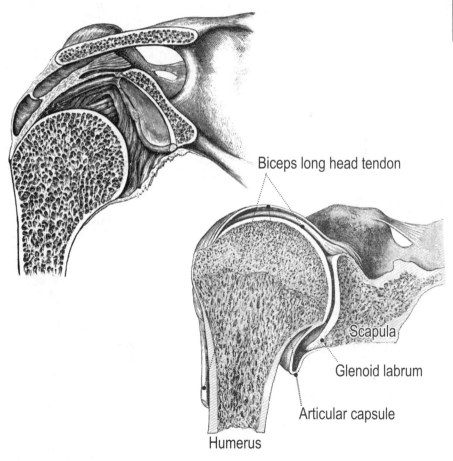

Biceps long head tendon

Scapula

Glenoid labrum

Articular capsule

Humerus

S = stabilization (indifferent hand), ● = contact, ⟶ = examiner force, ┈┈┈▷ = patient motion

Shoulder

Posterior Glide

Indications: ↓ GH posterior glide, adhesions, contracture, joint dysfunction

Position: patient supine

Contact: clinician contacts proximal humerus

Force: A-P pushing force at proximal humerus

Clinical notes: maneuver can be performed as a mobilization or manipulation - maneuver is contraindicated in cases of GH instability

Verbally check patient tolerance to pressure

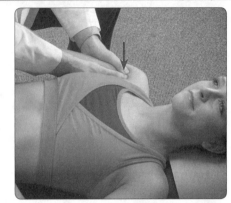

Posterior Glide 90° Flexion

Indications: ↓ GH posterior glide, adhesions, contracture, joint dysfunction

Position: patient supine with shoulder flexed to 90º & elbow fully flexed

Contact: clinician stabilizes posterior scapula & applies force through patients elbow

Force: A-P force through humerus

Clinical notes: maneuver can be performed as a mobilization or manipulation - maneuver is contraindicated in cases of GH instability

Verbally check patient tolerance to pressure

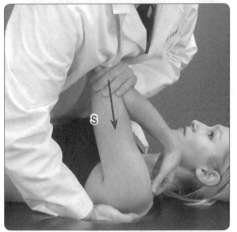

Anterior Glide

Indications: ↓ GH anterior glide, adhesions, contracture, joint dysfunction

Position: patient supine, or standing with hand on hip

Contact: clinician stabilizes anterior shoulder & asks patient to rapidly push elbow into the clinicians hand force through patients elbow

Force: P-A force through humerus

Clinical notes: maneuver can be performed as a mobilization or manipulation - maneuver is contraindicated in cases of GH instability

Verbally check patient tolerance to pressure

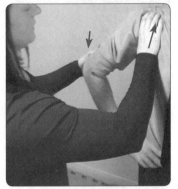

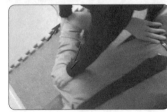

S = stabilization (indifferent hand),　● = contact,　──► = examiner force,　·······► = patient motion

Inferior-Anterior-Lateral Glide

Indications: combination of ↓ GH inferior, anterior lateral glide, adhesions, contracture

Position: patient supine

Contact: clinician contacts proximal humerus

Force: S-I, M-L, P-A pulling force at proximal humerus

Clinical notes: maneuver can be performed as a mobilization or manipulation - maneuver is contraindicated in cases of GH instability

Verbally check patient tolerance to pressure

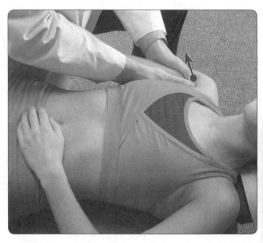

Anterior Glide 90° Abduction

Indications: ↓ GH anterior glide, adhesions, contracture

Position: patient supine or prone with shoulder abducted 90°

Contact: clinician contacts proximal humerus

Force: P-A force at proximal humerus

Clinical notes: maneuver can be performed as a mobilization or manipulation - maneuver is contraindicated in cases of GH instability

Verbally check patient tolerance to pressure, consider have patient's shoulder completely off the edge of table

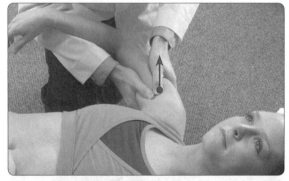

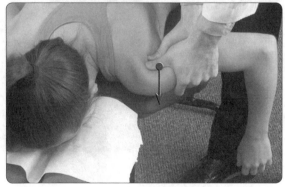

S = stabilization (indifferent hand), ● = contact, ——▶ = examiner force, ·········▶ = patient motion

Anterior Glide

Indications: ↓ GH anterior glide, adhesions, contracture

Position: patient supine

Contact: clinician contacts proximal humerus & stabilizes elbow

Force: P-A force at proximal humerus

Clinical notes: maneuver can be performed as a mobilization or manipulation - maneuver is contraindicated in cases of GH instability

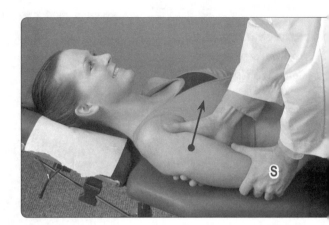

Anterior-Lateral Glide

Indications: ↓ GH anterior glide, adhesions, contracture

Position: patient supine

Contact: clinician contacts proximal humerus

Force: P-A pulling force at proximal humerus

Clinical notes: maneuver can be performed as a mobilization or manipulation - maneuver is contraindicated in cases of GH instability

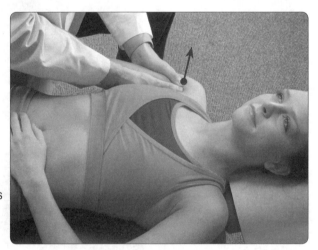

S = stabilization (indifferent hand), ● = contact, ⟶ = examiner force, ┈┈┈▶ = patient motion

Internal Rotation

Indications: ↓ GH internal rotation, adhesions, contracture

Position: patient supine with shoulder abducted 90° & internally rotated

Contact: clinician contacts proximal humerus

Force: internal rotation force at proximal humerus

Clinical notes: maneuver can be performed as a mobilization or manipulation - maneuver is contraindicated in cases of GH instability

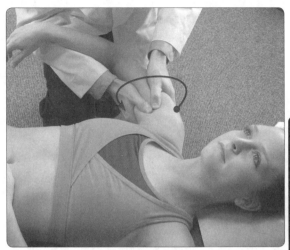

Shoulder

External Rotation

Indications: ↓ GH external rotation, adhesions, contracture

Position: patient supine with shoulder abducted 90° & externally rotated

Contact: clinician contacts proximal humerus

Force: external rotation force at proximal humerus

Clinical notes: maneuver can be performed as a mobilization or manipulation - maneuver is contraindicated in cases of GH instability

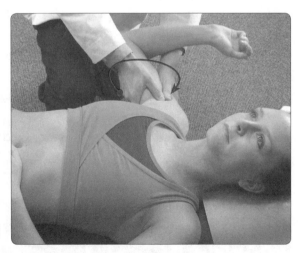

S = stabilization (indifferent hand),   ● = contact,   ⟶ = examiner force,   ┈┈┈▶ = patient motion

Inferior Glide

Indications: superior clavicle malposition, AC inferior glide restriction, non-acute AC separation

Position: patient seated or supine

Contact: soft thumb, thenar or hypothenar contact over lateral clavicle

Force: S-I depression force downward on clavicle

Clinical notes: use a soft contacts, verbally check patient tolerance to pressure

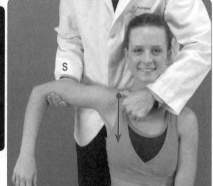
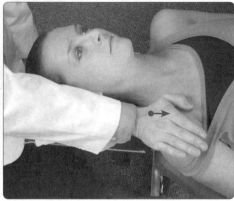

Superior Glide

Indications: superior clavicle malposition, AC inferior glide restriction

Position: patient seated or supine

Contact: soft thumb, digital or hypothenar contact over lateral clavicle

Force: I-S elevation force upward on clavicle

Clinical notes: use a soft contacts, verbally check patient tolerance to pressure

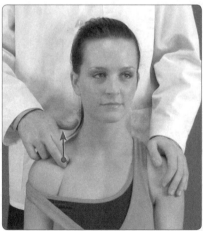

S = stabilization (indifferent hand),　● = contact,　——▶ = examiner force,　········▶ = patient motion

Posterior Glide

Indications: AC posterior glide restriction, anterior clavicle malposition

Position: patient supine with shoulder abducted ~80°

Contact: soft thumb or hypothenar contact over lateral clavicle

Force: A-P compression force toward floor on clavicle

Clinical notes: use a soft contacts, verbally check patient tolerance to pressure

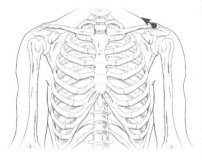

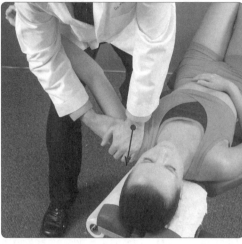

Shoulder

Anterior Glide

Indications: AC anterior glide restriction, posterior clavicle malposition

Position: patient supine with shoulder abducted ~80°

Contact: soft thumb or digital contact over lateral clavicle

Force: P-A force toward ceiling on clavicle

Clinical notes: use a soft contacts, verbally check patient tolerance to pressure

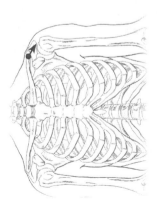

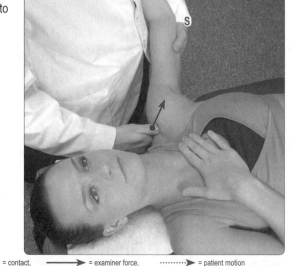

S = stabilization (indifferent hand), ● = contact, ⟶ = examiner force, ┈┈┈▶ = patient motion

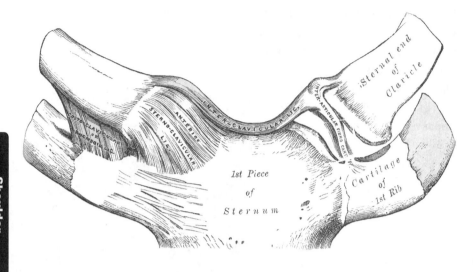

Posterior Glide

Indications: SC posterior glide restriction, anterior clavicle malposition

Position: patient supine or seated

Contact: soft thenar contact over medial clavicle

Force: A-P compression force

Clinical notes: use a soft contacts, verbally check patient tolerance to pressure

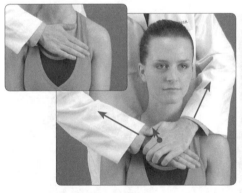

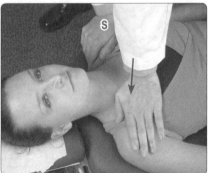

S = stabilization (indifferent hand),   ● = contact,   ——▶ = examiner force,   ·········▶ = patient motion

Anterior Glide

Indications: SC anterior glide restriction, posterior clavicle malposition

Position: patient supine or seated this shoulder flexed 90°

Contact: soft thumb digital contact (pincer grip) over medial clavicle

Force: P-A distraction force as the shoulder is horizontally abducted

Clinical notes: use a soft contacts, verbally check patient tolerance to pressure, anterior mobilization of the SC joint is often very difficult to perform due to tenderness, limiting shape & access of the anatomy

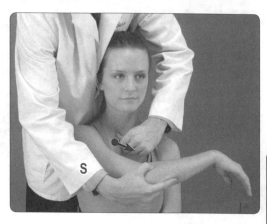

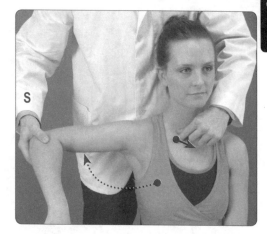

Inferior Glide

Indications: SC inferior glide restriction, SC elevation malposition

Position: patient seated or supine with shoulder and elbow flexed 90°

Contact: clinician contacts medial clavicle with thumb, thenar or hypothenar contact & stabilizes ipsilateral shoulder

Force: S-I force is applied

Clinical notes: maneuver can be performed as a mobilization or manipulation

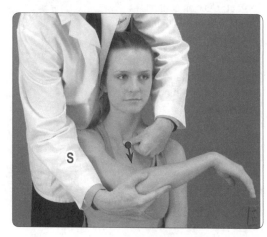

S = stabilization (indifferent hand),　● = contact,　——▶ = examiner force,　••••••••▶ = patient motion

Shoulder

Shoulder

Superior Glide

Indications: SC superior glide restriction, SC depression malposition

Position: patient seated or supine

Contact: clinician contacts medial clavicle with digits, thenar or hypothenar contact

Force: I-S force is applied

Clinical notes: maneuver can be performed as a mobilization or manipulation

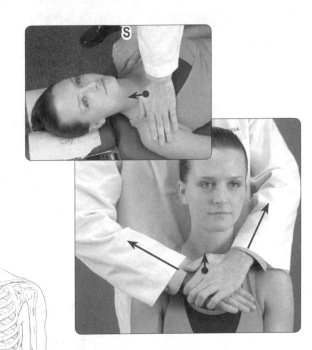

Lateral Distraction

Indications: SC lateral glide restriction, SC medial malposition

Position: patient seated or supine

Contact: clinician contacts medial clavicle with thenar or hypothenar contact

Force: M-L force is applied

Clinical notes: maneuver can be performed as a mobilization or manipulation

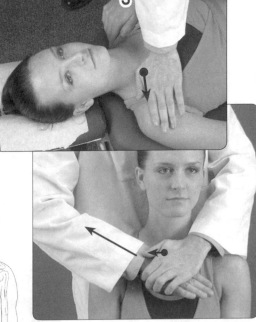

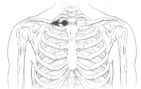

S = stabilization (indifferent hand), ● = contact, ——▶ = examiner force, ┈┈┈▶ = patient motion

Lateral Glide

Indications: scapular lateral glide restriction, medial scapula malposition

Position: patient side-lying

Contact: clinician contacts medial scapula with bilateral thumb or digital contact

Force: M-L force is applied

Clinical notes: maneuver can be performed as a mobilization or manipulation

To make scapula more prominent have patient place ipsilateral hand behind lumbar spine

Images show two variations (mobilization of up-side or down-side scapula and IASTM)

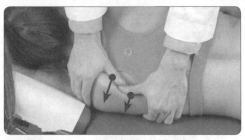

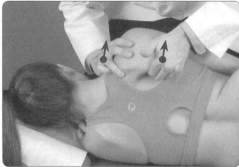

Shoulder

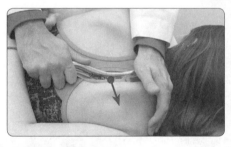

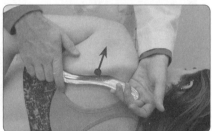

Medial Glide

Indications: scapular medial glide restriction, lateral scapula malposition

Position: patient side-lying

Contact: clinician contacts lateral scapula with bilateral thenar or palmar contact

Force: L-M force is applied over lateral scapula

Clinical notes: maneuver can be performed as a mobilization or manipulation

To make scapula more prominent have patient place ipsilateral hand behind lumbar spine

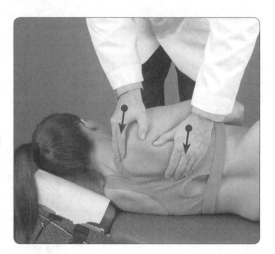

S = stabilization (indifferent hand), ● = contact, = examiner force, ┈┈┈▶ = patient motion

Downward Rotation

Indications: scapular downward rotation restriction, upward rotation scapula malposition

Position: patient seated or side-lying

Contact: clinician contacts superior lateral & inferior angle of scapula

Force: downward rotation force is applied to scapula

Clinical notes: maneuver can be performed as a mobilization or manipulation

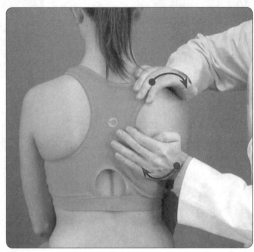

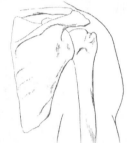

Upward Rotation

Indications: scapular upward rotation restriction, downward rotation scapula malposition

Position: patient seated or side-lying

Contact: clinician contacts lateral scapula (or proximal humerus) & inferior angle of scapula

Force: upward rotation force is applied to scapula

Clinical notes: maneuver can be performed as a mobilization or manipulation

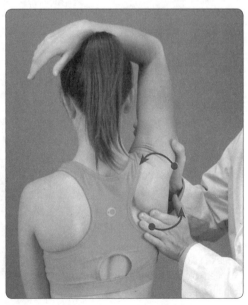

S = stabilization (indifferent hand),   ● = contact,   ——▶ = examiner force,   ·······▶ = patient motion

Distraction

Indications: scapular distraction restriction, anterior scapula malposition

Position: patient side-lying

Contact: clinician contacts anterior medial scapula (digital contact) & anterior GH joint

Force: upward rotation force is applied to scapula

Clinical notes: maneuver can be performed as a mobilization or manipulation

To make scapula more prominent have patient place ipsilateral hand behind lumbar spine

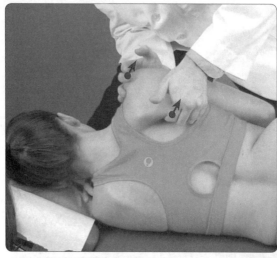

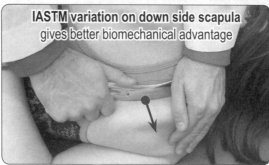

IASTM variation on down side scapula gives better biomechanical advantage

Inferior Glide

Indications: scapular inferior glide restriction, superior scapula malposition

Position: patient side-lying

Contact: clinician contacts scapula & GH joint

Force: S-I force is applied downward to scapula

Clinical notes: maneuver can be performed as a mobilization or manipulation

To make scapula more prominent have patient place ipsilateral hand behind lumbar spine

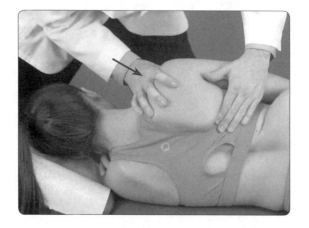

S = stabilization (indifferent hand), ● = contact, ⟶ = examiner force, ┈┈┈▷ = patient motion

1. Vizniak, NA. Clinical Cadaver Dissections. 1999-2018.
2. Taylor MH, Monroe LG. Physical Rehabilitation: Evidence-Based Examination, Evaluation and Intervention. Saunders. 2017.
3. Warlow C, Hughes R, Uitehaag B, Liberati A. Evidence-Based Neurology. Blackwell Publishing Limited, BMJI Books. 2007.
4. Malanga GA & Nadler. Musculoskeletal Physical Exam, An Evidence-Based Approach. Mosby. 2016.
5. Hoppenfield S. Physical Examination of the Spine & Extremities. Lippincott Williams & Wilkins. 1976.
6. Hoppenfield S. Orthopaedic Neurology: A Diagnostic Guide to Neurologic Levels. Lippincott Williams & Wilkins. 1977.
7. Spencer JW, Jacobs JJ. Complementary and Alternative Medicine: An Evidence-Based Approach. Mosby. 2003.
8. Jewell D. Guide to Evidence-Based Physical Therapy Practice. Jones Barlett Publishers Inc. 2007.
9. Iesel SW. Operative Orthopaedics: An Illustrative Approach. Lippincott Williams & Wilkins. 2008.
10. Bandiera G, Stiell IG, Wells GA, Clement C, DeMaio V.
11. Bak K, Fauni P. Clinical findings in competitive swimmers with shoulder pain. Am J Sports Med. 1 997;25:254-260.
12. Bennett WF. Specificity of the Speed's test: arthroscopic technique for evaluating the biceps tendon at the level of the bicipital groove. Arthroscopy. 1 998;14:789-796.
13. Calis M, Akgun K, Birtane M, Karacan I, Calis H, Tuzun F. Diagnostic values of clinical diagnostic tests in subacromial impingement syndrome. Ann Rheum Dis. 2000;59:44-47.
14. Chronopoulos E, Kim TK, Park HB, Ashenbrenner D, McFarland EG. Diagnostic value of physical tests for isolated chronic acromioclavicular lesions. Am J Sports Med. 2004;32:655-661.
15. Codman EA. Rupture of the supraspinatus tendon. 1 911. Clin Orthop Relat Res. 1990:3-26.
16. Crenshaw AH, Kilgore WE. Surgical treatment of bicipital tenosynovitis. J Bone Joint Surg Am. 1966;48:1 496-1502.
17. Field LD, Savoie FH, 3rd. Arthroscopic suture repair of superior labral detachment lesions of the shoulder. Am J Sports Med. 1993;21:783-790; discussion 790.
18. Gagey OJ, Gagey N. The hyperabduction test. J Bone Joint Surg Br. 2001 ;83:69-74.
19. Gerber C, Ganz R. Clinical assessment of instability of the shoulder. With special reference to anterior & posterior drawer tests. J Bone Joint Surg Br. 1984;66:551-556.
20. Gerber C, Hersche O, Farron A. Isolated rupture of the subscapularis tendon. J Bone Joint SurgAm. 1996;78:1015-1023.
21. Gerber C, Krushell RJ. Isolated rupture of the tendon of the subscapularis muscle. Clinical features in 16 cases. J Bone Joint Surg Br. 1991 ;73:389-394.
22. Gross ML, Distefano MC. Anterior release test. A new test for occult shoulder instability. Clin Orthop Relat Res. 1 997:105-108.
23. Guanche CA, Jones DC. Clinical testing for tears of the glenoid labrum. Arthroscopy. 2003;1 9:51 7-523.
24. Hamner DL, Pink MM, Jobe FW. A modification of the relocation test: arthroscopic findings associated with a positive test. J Shoulder Elbow Surg. 2000;9:263-267.
25. Hawkins RJ, Kennedy JC. Impingement syndrome in athletes. Am J Sports Med. 1 980;8:151-158.
26. Hertel R, Ballmer FT, Lombert SM, Gerber C. Lag signs in the diagnosis of rotator cuff rupture. J Shoulder Elbow Surg. 1 996;5:307-31 3.
27. Hertel R, Lambert SM, Ballmer FT. The deltoid extension lag sign for diagnosis & grading of axillary nerve palsy. J Shoulder Elbow Surg. 1998;7:97-99.
28. Holtby R, Razmjou H. Accuracy of the Speed's & Yergason's tests in detecting biceps pathology & SLAP lesions: comparison with arthroscopic findings. Arthroscopy. 2004;20:231-236.
29. Itoi E, Kido I, Sano A, Urayama M, Sato K. Which is more useful, the "full can test" or the "empty can test," in detecting the torn supraspinatus tendon? Am J Sports Med. 1 999;27:65-68.
30. Jacob AK, Sallay P1. Therapeutic efficacy of corticosteroid injections in the acromioclavicular joint. Biomed Sci Instrum. 1997; 34:380-385.
31. Jobe P, Kvitne RS, Giangarra CE. Shoulder pain in the overhand or throwing athlete: the relationship of anterior instability & rotator cuff impingement. Orthop Rev. 1989;18:963-975.
32. Jobe FW, Moynes DR. Delineation of diagnostic criteria & a rehabilitation program for rotator cuff injuries. Am I Sports Med. 1 982;10:336-339.
33. Kelly BT, Kadrmas WR, Speer KP. The manual muscle examination for rotator cuff strength: an electromyographic investigation. Am J Sports Med. 1 996;24:581 -588.
34. Kessel L, Watson M. The painful arc syndrome. Clinical classification as a guide to management. J Bone Joint Surg Br. 1977;59:166-172.
35. Kibler WB. Specificity & sensitivity of the anterior slide test in throwing athletes with superior glenoid labral tears. Arthroscopy. 1995;11:296-300.
36. Kim KH, Cho JG, Lee KO, et al. Usefulness of physical maneuvers for prevention of vasovagal syncope. Circ J. 2005;69:1084-1088.
37. Kim SH, Ha KI, Ahn JH, Kim SH, Choi HJ. Biceps load test II: a clinical test for SLAP lesions of the shoulder. Arthroscopy. 2001;17:160-1 64.
38. Kim SH, Ha KI, Han KY. Biceps load test: a clinical test for superior labrum anterior & posterior lesions in shoulders with recurrent anterior dislocations. Am J Sports Med. 1999; 27:300-303.
39. Kim SH, Park JS, Jeong WK, Shin 5K. The Kim test: a novel test for posteroinferior labral lesion of the shoulder-a comparison to the jerk test. Am J Sports Med. 2005;33:1 188-1192.
40. Litaker D, Pioro M, El Bilbeisi H, Brems J. Returning to the bedside: using the history & physical examination to identify rotator cuff tears. J Am Geriatr Soc. 2000;48:1 633-1 637.
41. Liu SH, Henry MH, Nuccion SL. A prospective evaluation of a new physical examination in predicting glenoid labral tears. Am J Sports Med. 1996;24:721-725.
42. Lo 1K, Nonweiler B, Woolfrey M, Litchfield R, Kirkley A. An evaluation of the apprehension, relocation, & surprise tests for anterior shoulder instability. Am J Sports Med. 2004;32:301 -307.
43. Lyons AR, Tomlinson JE. Clinical diagnosis of tears of the rotator cuff. J Bone Joint Surg Br. 1992;74:414-415.
44. MacDonald PB, Clark P, Sutherland K. Ananalysis of the diagnostic accuracy of the Hawkins & Neer subacromial impingement signs. J Shoulder Elbow Surg. 2000;9:299-301.
45. McFarland EG, Kim TK, Savino RM. Clinical assessment of three common tests for superior labral anterior-posterior lesions. Am J Sports Med. 2002;30:810-815.
46. McLaughlin H. On the frozen shoulder. Bull Hosp Joint Dis. 1951;12:383-393.
47. Meister K, Buckley B, Batts J. The posterior impingement sign: diagnosis of rotator cuff & posterior labral tears secondary to internal impingement in overhand athletes. AmJ Orthop. 2004;33:41 2-415.
48. Mimori K, Muneta T, Nakagawa T, Shinomiya K. A new pain provocation test for superior labral tears of the shoulder. Am J Sports Med. 1 999;27:137-142.
49. Morgan CD, Burkhart SS, Palmeri M, Gillespie M. Type II SLAP lesions: three subtypes & their relationships to superior instability & rotator cuff tears. Arthroscopy. 1 998;1 4:55 3-565.
50. Murrell GA, Walton JR. Diagnosis of rotator cuff tears. Lancet. 2001;357:769-770.
51. Myers TH, Zemanovic JR, Andrews JR. The resisted supination external rotation test: a new test for the diagnosis of superior labral anterior posterior lesions. Am J Sports Med. 2005;33:1315-1320.
52. Nakagawa S, Yoneda M, Hayashida K, Obata M, Fukushima S, Miyazaki Y. Forced shoulder abduction & elbow flexion test: a new simple clinical test to detect superior labral injury in the throwing shoulder. Arthroscopy. 2005;21 :1290-1295.
53. O'Brien SJ, Pagnani MJ, Fealy 5, McGlynn SR, Wilson JB. The active compression test: a new & effective test for diagnosing labral tears & acromioclavicular joint abnormality. Am J Sports Med. 1 998;26:610-613.
54. Ostor AJ, Richards CA, Prevost AT, Hazieman BL, Speed CA. Interrater reproducibility of clinical tests for rotator cuff lesions. Ann Rheum Dis. 2004;63:1288-1292.
55. Parentis MA, Mohr KJ, ElAttrache NS. Disorders of the superior labrum: review & treatment guidelines. Clin Orthop Relat Res. 2002:77-87.
56. Park HB, Yokota A, Gill HS, El Rassi G, McFarland EG. Diagnostic accuracy of clinical tests for the different degrees of subacromial impingement syndrome. J Bone Joint Surg Am. 2005;87:1 446-1455.
57. Rowe CR, Zarins B. Recurrent transient subluxation of the shoulder. J Bone Joint Surg Am. 1981 ;63:863-872.
58. Silliman JF, Hawkins Ri. Current concepts & recent advances in the athlete's shoulder. Clin Sports Med. 1991;1 0:693-705.
59. Snyder Sj, Karzel RP, Del Pizzo W, Ferkel RD, Friedman MJ. SLAP lesions of the shoulder. Arthroscopy. 1990;6:274-279.
60. So. Speer KP, Hannafin JA, Aitchek DW, Warren RF. An evaluation of the shoulder relocation test. Am J Sports Med. 1994;22:177-183.
61. Stetson WB, Templin K. The crank test, the O'Brien test, & routine magnetic resonance imaging scans in the diagnosis of labral tears. Am J Sports Med. 2002;30:806-809.
62. Walch G, Boulahia A, Calderone S, Robinson AH. The "dropping" & "hornblower's" signs in evaluation of rotator-cuff tears. I Bone Joint Surg Br. 1998;80:624-628.
63. Walton J, Mahajan S, Paxinos A, et al. Diagnostic values of tests for acromioclavicular joint pain. J Bone Joint Surg Am. 2004;86-A:807-81 2.
64. Wolf EM, Agrawal V. Transdeltoid palpation (the rent test) in the diagnosis of rotator cuff tears. J Shoulder Elbow Surg. 2001 ;1 0:470-473.
65. Yergason R. Supination sign. J Bone Joint Surg. 1931;13:160-165.
66. Zaslav KR. Internal rotation resistance strength test: a new diagnostic test to differentiate intra-articular pathology from outlet (Neer) impingement syndrome in the shoulder. J Shoulder Elbow Surg. 2001;1 0:23-27.
67. Chao , s et al. An Electromyographic Assessment of the "Bear Hug": An Examination for the Evaluation of the Subscapularis Muscle. Journal of Arthroscopic & Related Surgery. 2008

Shoulder Quiz (answer page)

1. What are the joint type classifications for this region - GH & AC? (243) _____

2. What are the GH surface shapes for this region (convex/concave)? (243)

3. What is the normal ROM for _____?
   - Flexion/Ext.: _____, _____
   - Abduction/Add: _____, _____
   - Rotation (ext./int) _____, _____

4. What is the GH resting position? _____

5. What is the GH joint tight packed position?

6. What ligaments resist abduction? (241)

7. What muscles cause flexion to occur? (243)

8. What tissues are stretched with flexion? (247)

9. What is the ratio of scapular to GH movement during shoulder abduction? (244) _____

10. Can you palpate _____? (238)

S = stabilization (indifferent hand),   ● = contact,   ➝ = examiner force,   ·····▷ = patient motion

prohealthsys.com

Learning Objectives

After completing this chapter, students will be able to:

1. Perform a regional exam and differentiate common pathologies of the region

2. Identify and palpate body region bony landmarks, ligaments and muscles

3. Discuss regional kinematics and joint organ biomechanics

4. Demonstrate regional AROM, PROM & goniometry, stretch and strengthen protocols

5. Recognize and execute steps of effective mobilization and joint-play including indications, position, contact, force and relevant clinical notes

6. Perform supine, prone, seated assessment and mobilizations including

   - Pin & stretch & MET
   - Long axis distraction
   - Lateral/medial glides & gapping
   - Humeral-ulnar glides, flex/extension restrictions
   - Radial-ulnar glides

Elbow

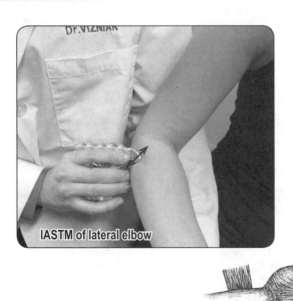

IASTM of lateral elbow

> **Follow HIP-MNRS** (see Yellow "Physical Assessment" text for specific details or review)
> History, Inspection, Palpation - Motion, Neurovascular screen, Referred pain, Special tests

Special history considerations
- Specific mechanism of injury & forces involved?
  - Did you fall on outstretched hand?
- Any numbness, tingling or weakness?
- Type of work, typical posture?

Standing or sitting

Inspection
- Asymmetry, bruising, bumps, color, swelling, height, head tilt, winging of scapula
- Posture of neck, body, shoulder
- Carrying angle

Fracture screen (if indicated)
1. Older than 55? Torsion Test
2. Bony tenderness on palpation
3. Percussion, tuning fork (128 Hz)
4. Ultrasound

Palpation (may be done after ROM assessment)

medial epicondyle	extensor tendon
ulnar groove	anconeus
medial collateral lig.	brachioradialis
common flexor tendon	ext. carpi ulnaris
flexor carpi ulnaris	ext. carpi rad. longus
palmaris longus	ext. carpi rad. brevis
flexor carpi radialis	extensor digitorum
pronator teres	supinator
biceps tendon/aponeur	triceps tendon
head of radius	triceps muscle
radial tunnel	olecranon
lateral epicondyle	olecranon bursa
lateral collateral lig.	cubital fossa
brachial artery	brachialis

Functional assessment (ADLs)
- Elbow flexion extension

AROM
Flexion	**150°**
Extension	**0° to -5°**
Pronation	**90°**
Supination	**90°**

PROM & Joint Play (if lacking AROM in any motion)

Myotomes (resisted isometric movements)
- Shoulder elevation (C4, XI)
- Deltoid (**C5**, C6 - axillary)
- Brachioradialis (C5, C6 - radial)
- Biceps (C5, **C6** - musculocutaneous)
- Triceps (C6, **C7**, C8, T1 - radial)
- Wrist extensors (**C6**, C7, C8 - radial)
- Wrist flexors (C6, **C7** - median/ulnar)
- Finger flexors (C7, **C8**, T1 - ulnar/median)
- Interossei (C7, C8, **T1** - ulnar)

Neurovascular screen
- *Sensory:* light touch, two point discrimination, Vibration (3rd digit), Tinel's
- *DTR's:*
  - Biceps (C5)
  - Brachioradialis (C6)
  - Triceps (C7)
- Girth measurements
- Grip strength (Dynamometer)
- Radial & brachial pulse, blanching, temperature

Orthopedic tests (as indicated)
Screening
- Valgus stress (0°) – forearm supinated
- Valgus stress (30°)
- Varus stress (0°) – forearm pronated
- Varus stress (30°)

Lateral epicondylitis
- Cozen's test
- Mill's Test
- Middle finger test
- Book lift test

Medial epicondylitis
- Reverse Cozen's
- Reverse Mill's

Pronator Teres/Median nerve
- Tinel's (wrist)
- Tinel's (elbow)
- Elbow flexion test
- Pronator stretch test
- Sustained flexion test

Wrist, shoulder & cervical spine screen

Diagnostic imaging (if indicated)

 youtube: Elbow Exam Brief Vizniak

Elbow	Clinical notes
Lateral epicondylitis	*Hx:* repetitive motions (gripping, hammering, lifting, tennis backhand) *SSx:* tender to palpation over lateral epicondyle/common extensor tendon; ↑ elbow pain with resisted wrist extension; (+) Mill's, Cozen's Test *DDx:* cervical radiculopathy, posterior interosseous nerve entrapment
Medial epicondylitis	*Hx:* repetitive motions (gripping, lifting, golfing) *SSx:* tender to palpation over medial epicondyle/common flexor tendon; ↑ elbow pain with resisted wrist flexion; (+) reverse Mill's, reverse Cozen's Test *DDx:* cervical radiculopathy
Pulled (Toddler's) **Elbow**	*Hx:* child (age 1-4) swung by arms or arm tugged "hurry up Sally" *SSx:* pain & apprehension, child is unwilling to straighten elbow *DDx:* elbow or wrist fracture (usually more significant trauma)
Pronator teres syndrome	*Hx:* repetitive motions (gripping with pronation), tingling & weakness in hand *SSx:* tender to palpation over mid pronator teres; ↑ hand symptoms with palpation of pronator teres, weakness in wrist flexion; (+) Tinel's (possible) *DDx:* cervical radiculopathy, carpal tunnel syndrome - Remember the median nerve travels between the 2 heads of pronator teres
UCL rupture	*Hx:* prior elbow dislocation, throwing injury or chronic overload (throwing athlete) *SSx:* tenderness to palpation of UCL; (+) valgus stress test *DDx:* olecranon bursitis, osteocondritis dessicans, fracture

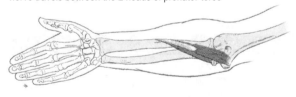

↑ = increase, ↓ = decrease, Hx = history, SSx = signs & symptoms, DDx = differential diagnosis
see blue 'Orthopedic Conditions' and yellow 'Physical Assessment' texts for more details

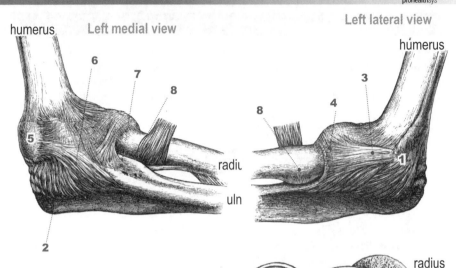

Left medial view

humerus
6
7
8
5
radiu
uln
2

Left lateral view

húmerus
3
4
8
1

Posterior view right elbow
(radius removed from annular ligament)

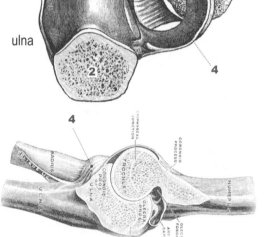

radius
ulna
4
2
4

Elbow joint

1. Lateral epicondyle
2. Olecranon
3. Radial collateral ligament
4. Annular ligament
5. Medial epicondyle
6. Ulnar collateral ligament
7. Ulnar tuberosity
8. Radial tuberosity

Ligament	Attaches (origin/insertion)	Function
Annular	Anterior margin of radial notch to posterior margin of radial notion	Surrounds and supports head of radius; holds radius in joint
Radial collateral	Lateral epicondyle to annular ligament	Supports lateral joint (resists varus forces)
Ulnar collateral Posterior, Transverse, Anterior	Medial epicondyle, olecranon process to coronoid process	Supports medial joint (resists valgus forces - throwing, falling)

Elbow

Joint type: synovial
Hinge (humeroulnar & humeroradial)
Pivot (proximal radioulnar)

Articular surfaces
Humeroulnar: *concave* (trochlear notch of ulna) *on convex* (trochlea of humerus)
Humeroradial: *concave* (radial head) *on convex* (capitilum of humerus)
Proximal radioulnar: *convex* (radial head) *on concave* (radial notch of ulna)

Active range of motion (elbow)
Flexion .... 150°
Extension .... 0° to -5°
Pronation .... 80°-90°
Supination .... 90°

Main muscle actions
Flexion: brachialis, biceps brachii, brachioradialis
Extension: triceps brachii, anconeus
Pronation: pronator teres, pronator quadratus
Supination: biceps brachii, supinator

Resting position
Humeroulnar: 70° flexion
Humeroradial: full extension & supination
Proximal radioulnar: 70° flexion, 35° supination

Close packed position
Humeroulnar: full extension
Humeroradial: 90° flexion, 5° supination
Proximal radioulnar: 5° supination, 90° flexion

Capsular pattern of restriction
Humeroulnar: flexion > extension
Humeroradial: flexion > extension
Proximal radioulnar: supination = pronation limited

Normal end feel
Flexion: soft tissue or bony approximation
Extension: bony approximation
Pronation: bony approx. or ligamentous
Supination: ligamentous

Abnormal end feel
Boggy → joint effusion
Early myospasm → acute injury
Late myospasm → instability
Springy block → loose body (osteochondritis dissecans)

Open kinetic chain
Humeroulnar & humeroradial:
Flexion: radius & ulna roll & glide posterior on humerus
Extension: radius & ulna roll & glide anterior on humerus
Proximal radioulnar:
Pronation: radius spins medially on ulna
Supination: radius spins laterally on ulna

Closed kinetic chain
Humeroulnar & humeroradial:
Flexion: humerus roll & glide anterior on radius & ulna
Extension: humerus roll & glide posterior on radius & ulna
Proximal radioulnar:
Pronation: ulna spins laterally on radius
Supination: ulna spins medially on radius

Carrying angle of the elbow
Normal = 5°-15° - angle permits the forearms to clear the hips in swinging movements during walking & is important when carrying objects
Cubital valgus - angle greater than 15°
Cubital varus - angle less than 5°

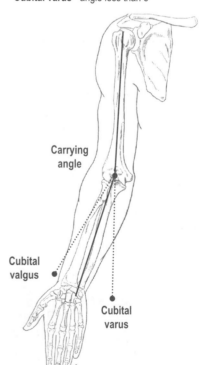

Carrying angle

Cubital valgus

Cubital varus

Elbow

Range of Motion	Ulnohumeral Joint uniaxial, hinge	Radiohumeral Joint uniaxial, hinge
Flexion ....150° Extension ....0° to -5° Pronation ....90° Supination ......90°	**Resting position** 70° flexion, 10° supination **Tight packed position** Extension with supination **Capsular pattern** Flexion, extension	**Resting position** Full extension & supination **Tight packed position** 90° flexion, 5° supination **Capsular pattern:** flexion, extension

The proximal radioulnar joint is considered a uniaxial pivot joint

Elbow AROM

Compare bilaterally, examiner should make an introduction statement:
"Try and move as far as possible, if any of the actions or movements are painful or uncomfortable please let me know, do not do any action you feel will cause you further injury."

Flexion (150°-160°)
Muscles Activated: brachialis, biceps brachii, brachioradialis
Tissue Stretched: triceps brachii, posterior elbow joint capsule, ulnar nerve
Tissue Compressed: forearm flexors, median nerve, anterior joint capsule

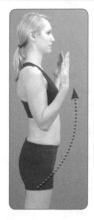
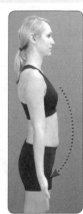

Extension (0° to -5°)
Muscles Activated: triceps brachii, anconeus
Tissue Stretched: brachialis, biceps brachii, brachioradialis, median nerve
Tissue Compressed: posterior joint capsule

Supination (80°-100°)
Muscles Activated: biceps brachii, supinator
Tissue Stretched: pronator teres, pronator quadratus

Pronation (80°-100°)
Muscles Activated: pronator teres, pronator quadratus
Tissue Stretched: biceps brachii, supinator, brachioradialis

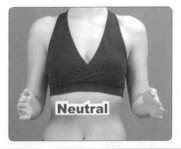

Neutral

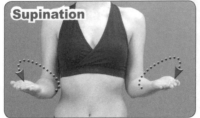

Supination

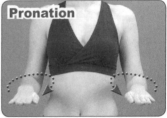

Pronation

prohealthsys

PROM

Flexion (> 150°-160°)
Tissue Stretched: triceps brachii, posterior elbow joint capsule, ulnar nerve
Tissue Compressed: forearm flexors, median nerve, anterior joint capsule

Extension (> 0° to -5°)
Tissue Stretched: brachialis, biceps brachii, brachioradialis, median nerve
Tissue Compressed: posterior joint capsule

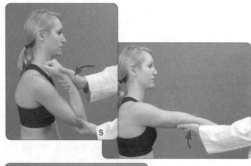

Supination (> 80°-100°)
Tissue Stretched: pronator teres, pronator quadratus
Tissue Compressed:

Pronation (> 80°-100°)
Tissue Stretched: biceps brachii, supinator, brachioradialis
Tissue Compressed:

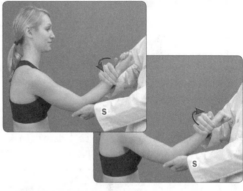

Elbow Muscle Testing

Flexion
Muscles Activated: brachialis, biceps brachii, brachioradialis

Extension
Muscles Activated: triceps brachii, anconeus

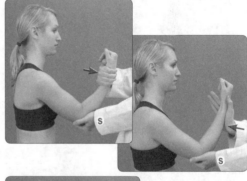

Supination
Muscles Activated: biceps brachii, supinator

Pronation
Muscles Activated: pronator teres, pronator quadratus

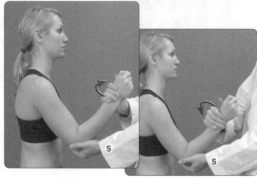

Elbow

Stretch: deliberate lengthening of muscles & fascia, in order to increase muscle flexibility and/or joint range of motion (stretches develop passive tension); **it is crucial to ask patients to demonstrate the stretches they are performing to ensure proper technique & injury avoidance**
Stretches should be held for 15-30 seconds & performed after a mild warm up

Self Stretch 1
- Flex elbow and place behind head, keep neck in neutral position & apply pressure with opposite hand

Self Stretch 2
- Place towel behind back & pull downward with lower hand; for more stretch place the raised elbow against the wall

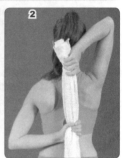
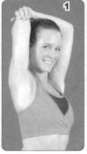

Elbow strengthening

Exercises demonstrated in this text may be performed at home with weights, therapy bands, soup cans, pots or any other device that can provide muscle resistance.
KIS - Keep it simple. Exercises & stretches should be easy to do & easy to remember (**show patients how to do it, have them demonstrate it & give handouts with pictures to use at home**)

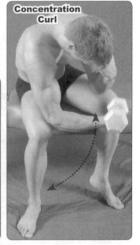
Concentration Curl

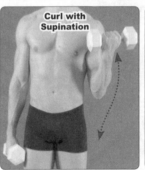
Curl with Supination

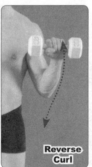
Reverse Curl

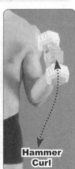
Hammer Curl

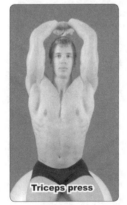
Triceps press

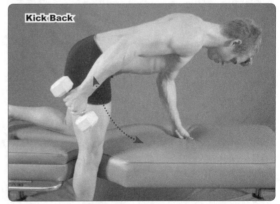
Kick Back

S = stabilization (indifferent hand), ● = contact, ——➤ = examiner force, ·········➤ = patient motion

Elbow

Pin & Stretch treatments can be adapted & applied to any myofascial structure if the clinician has a detailed understanding of basic anatomy & biomechanics
1. Clinician places muscle in shortened position & pins specific myofascial fibers with other hand
2. Patient is then passively moved to lengthen muscle while pinning force is maintained
3. Hold at tension for ~10 seconds or until myofascial release is felt; repeat & reassess as needed

Triceps Deep Head Pin & Stretch

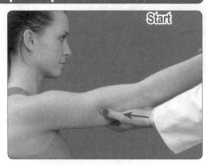
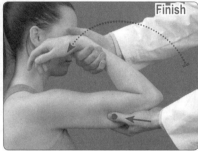

Brachialis Pin & Stretch

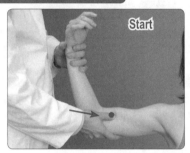
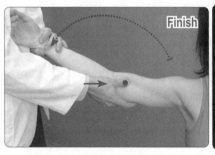

With good anatomy & biomechanical understanding, MET can be adapted to any patient
1. Clinician gently stretches patient into direction of restriction or decreased range of motion
2. Patient gently (~10% of maximum) contracts in exact opposite motion
3. Clinician resists & patient holds contraction for 3-7 seconds, then patient completely relaxes
4. On relaxation, clinician moves to new resistive barrier; repeat 3-5 times & reassess

Elbow Extension Restriction MET

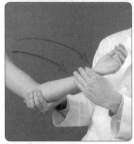
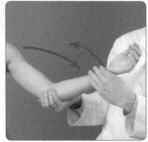
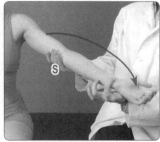

Extension tissue resistance | Patient contracts ~10% in flexion | Clinician finds new end range

S = stabilization (indifferent hand), ● = contact, ——➤ = examiner force, ······➤ = patient motion

Long Axis Distraction

Indications: compression injury, elbow stiffness & adhesion formation

Position: patient seated or supine with elbow flexed ~45°; clinician standing in front of patient

Contact: clinician places web of stabilization hand over anterior distal humerus and grasps ipsilateral distal radius & ulna with other hand

Force: tissue force is S-I; develop tension by gently pulling the distal forearm away from the patient

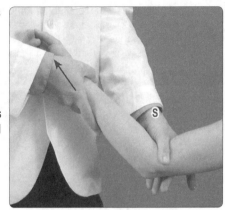

Lateral Glide & Gapping

Indications: restricted lateral glide

Position: patient supine or seated; clinician at head of table

Contact: clinician places

Force: tissue force is L-M; develop tension by gently pushing the affected segment laterally

Clinical notes: this is also the same movement as a 'valgus stress test' at the elbow to check for ulnar collateral ligament damage

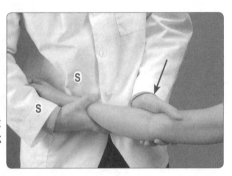

Medial Glide & Gapping

Indications: restricted lateral glide

Position: patient supine or seated; clinician at head of table

Contact: clinician places

Force: tissue force is M-L; develop tension by gently pushing the affected segment laterally

Clinical notes: this is also similar to the movement of a 'varus stress test' at the elbow to check for radial collateral ligament damage

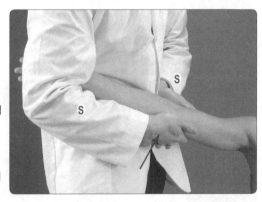

S = stabilization (indifferent hand), ● = contact, ——➤ = examiner force, ·······➤ = patient motion

Elbow

prohealthsys

Anterior Glide Radius on Ulna

Indications: restricted anterior glide of radius

Position: patient seated, standing, supine or prone

Contact: clinician uses thumb contact over posterior radial head & neck

Force: tissue force is P-A

Clinical notes: variation (lower image) shows hypothenar contact over posterior radial head & neck

Maneuver can be performed as a mobilization or manipulation; some clinicians recommend performing manipulation while pronating the patients forearm

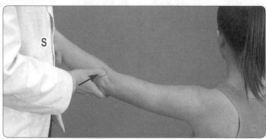

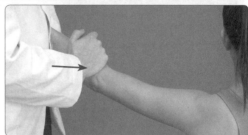

Posterior Glide of Radius on Ulna

Indications: restricted posterior glide of radius

Position: patient seated or supine

Contact: clinician uses thumb contact over posterior radial head & neck

Force: tissue force is A-P

Clinical notes: variation (lower image) shows hypothenar contact over posterior radial head & neck

Maneuver can be performed as a mobilization or manipulation; some clinicians recommend performing manipulation while pronating the patients forearm

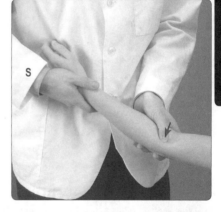

Elbow

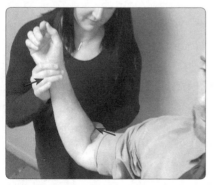

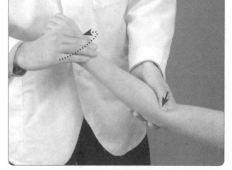

S = stabilization (indifferent hand), 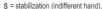 ● = contact, = examiner force, 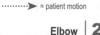 = patient motion

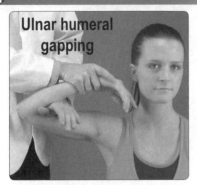

Ulnar humeral gapping

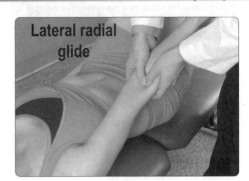

Lateral radial glide

1. Vizniak, NA. Human Cadaver Dissection. 1999-2018
2. Jewell D. Guide to Evidence-Based Physical Therapy Practice. Jones Barlett Publishers Inc. 2017.
3. Iesel SW. Operative Orthopaedics: An Illustrative Approach. Lippincott Williams & Wilkins. 2008.
4. Abbott LC, Saunders JB. Acute traumatic dislocation of tendon of long head of biceps brachii: report of cases with operative findings. Surgery 1939;6:817-840.
5. Abrams WB, Berkow R: The Merck manual of geriatrics, Rahway, NJ, 1990, Merck Sharp & Dohme Research Laboratories.
6. Adams JC, Hamblen DL: Outline oforthopaedics, ed II, Edinburgh, 1990, Churchill Livingstone.
7. Adams, I.e.: Outline of Orthopaedics. London, E & S Livingstone, 1968.
8. Adson AW, Coffey JR. Cervical rib. Ann Surg 1927;85:839-857.
9. Adson AW. Cervical ribs: symptoms, differential diagnosis & indications for section of the insertion of the scalenus anticus muscle. J Coil Int Surg 1951;106:546.
10. Adson, A.W. & 1.R. Coffey: Cervical rib: A method of anterior approach for relief of symptoms by division of the scalenus anticus. Ann. Surg. 85:839-857, 1927.
11. Alario AJ: Practical guide to the care of the pediatric patient, St Louis, 1997, Mosby.
12. Alien. E.V.: Thromboangiitis obliterans: Methods of diagnosis of chronic occlusive arterial lesions distal to the wrist with illustrative cases. Am. 1. Med. Sci. 178:237-244, 1929.
13. Allison D, Strickland N: Acronyms & synonyms in medical imaging, Oxford, 1996, ISIS Medical Media.
14. American Medical Association: Guides to the evaluation of permanent impairment, ed 4, Chicago, 1993, American Medical Association.
15. American Orthopaedic Association: Manual of Orthopaedic Surgery. Chicago, 1972.
16. Anderson KN, Anderson LE: Mosby's pocket dictionary of medicine, nursing, & allied health, ed 2, St Louis, 1994, Mosby.
17. Anderson, I.E.: Grant's Atlas of Anatomy. Baltimore, Williams & Wilkins, 1983.
18. Docherty MA, Schwab RA, Ma OJ. Can elbow extension be used as a test of clinically significant injury? South Med J. 2002;95:539-541.
19. Andrews,).A., L.A. Timmerman, & K.E. Wilk: Baseball. In Pettrone, F.A. (ed.): Athletic Injuries of the Shoulder. New York, McGraw-Hill Inc., 1995.
20. Arntz CT, Jackins S, Matsen FA III. Prosthetic replacement of the shoulder for the treatment of defects in rotator cuff & the surface of the glenohumeral joint, J Bone Joint Surg 75A:485, 1993.
21. Baker, C.L, & S.H. Liu: Neurovascular injuries to the shoulder. 1. Orthop. Sports Phys. Ther. 18:360-364, 1993.
22. Ballinger PW: Merrill's atlas of radiographic positions & radiologic procedures, vol 1-3, ed 8, St Louis, 1995, Mosby.
23. Bankart ASB: Recurrent or habitual dislocation of the shoulder joint. Br Med J 1923; 2: 1132-1133.
24. Barabis J: Therapist's management of thoracic outlet syndrome. In Hunter JM, Schneider LH, Mackin EJ, Callahan AB, editors: Rehabilitation of the hand: surgery & therapy, ed 3, St Louis, 1990, Mosby.
25. Barkauskas VH, Stoltenberg-Allen K, Baumann LC, Darling-Fisher C: Health & physical assessment, ed 2, St Louis, 1998, Mosby.
26. Bassett, L.W., R.H. Gold, & L.L. Seeger: MRI Atlas of the Musculoskeletal System. London, Martin Dunitz Ltd., 1989.
27. Bateman JE: The diagnosis & treatment of ruptures of the rotator cuff, Surg Clin North Am 43:1523, 1963.
28. Bateman, I.E.: The Shoulder & Neck, 2nd ed. Philadelphia, W.B. SaundersCo., 1978.
29. Beetham, W.P., H.F. Policy, C.H. Slocum, & W.F. Weaver: Physical Examination of the joints. Philadelphia, W.B. Saunders Co., 1965.
30. Bernageau, 1.: Roentgenographic assessment of the rotator cuff. Clin. Orthop. 254:87-91, 1990.
31. Berquist T: MRI of the musculoskeletal system, ed 3, Philadelphia, 1996, JB Lippincott.
32. Bigg-Wither, G., & P. Kelly: Diagnostic imaging in musculoskeletal physiotherapy. In Refshauge, K... & E. Gass (eds.): Musculoskeletal Physiotherapy. Oxford, Butterworth-
33. Bigliani, L.U., I.B. Tucker, E.L. Flatow, L.I. Soslowsky, & V.C. Mow: The relationship of

Elbow Quiz (answer page)

1. What are the joint type classifications for this region? (275) _____

2. What are the joint surface shapes for this region (convex/concave)? (275)

   _____

3. What is the normal ROM for _____?
   - Flexion/Ext.: _____, _____
   - Rotation (pron/sup) _____, _____

4. What is the elbow resting position? _____

5. What is the elbow joint tight packed position?

   _____

6. What ligaments resist abduction? (275)

   _____

7. What muscles cause flexion to occur? (275)

   _____

8. The normal carrying angle of the elbow? (275)

   _____

9. During open chain elbow flexion the radius & ulna glide _____ on the humerus? (275)

10. Can you palpate _____ ? (272)

Learning Objectives

After completing this chapter, students will be able to:

1. Perform a regional exam and differentiate common pathologies of the region

2. Identify and palpate body region bony landmarks, ligaments and muscles

3. Discuss regional kinematics and joint organ biomechanics

4. Demonstrate regional AROM, PROM & goniometry, stretch and strengthen protocols

5. Recognize and execute steps of effective mobilization and joint-play including indications, position, contact, force and relevant clinical notes

6. Perform supine, prone, seated assessment and mobilizations including

   - Carpal glides & distraction
   - Radial ulnar glides & distraction
   - Carpal-metacarpal glides & distraction
   - Interphalangeal glides, distraction and rotation

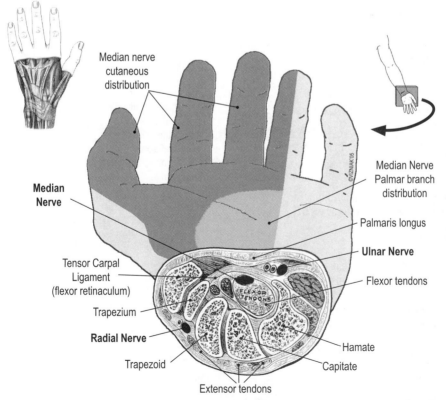

Median nerve cutaneous distribution

Median Nerve

Tensor Carpal Ligament (flexor retinaculum)

Trapezium

Radial Nerve

Trapezoid

Extensor tendons

Median Nerve Palmar branch distribution

Palmaris longus

Ulnar Nerve

Flexor tendons

Hamate

Capitate

Forearm, Wrist & Hand

> **Follow HIP-MNRS** (see Yellow "Physical Assessment" text for specific details or review)
> History, Inspection, Palpation - Motion, Neurovascular screen, Referred pain, Special tests

Special history considerations
- Specific mechanism of injury & forces involved?
  - Did you fall on outstretched hand (FOOSH)?
- Any numbness, tingling or weakness?
- Type of work, typical posture?

Inspection
- Asymmetry, bruising, bumps, color, swelling, height, head tilt
- Posture of neck, body, shoulder

Fracture screen (if indicated)
1. Older than 55? Isometric Test
2. Bony tenderness on palpation
3. Percussion, tuning fork (128 Hz), Ultrasound

Palpation (may be done after ROM assessment)

Wrist flexors	Middle finger (#3)
Pronator teres	Ring finger (#4)
Wrist extensors	Little finger (#5)
Supinator	Scaphoid
Thumb extensors	Lunate
Interossei	Triquetrum, Pisiform
Thenar pad	Lister's tubercle
Hypothenar pad	Hamate
Carpal tunnel	Capitate
Tunnel of Guyon	Trapezoid
Anatomic snuff box	Trapezium
Metacarpals	Ulnar/radial styloids
Thumb (#1)	Triangular fibrocartilage
Index finger (#2)	Collateral ligaments

Functional assessment (ADL)
- Handshake with grip strength

AROM
Wrist
  Flexion ....80°
  Extension ....70°
  Ulnar Flexion ....30°
  Radial Flexion ....20°
Fingers
  Flexion (MP) ......90°
  Extension (MP) ....40°
  Abduction ....20°
  Adduction ....20°

PIP joint
Flexion ....70°
Extension ......0°

DIP joint
Flexion ....80°
Extension ....20°

PROM & Joint Play (if lacking AROM in any motion)

Myotomes (resisted isometric movements)
- Brachioradialis (C5, C6 - radial)
- Biceps (C5, **C6** - musculocutaneous)
- Triceps (C6, **C7**, C8, T1 - radial)
- Wrist extensors (**C6**, C7, C8 - radial)
- Wrist flexors (C6, **C7** - median/ulnar)
- Finger flexors (C7, **C8**, T1 - ulnar/median)
- Interossei (C7, C8, **T1** - ulnar)

Neurovascular screen
- *Sensory:* light touch, two point discrimination, Vibration (3rd digit), Tinel's
- *DTR's:* Biceps (C5), Brachioradialis (C6)
  - Triceps (C7)
- Grip strength (Dynamometer)
- Radial & brachial pulse, blanching, temperature

Orthopedic tests (as indicated)
  Carpal tunnel syndrome
  - Phalen's
  - Tinel's / Median nerve compression test
  - Flick maneuver
  Ulnar neuropathy
  - Tinel's at wrist & elbow
  - Froment's test
  - Wartenberg's test
  Vascular disorder
  - Allen's test, capillary refill
  Tenosynovitis
  - Finkelstein's test
  Instability
  - Valgus/varus stress
  - Lunatotriquetral ballotement
  - Watson's test; Thumb abduction stress test
  TFC tear
  - Press test; TFC dorsal glide test
  Contracture
  - Bunnel-Littler test
  Fracture
  - Scaphoid fracture test

Elbow, shoulder & cervical spine screen

Diagnostic imaging (if indicated)

Joint type: synovial
Gliding (intercarpal)
Ellipsoid (radiocarpal & ulnocarpal)
Pivot (distal radioulnar)
Saddle (trapeziometacarpal)

Main muscle actions
Wrist flexion: flexor carpi radialis & flexor carpi ulnaris, palmaris longus
Wrist extension: extensor carpi radialis longus & brevis, extensor carpi ulnaris, extensor digitorum
Radial flexion (abduction): extensor carpi radialis longus/brevis, flexor carpi radialis
Ulnar flexion (adduction): flexor & extensor carpi ulnaris
Finger flexion: flexor digitorum profundus, superficialis, lumbricals
Thumb flexion: flexor pollicis longus & brevis
Finger extension: extensor digitorum

Thumb extension: extensor pollicis longus & brevis
Abduction: dorsal interossei
Adduction: palmar interossei

Normal joint end feels
Radiocarpal flex/ext: firm ligamentous
Radiocarpal add/abd: bony

CMC thumb: elastic
MCP extension: elastic / ligamentous
MCP flexion: firm / ligamentous
MCP thumb: firm / bony

PIP flexion: firm / bony
PIP extension: firm / ligamentous
DIP flexion: firm / ligamentous / elastic
DIP extension: firm / ligamentous / elastic

Wrist/Hand	Clinical notes
Carpal tunnel syndrome	*Hx:* insidious onset; paresthesia into hand; loss of digital dexterity *SSx:* (+) Tinel's, Phalen's test; ↓ sensation over median nerve distribution in hand *DDx:* pronator teres syndrome, thoracic outlet syndrome, C6-C7 radiculopathy
de Quervain's tenosynovitis	*Hx:* aching pain above radial styloid; worse with wrist & thumb movements *SSx:* (+) Finkelstein's test; audible squeaking sound with wrist movement *DDx:* scaphoid fracture, osteoarthrosis
Gamekeeper's thumb	*Hx:* traumatic extension or abduction of thumb; pain over ulnar side of MCP joint *SSx:* (+) thumb abduction test; UCL instability *DDx:* scaphoid fracture, Bennett fracture, osteoarthrosis
Wrist Sprain	*Hx:* traumatic extension or flexion of wrist (FOOSH) *SSx:* palpable tenderness over ligaments, limited AROM & PROM (+) bracelet test *DDx:* scaphoid fracture, TFC tear, rheumatoid or septic arthritis
Ganglion cyst	*Hx:* painful or painless lump or mass on wrist, weight bearing aggravates (push-up) *SSx:* palpable, solid mass, may be tender to palpation *DDx:* infection, carpal subluxation
Lunate dislocation	*Hx:* FOOSH (fall on out stretched hand) or impact trauma to hand *SSx:* tenderness in wrist in line with 3rd metacarpal; visible on x-ray (spilled tea cup) *DDx:* lunate or scaphoid fracture, osteoarthrosis
Scaphoid fracture	*Hx:* FOOSH (fall on out stretched hand) or impact trauma to hand *SSx:* pain in anatomical snuff box with radial flexion; (+) scaphoid fracture test *DDx:* lunate dislocation, osteoarthrosis
TFC Tear	*Hx:* FOOSH (fall on out stretched hand) or impact trauma to hand with twisting *SSx:* local pain with ROM; possible ↓ ROM & grip strength; (+) TFC dorsal glide *DDx:* lunate dislocation, ulnar styloid fracture, osteoarthrosis

↑ = increase, ↓ = decrease, Hx = history, SSx = signs & symptoms, DDx = differential diagnosis, (+) = positive, TFC = triangular fibrocartilage
FOOSH = Fall On Out Stretched Hand - see blue 'Orthopedic Conditions' and yellow 'Physical Assessment' texts for more details

Forearm, Wrist & Hand

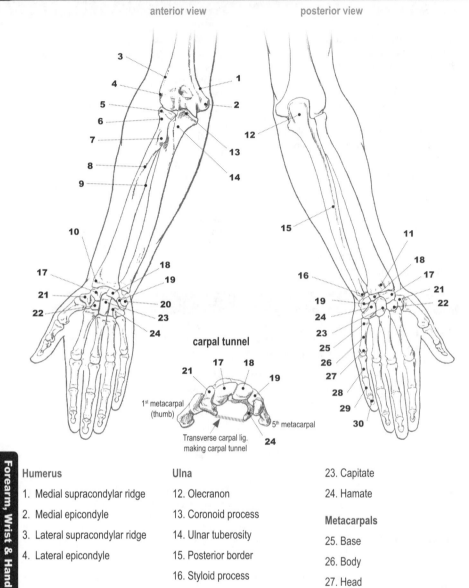

anterior view   posterior view

carpal tunnel

1st metacarpal (thumb)

5th metacarpal

Transverse carpal lig. making carpal tunnel

Humerus

1. Medial supracondylar ridge
2. Medial epicondyle
3. Lateral supracondylar ridge
4. Lateral epicondyle

Radius

5. Head
6. Neck
7. Radial / bicipital tuberosity
8. Oblique line
9. Interosseous border
10. Styloid process
11. Dorsal (Lister's) tubercle

Ulna

12. Olecranon
13. Coronoid process
14. Ulnar tuberosity
15. Posterior border
16. Styloid process

Carpals

17. Scaphoid
18. Lunate
19. Triquetrum
20. Pisiform
21. Trapezium
22. Trapezoid

23. Capitate
24. Hamate

Metacarpals

25. Base
26. Body
27. Head

Phalanges

28. Proximal
29. Middle
30. Distal

Forearm, Wrist & Hand

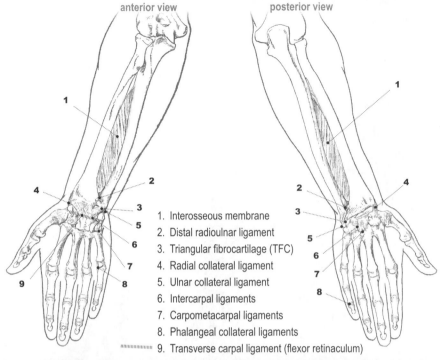

anterior view   posterior view

1. Interosseous membrane
2. Distal radioulnar ligament
3. Triangular fibrocartilage (TFC)
4. Radial collateral ligament
5. Ulnar collateral ligament
6. Intercarpal ligaments
7. Carpometacarpal ligaments
8. Phalangeal collateral ligaments
9. Transverse carpal ligament (flexor retinaculum)

Ligament	Attaches (origin/insertion)	Function
Interosseous membrane	Shafts of radius & ulna	Resists separation of radius & ulna, attachment point for forearm muscles
Radial Collateral	Radius to scaphoid, trapezium	Supports lateral side of wrist (resists valgus forces)
Ulnar Collateral	Ulna to pisiform, triquetrum	Supports medial side of wrist (resists varus forces)
Dorsal Radiocarpal	Lower end of radius to scaphoid, lunate, triquetrum	Connects radius to carpals; supports posterior side of wrist
Palmar Intercarpal	Scaphoid to lunate, triquetrum	Holds carpals together
Palmar Plates	Across anterior joint of MP, PIP, DIP	Supports anterior MP, PIP, & DIP joint
Palmar Radiocarpal	Lower radius to scaphoid, lunate, triquetrum	Connects radius to carpals; supports anterior side of wrist
Dorsal Intercarpal	First row of carpals to second row of carpals	Holds carpals together
Deep Transverse	MP of finger to MP of adjacent finger	Taught in finger flexing, disallowing abduction
Collateral	Phalanx to phalanx, sides of MCP, PIP & DIP joints	Supports sides of fingers; resists varus/valgus force

Forearm, Wrist & Hand

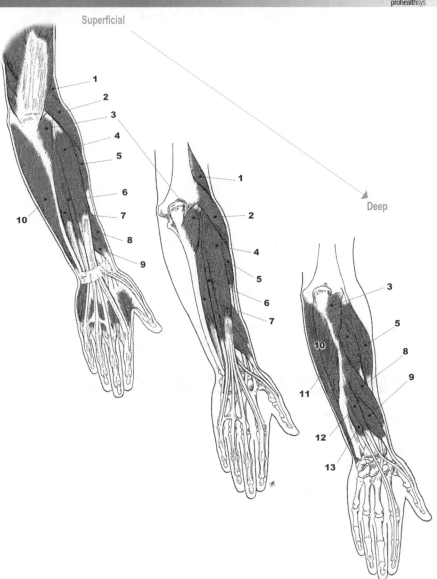

Superficial

Deep

1. Brachioradialis
2. Extensor carpi radialis longus
3. Anconeus
4. Extensor digitorum
5. Extensor carpi radialis brevis
6. Extensor digiti minimi
7. Extensor carpi ulnaris
8. Abductor pollicis longus
9. Extensor pollicis brevis
10. Flexor carpi ulnaris
11. Supinator
12. Extensor pollicis longus
13. Extensor indicis

Forearm, Wrist & Hand

prohealthsys

1. Brachioradialis
2. Pronator teres (superficial head)
3. Flexor carpi radialis
4. Palmaris longus
5. Flexor carpi ulnaris
6. Flexor digitorum superficialis
7. Flexor digitorum profundus
8. Flexor pollicis longus
9. Pronator teres (deep head)
10. Supinator
11. Pronator quadratus
12. Thenar muscles
13. 1st Dorsal interosseus
14. Hypothenar muscles

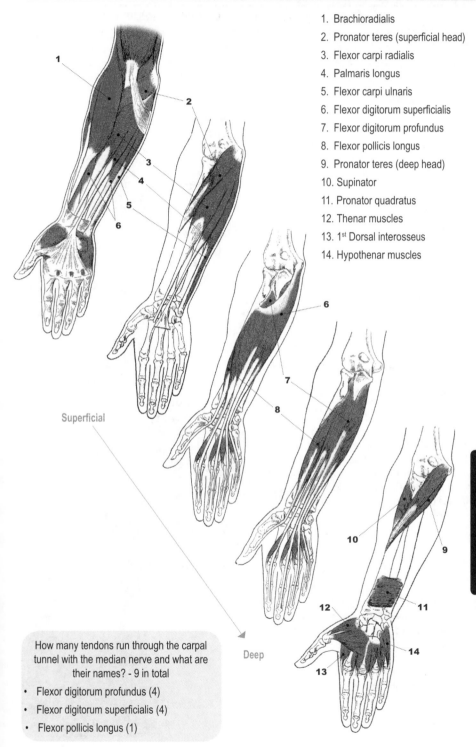

Superficial

Deep

Forearm, Wrist & Hand

How many tendons run through the carpal
tunnel with the median nerve and what are
their names? - 9 in total

- Flexor digitorum profundus (4)
- Flexor digitorum superficialis (4)
- Flexor pollicis longus (1)

prohealthsys

Compare bilaterally, start with unaffected side for PROM & MMT
Prior to assessing ROM the examiner should make an introduction statement:
"Try and move as far as possible, if any of the actions or movements are painful or uncomfortable please let me know, do not do any action you feel will cause you further injury."

AROM

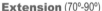

Flexion (75°-90°)
Muscles Activated: flexor carpi radialis & flexor carpi ulnaris, palmaris longus, flexor digitorum superficialis & profundus
Tissue Stretched: extensor carpi radialis longus & brevis, extensor carpi ulnaris, extensor digitorum, posterior carpal ligaments
Tissue Compressed: carpal tunnel & median nerve

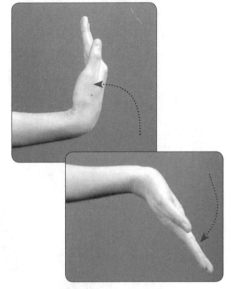

Extension (70°-90°)
Muscles Activated: extensor carpi radialis longus & brevis, extensor carpi ulnaris, extensor digitorum
Tissue Stretched: flexor carpi radialis & flexor carpi ulnaris, palmaris longus, flexor digitorum superficialis & profundus
Tissue Compressed: posterior carpal ligaments

Abduction (radial flexion) (15°-25°)
Muscles Activated: extensor carpi radialis longus/ brevis, flexor carpi radialis
Tissue Stretched: flexor & extensor carpi ulnaris, medial carpal ligament, triangular fibrocartilage
Tissue Compressed: lateral carpal ligaments, scaphoid & trapezium

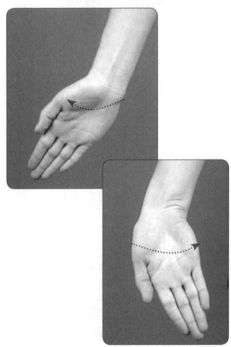

Adduction (ulnar flexion) (20°-35°)
Muscles Activated: flexor & extensor carpi ulnaris
Tissue Stretched: extensor carpi radialis longus/ brevis, flexor carpi radialis, lateral carpal ligaments
Tissue Compressed: medial carpal ligaments, hamate & triquetrum, TFC

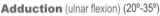
Forearm, Wrist & Hand

prohealthsys

PROM

Flexion (> 75º-90º)
Tissue Stretched: extensor carpi radialis longus & brevis, extensor carpi ulnaris, extensor digitorum, anterior carpal ligaments
Tissue Compressed: carpal tunnel & median nerve

Extension (> 70º-90º)
Tissue Stretched: flexor carpi radialis & flexor carpi ulnaris, palmaris longus, flexor digitorum superficialis & profundus
Tissue Compressed: posterior carpal ligaments

Abduction (radial flexion) (> 15º-25º)
Tissue Stretched: flexor & extensor carpi ulnaris, medial carpal ligament, triangular fibrocartilage
Tissue Compressed: lateral carpal ligaments, scaphoid & trapezium

Adduction (ulnar flexion) (> 20º-35º)
Tissue Stretched: extensor carpi radialis longus/brevis, flexor carpi radialis, lateral carpal ligaments
Tissue Compressed: medial carpal ligaments, hamate & triquetrum, TFC (triangular fibrocartilage)

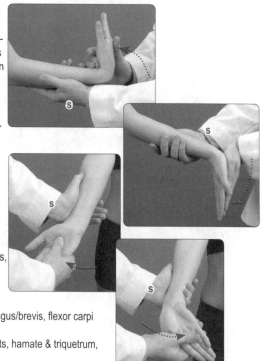

Wrist Goniometry

Flexion (normal 80º-90º)
- Patient seated, forearm supinated
- Fulcrum aligned with midcarpal joint
- Stationary arm in line with ulna; moving arm is parallel to the fifth metacarpal
- Ask patient to flex wrist

Extension (normal: 70º-90º)
- Same as flexion except ask patient to extend wrist

Abduction (radial flexion) (15º)
- Patient seated, forearm supinated
- Fulcrum aligned over mid-carpal joint
- Stationary arm in midline forearm; moving arm parallel to the 3rd metacarpal
- Ask patient to abduct wrist

Adduction (ulnar flexion) (30º-45º)
- Same as abduction except, ask patient to adduct wrist

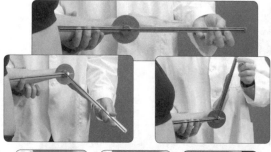
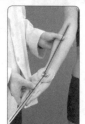
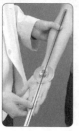
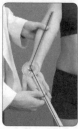

Forearm, Wrist & Hand

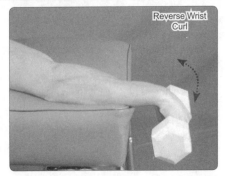

Wrist Curl

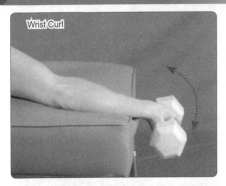

Reverse Wrist Curl

Pronator Twist

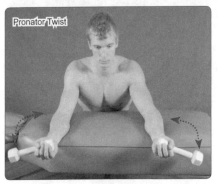

Supinator Twist

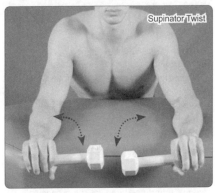

Finger Curl

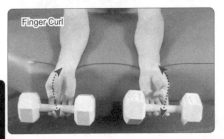

Wrist Hammer Curl

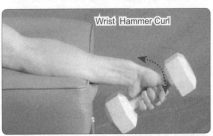

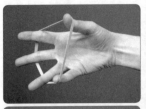

Elastic Band
Exercises

Grip strength
(squeeze tennis
ball or racket
ball)

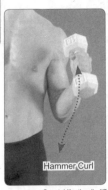

Hammer Curl

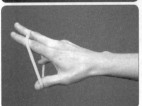

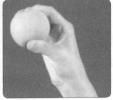

S = stabilization (indifferent hand), ● = contact, ⟶ = examiner force, ┄┄► = patient motion

Forearm, Wrist & Hand

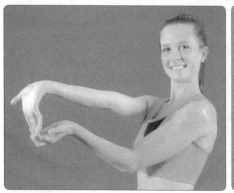

Flexor Stretch:
- Elbow straight, wrist extended, use opposite hand to pull fingers back

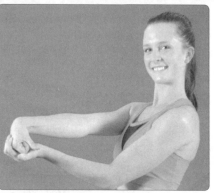

Extensor Stretch:
- Elbow straight, wrist flexed & hand in a fist, use opposite hand to apply flexion pressure

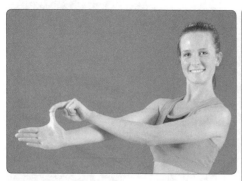

Thumb Extension Stretch:
- Elbow straight, wrist extended, use opposite hand to pull distal phalanx of thumb into extension

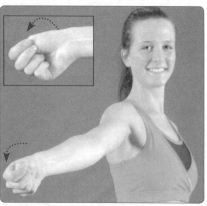

Thumb Flexion Stretch

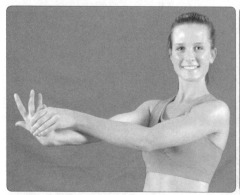

Self Stretch:
- Elbow straight, wrist flexed & supinated, use opposite hand to apply flexion pressure over the hand

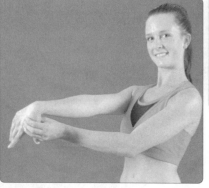

Self Stretch:
- Elbow straight, wrist flexed & pronated, use opposite hand to apply pressure over wrist

S = stabilization (indifferent hand), ● = contact, ———▶ = examiner force, **Patient handouts**

Forearm, Wrist & Hand

Pin & Stretch treatments can be adapted & applied to any myofascial structure if the clinician has a detailed understanding of basic anatomy & biomechanics

1. Clinician places muscle in shortened position & pins specific myofascial fibers with other hand
2. Patient is then passively moved to lengthen muscle while pinning force is maintained
3. Hold at tension for ~10 seconds or until myofascial release is felt; repeat & reassess as needed

Flexor Carpi Ulnaris

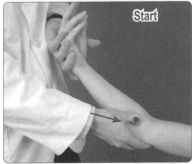

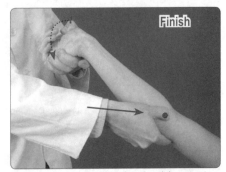

- Elbow slightly flexed, wrist neutral; pin origin
- Elbow straight, extend wrist; pin origin

Extensor Carpi Radialis Brevis

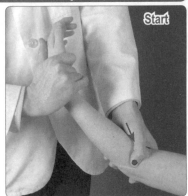

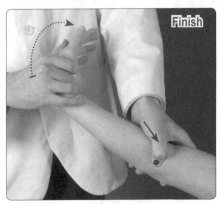

- Wrist neutral; pin origin
- Flex wrist; pin origin

Extensor Indicis

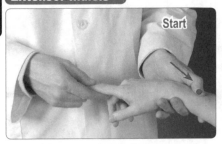

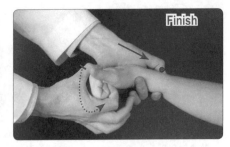

- Finger straight, wrist neutral; pin origin
- Flex finger (also consider flexing wrist); pin origin

S = stabilization (indifferent hand), ● = contact, ⟶ = examiner force, ┄┄┄▶ = patient motion

Forearm, Wrist & Hand

With good anatomy & biomechanical understanding, MET can be adapted to any patient

1. Clinician gently stretches patient into direction of restriction or decreased range of motion
2. Patient gently (10% of maximum) contracts in exact opposite motion
3. Clinician resists & patient holds contraction for 3-7 seconds, then patient completely relaxes
4. On relaxation, clinician moves to new resistive barrier; repeat 3-5 times & reassess

Wrist Extension Restriction MET

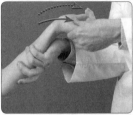
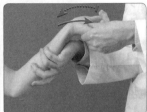
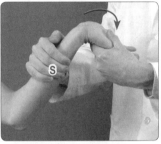

Extension tissue resistance   Patient contracts ~10% in flexion

Clinician finds new end range

Wrist Flexion Restriction MET

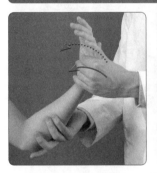
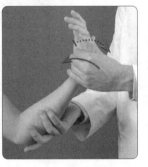
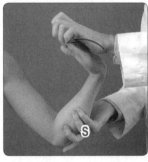

Flexion tissue resistance   Patient contracts ~10% in extension   Clinician finds new end range

Wrist Supination Restriction MET

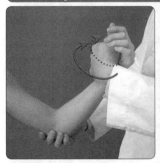
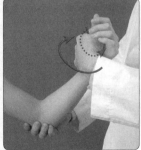
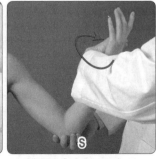

Supination tissue resistance   Patient contracts ~10% in pronation   Clinician finds new end range

S = stabilization (indifferent hand),   ● = contact,   ⟶ = examiner force,   ⋯⋯▷ = patient motion

Forearm, Wrist & Hand

prohealthsys

Posterior & Anterior Carpal Glide

Indications: restricted anterior or posterior carpal glide

Position: patient seated, standing, supine or prone with wrist in neutral position

Contact: clinician uses a web thumb grip

Force: A-P or P-A for is applied to mobilize carpals in desired direction

Clinical notes: not that this is a general carpal mobilization, by using an digital/thumb contact individual carpal bones may be mobilized

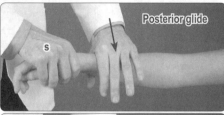

Posterior glide

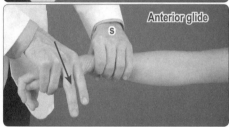

Anterior glide

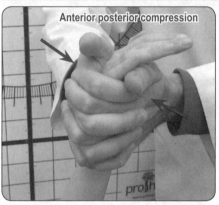

Anterior posterior compression

Direct bilateral wrist/hand compression offers one of the best mobilizations - most patients love having this done!

Carpal Mobilization

Indications: restricted anterior or posterior carpal glide

Position: patient seated, standing, supine or prone with wrist in neutral position

Contact: pincer grip (anterior & posterior stabilization) over adjacent carpal bones

Force: A-P or P-A for is applied to mobilize carpals in desired direction

Clinical notes: not that this is a general carpal mobilization, by using an digital/thumb contact individual carpal bones may be mobilized individually

Caution is warranted for compression of the median nerve with A-P pressure over the lunate

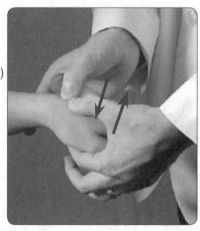

S = stabilization (indifferent hand), ● = contact, ——————▶ = examiner force, ·········▶ = patient motion

Forearm, Wrist & Hand

Specific Mobilization Vatiations

Clinical notes: below are sample of variations that may be applied
to specific carpal bone restrictions or malpositions

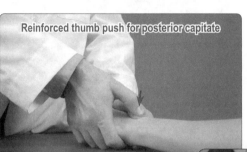
Reinforced thumb push for posterior capitate

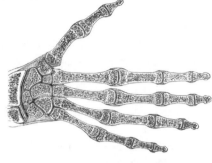

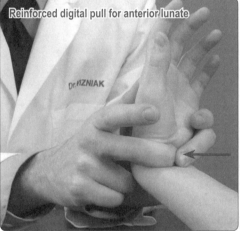
Reinforced digital pull for anterior lunate

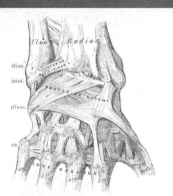

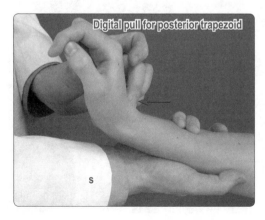
Digital pull for posterior trapezoid

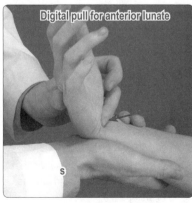
Digital pull for anterior lunate

Forearm, Wrist & Hand

S = stabilization (indifferent hand), ● = contact, ⟶ = examiner force, ·········▷ = patient motion

prohealthsys

Long Axis Distraction & Compression

Indications: restricted distraction or compression of carpals

Position: patient seated, standing, supine or prone with wrist in neutral position

Contact: clinician uses a web thumb grip contact

Force: long axis distraction or compression is applied to mobilize carpals in desired direction

Clinical notes: by using an digital/thumb contact individual carpal bones may be mobilized; maneuver can be performed as a mobilization or manipulation

Variation - examiner applies lateral compressive force around the distal radius & ulna (at the location of patient wearing a bracelet)

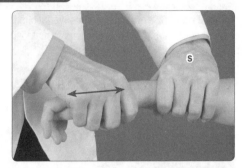

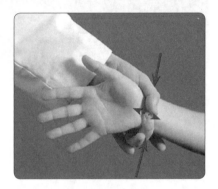

Valgus & Varus Glide

Indications: restricted wrist abduction or adduction

Position: patient seated, standing, supine or prone with wrist in neutral position

Contact: clinician stabilizes proximal wrist

Force: valgus (M-L) or varus (L-M) applied to mobilize carpals in desired direction

Clinical notes: maneuver can be performed as a mobilization or manipulation - these motions are essentially the same as passive ROM assessment

Remember for a valgus movement the distal part of the joint moves laterally

A varus load may cause medial wrist pain in the presence of a triangular fibrocartilage tear

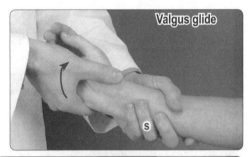

Valgus glide

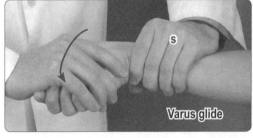

Varus glide

S = stabilization (indifferent hand), ● = contact, ⟶ = examiner force, ·····▷ = patient motion

Forearm, Wrist & Hand

Carpal Lateral Distraction

Indications: restricted lateral carpal glide

Position: patient seated, standing, supine or prone with wrist in neutral position

Contact: clinician uses bilateral thenar contact

Force: lateral distraction force is applied to mobilize carpals in desired direction

Clinical notes: not that this is a general carpal mobilization, by using an digital/thumb contact individual carpal bones may be mobilized

Instrument assisted mobilization may also offer specific treatment - excessive treatment may damage the median nerve and the patient may experience numbness tingling or weakness

In patients with carpal tunnel syndrome this method may be used to help stretch the flexor retinaculum

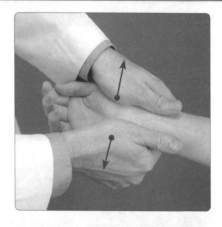

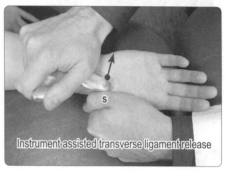

Instrument assisted transverse ligament release

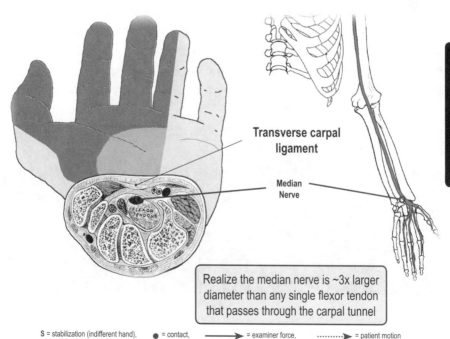

Transverse carpal ligament

Median Nerve

Realize the median nerve is ~3x larger diameter than any single flexor tendon that passes through the carpal tunnel

Forearm, Wrist & Hand

S = stabilization (indifferent hand),   ● = contact,   ⟶ = examiner force,   ·········▷ = patient motion

Distraction & Compression

Indications: restricted digital distraction or static malposition

Position: patient seated, standing, supine or prone with wrist in neutral position

Contact: clinician stabilizes bones on either side of joint

Force: distraction or compression force is applied to mobilize in desired direction

Clinical notes: maneuver can be performed as a mobilization or manipulation

Note that mobilization & manipulation are contraindicated following significant trauma (fracture risk) or moderate to severe local joint inflammation (RA, septic arthritis, etc.)

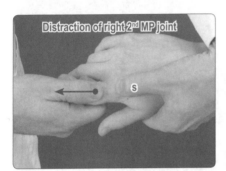

Distraction of right 2nd MP joint

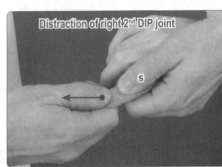

Distraction of right 2nd DIP joint

A-P & P-A Glide

Indications: restricted digital A-P or P-A glide or static malposition

Position: patient seated, standing, supine or prone with wrist in neutral position

Contact: clinician stabilizes bones on either side of joint

Force: A-P or P-A force is applied to mobilize in desired direction

Clinical notes: maneuver can be performed as a mobilization or manipulation

Note that mobilization & manipulation are contraindicated following significant trauma (fracture risk) or moderate to severe local joint inflammation (RA, septic arthritis, etc.)

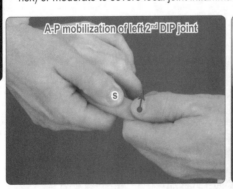

A-P mobilization of left 2nd DIP joint

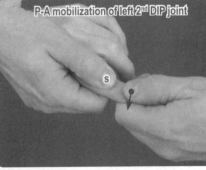

P-A mobilization of left 2nd DIP joint

Forearm, Wrist & Hand

M-L & L-M Glide

Indications: restricted digital M-L or L-M glide or static malposition

Position: patient seated, standing, supine or prone with wrist in neutral position

Contact: clinician stabilizes bones on either side of joint

Force: M-L or L-M force is applied to mobilize in desired direction

Clinical notes: maneuver can be performed as a mobilization or manipulation

Note that mobilization & manipulation are contraindicated following significant trauma (fracture risk) or moderate to severe local joint inflammation (RA, septic arthritis, etc.)

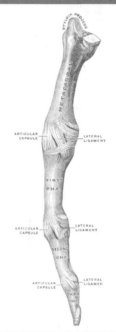

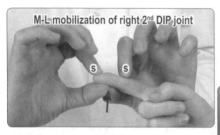

M-L mobilization of right 2nd DIP joint

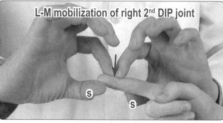

L-M mobilization of right 2nd DIP joint

Rotation

Indications: restricted rotation or rotational malposition

Position: patient seated, standing, supine or prone with wrist in neutral position

Contact: clinician stabilizes bones on either side of joint

Force: rotational force is applied to mobilize in desired direction

Clinical notes: maneuver can be performed as a mobilization or manipulation

Note that mobilization & manipulation are contraindicated following significant trauma (fracture risk) or moderate to severe local joint inflammation (RA, septic arthritis, etc.)

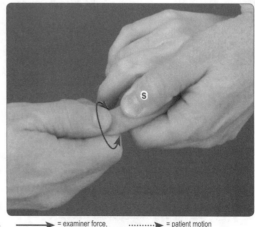

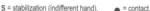
S = stabilization (indifferent hand), ● = contact, ⟶ = examiner force, ·······▷ = patient motion

Forearm, Wrist & Hand

1. Vizniak. Human Cadaver Dissection. 1999-2018.
2. McGee S. Evidence-Based Physical Diagnosis. Saunders. 2017.
3. Magee D. Orthopedic Physical Assessment, 5th Edition. Saunders. 2008.
4. Taylor MH, Monroe LG. Physical Rehabilitation: Evidence-Based Examination, Evaluation and Intervention. Saunders. 2007.
5. Warlow C, Hughes R, Uitehaag B, Liberati A. Evidence-Based Neurology. Blackwell Publishing Limited, BMJI Books. 2007.
6. Malanga GA & Nadler. Musculoskeletal Physical Exam, An Evidence-Based Approach. Mosby. 2006.
7. Hoppenfield S. Physical Examination of the Spine & Extremities. Lippincott Williams & Wilkins. 1976.
8. Hoppenfield S. Orthopaedic Neurology: A Diagnostic Guide to Neurologic Levels. Lippincott Williams & Wilkins. 1977.
9. Spencer JW, Jacobs JJ. Complementary and Alternative Medicine: An Evidence-Based Approach. Mosby. 2003.
10. Jewell D. Guide to Evidence-Based Physical Therapy Practice. Jones Barlett Publishers Inc. 2007.
11. Iesel SW. Operative Orthopaedics: An Illustrative Approach. Lippincott Williams & Wilkins. 2008.
12. Ahn DS. Hand elevation: a new test for carpal tunnel syndrome. Ann Plast Surg. 2001;46:120-124.
13. Alexander RD, Catalano LW, Barron OA, Glickel SZ. The extensor pollicis brevis entrapment test in the treatment of de Quervain's disease. J Hand Surg [Am]. 2002;27:81 3-81 6.
14. Amirfeyz R, Gozzard C, Leslie Ii. Hand elevation test for assessment of carpal tunnel syndrome. J Hand Surg [Br]. 2005;30:361 -364.
15. Atroshi I, Breidenbach WC, McCabe Si. Assessment of the carpal tunnel outcome instrument in patients with nerve-compression symptoms. J Hand Surg Am]. 1997;22:222-227.
16. Bland JD. The value of the history in the diagnosis of carpal tunnel syndrome. J Hand Surg [Br]. 2000;25:445-450.
17. Borg K, Lindblom U. Diagnostic value of quantitative sensory testing (QST) in patients with carpal tunnel syndrome. Acta Neurol Scand. 1988; 78:537-541.
18. Borg K, Lindblom U. Increase of vibration threshold during wrist flexion in patients with carpal tunnel syndrome. Pain. 1986;26:211-219.
19. Buch-Jaeger N, Foucher G. Correlation of clinical signs with nerve conduction tests in the diagnosis of carpal tunnel syndrome. J Hand Surg [Br.]. 1 994;1 9:720-724.
20. Buehler Mi, Thayer DT. The elbow flexion test. A clinical test for the cubital tunnel syndrome. C/in Orthop Re/at Res. 1988;21 3-216.
21. Burke DT, Burke MA, Bell R, Stewart GW, Mehdi RS, Kim Hi. Subjective swelling: a new sign for carpal tunnel syndrome. Am J Phys Med Rehab. 1999;78:504-508.
22. Buterbaugh GA, Brown TR, Horn PC. Ulnar-sided wrist pain in athletes. Clin Sports Med. 1998;1 7:567-583.
23. Cherniack MG, Moalli D, Viscolli C. A comparison of traditional electrodiagnostic studies, electroneurometry, & vibrometry in the diagnosis of carpal tunnel syndrome. J Hand Surg [Am]. 1 996;21 :122-131.
24. Cozen L. The painful elbow. Ind Med Surg. 1962;31 :369-371.
25. de Krom MC, Knipschild PC, Kester AD, Spaans F. Efficacy of provocative tests for diagnosis of carpal tunnel syndrome. Lancet. 1990;335:393-395.
26. Docherty MA, Schwab RA, Ma OJ. Can elbow extension be used as a test of clinically significant injury? South Med J. 2002;95:539-541.
27. Durkan JA. The carpal-compression test: an instrumented device for diagnosing carpal tunnel syndrome. Orthop Rev. 1994;23:522-525.
28. Durkan iA. A new diagnostic test for carpal tunnel syndrome. 1 Bone Joint Surg Am. 1991;73:535-538.

29. Easterling Ki, Wolfe SW. Scaphoid shift in the uninjured wrist. J Hand Surg [Am]. 1 994;19:604-606.
30. Edwards A. Phalen's test with carpal compression: testing in diabetics for the diagnosis of carpal tunnel syndrome. Orthopedics. 2002;25:519-520.
31. Etson RA. Rupture of the central slip of the extensor hood of the finger: a test for early diagnosis. I Bone Joint Surg Br. 1986;68:229-231.
32. Fertl E, Wober C, Zeitlhofer J. The serial use of two provocative tests in the clinical diagnosis of carpal tunnel syndrome. Acta Neurol Scand. 1998;98:328-332.
33. Finkelstein H. Stenosing tenovaginatis at the radial styloid process. J Bone Joint Surg 1 930;12:9-540.
34. Gellman H, Gelberman RH, Tan AM, Botte MJ. Carpal tunnel syndrome: an evaluation of the provocative diagnostic tests. / Bone Joint Surg Am. 1986;68:735-737.
35. Gelmers HJ. The significance of Tinel's sign in the diagnosis of carpal tunnel syndrome. Acta Neurochir (Wien). 1 979;49:255-258.
36. Gerr F, Letz R. The sensitivity & specificity of tests for carpal tunnel syndrome vary with the comparison subjects. I Hand Surg [Br]. 1998; 23:151-1 55.
37. Gerr F, Letz R, Harris-Abbott D, Hopkins LC. Sensitivity & specificity of vibrometry for detection of carpal tunnel syndrome. I Occup Environ Med. 1995;37:1108-1115.
38. Golding DN, Rose DM, Selvarajah K. Clinical tests for carpal tunnel syndrome: an evaluation. Br] Rheumatol. 1 986;25:388-390.
39. Gonzalez del Pino J, Delgado-Martinez AD, Gonzalez I, Lovic A. Value of the carpal compression test in the diagnosis of carpal tunnel syndrome. J Hand Surg [Br]. 1 997;22:38-41.
40. Gunnarsson LG, Amilon A, Hellstrand P, Leissner P, Philipson L. The diagnosis of carpal tunnel syndrome: sensitivity & specificity of some clinical & electrophysiological tests. J Hand Surg [Br]. 1997;22:34-37.
41. Gupta SK, Benstead Ti. Symptoms experienced by patients with carpal tunnel syndrome. Can J Neuro Sci. 1997;24:338-342.
42. Hansen PA, Micktesen P, Robinson LR. Clinical utility of the flick maneuver in diagnosing carpal tunnel syndrome. Am J Phys Med Rehab. 2004;83:363-367.
43. Helter L, Ring H, Costeff H, Solzi P. Evaluation of Tinel's & Phalen's signs in diagnosis of the carpal tunnel syndrome. Ear Neuro. 1 986;25:40-42.
44. Heyman P, Gelberman RH, Duncan K, Hipp JA. Injuries of the ulnar collateral ligament of the thumb metacarpophalangeal joint. Biomechanical & prospective clinical studies on the usefulness of valgus stress testing. Clin Orthop Relat Res. 1993:165-171.
45. Johnson RP, Carrera CF. Chronic capitolunate instability. J Bone Joint Surg Am. 1986;68:1164-1176.
46. Karl AI, Carney ML, Kaul MP. The lumbrical provocation test in subjects with median inclusive paresthesia. Arch Phys Med Rehab. 2001 ;82:935-937.
47. Katz JN, Larson MC, Sabra A, et at. The carpal tunnel syndrome: diagnostic utility of the history & physical examination findings. Ann Intern Med. 1 990;112:321-327.
48. Katz JN, Stirrat CR. A self-administered hand diagram for the diagnosis of carpal tunnel syndrome. J Hand Surg [Am]. 1990;15:360-363.
49. Kaul MP, Pagel KJ, Dryden JD. Lack of predictive power of the "tethered" median stress test in suspected carpal tunnel syndrome. Arch Phys Med Rehab 2000;81:348-350.
50. Kaul MP, Pagel KJ, Wheatley Mi, Dryden JD. Carpal compression test & pressure provocative test in veterans with median-distribution paresthesias. Muscle Nerve. 2001 ;24:107-111.
51. Koris M, Gelberman RH, Duncan K, Boublick M, Smith B. Carpal tunnel syndrome. Evaluation of a quantitative provocational diagnostic test. Clin Orthop Relat Res. 1990:157-161.

52. Kuhlman KA, Hennessey WJ. Sensitivity & specificity of carpal tunnel syndrome signs. Am J Phys Med Rehab. 1997;76:451-457.
53. LaBan MM, Friedman NA, Zemenick GA. "Tethered" median nerve stress test in chronic carpal tunnel syndrome. Arch Phys Med Reha. 1986;67:803-804.
54. Laioie AS, McCabe Si, Thomas B, Edgelt SE. Determining the sensitivity & specificity of common diagnostic tests for carpal tunnel syndrome using latent class analysis. Plast Reconstr Surg. 2005;116:502-507.
55. Lane LB. The scaphoid shift test. J Hand Surg [Am]. 1993;18:366-368.
56. LaStayo P, Howell j. Clinical provocative tests used in evaluating wrist pain: a descriptive study. J I-Iand Ther. 1 995;8:10-17.
57. Lester B, Halbrecht i1 Levy IM, Gaudinez R. "Press test" for office diagnosis of triangular fibrocartilage complex tears of the wrist. Ann Plast Surg. 1995;35:41-45.
58. MacDermid iC, Kramer JF, Roth JH. Decision making in detecting abnormal Semmes-Weinstein monofilament thresholds in carpal tunnel syndrome. J Hand Ther. 1994;7:1 58-1 62.
59. Molitor Pi. A diagnostic test for carpal tunnel syndrome using ultrasound. J Hand Surg [Br]. 1988;13:40-41.
60. Mondelli M, Passero 5, Giannini F. Provocative tests in different stages of carpal tunnel syndrome. C/in Neurol/ Neurosurg. 2001;103:178-183.
61. Mossman SS, Blau JN. Tinel's sign & the carpal tunnel syndrome. Br Med J(Clin Res Ed). 1987;294:680.
62. Novak CB, Lee CW, Mackinnon SE, Lay L. Provocative testing for cubital tunnel syndrome. J Hand Surg [Am]. 1994;19:817-820.
63. O'Driscoll SW, Bell DF, Morrey BF. Posterolateral rotatory instability of the elbow. J Bone Joint Surg Am. 1991;73:440-446.
64. O'Driscoll SW, Lawton RL, Smith AM. The "moving valgus stress test" for medial collateral ligament tears of the elbow. Am J Sports Med. 2005;33:231-239.
65. O'Gradaigh D, Merry P. A diagnostic algorithm for carpal tunnel syndrome based on Bayes's theorem. Rheumatology (Oxford). 2000; 39:1040-1041.
66. Pagel Ki, Kaul MP, Dryden JD. Lack of utility of Semmes-Weinstein monofilament testing in suspected carpal tunnel syndrome. Am J Phys Med Rehab. 2002;81:597-600.
67. Paley D, McMurtry R. Median nerve compression test in carpal tunnel syndrome diagnosis: reproduces signs & symptoms in affected wrist. Orthop Rev. 1985;14:41-45.
68. Patel MR, Bassini L. A comparison of five tests for determining hand sensibility. J Reconstr Microsurg. 1 999;15:523-526.
69. Phalen CS. The carpal-tunnel syndrome: seventeen years' experience in diagnosis & treatment of six hundred fifty-four hands. J Bone Joint Surg Am. 1966;48:211-228.
70. Pryse-Phillips WE. Validation of a diagnostic sign in carpal tunnel syndrome. J Neurol Neurosurg Psychiatry. 1984;47:870-872.
71. Radecki P. A gender specific wrist ratio & the likelihood of a median nerve abnormality at the carpal tunnel. Am J Phys Med Rehab. 1994;73:157-162.
72. Rayan CM, Jensen C, DukeJ. Elbow flexion test in the normal population. J Hand Surg [Am]. 1992;1 7:86-89.
73. Reagan DS, Linscheid RL, Dobyns JH. Lunotriquetral sprains. J Hand Surg [Am]. 1984;9:502-514.
74. Ruland RT, Dunbar RP, Bowen JD. The Biceps squeeze test for diagnosis of distal Biceps tendon ruptures. Clin Orthop Relat Res. 2005:128-131.
75. Seror P. Phalen's test in the diagnosis of carpal tunnel syndrome. J Hand Surg [Br] 1 988;13:383-385.
76. Seror P. Tinel's sign in the diagnosis of carpal tunnel syndrome. J Hand Surg [Br]. 1987;12:364-365.
77. Spindler HA, Dellon AL. Nerve conduction studies & sensibility testing in carpal tunnel syndrome. J Hand Surg [Am]. 1982;7:260-263.
78. Stewart iD, Eisen A. Tinel's sign & the carpal tunnel syndrome. Br

Wrist & Hand Quiz (answer page)

1. What are the joint type classifications for this region? (285) _____

2. What are the joint surface shapes for this region (convex/concave)? (275)

_____

3. What is the normal ROM for _____?
   - Wrist Flexion/Ext.: _____, _____
   - Rotation (pron/sup) _____, _____

4. What is the wrist resting position? _____

5. What is the wrist joint tight packed position?

_____

6. What ligaments resist abduction? (287)

_____

7. What muscles cause flexion to occur? (285)

_____

8. What does FOOSH stand for? (285)

_____

9. What the 9 tendons that travel through the carpal tunnel with the median nerve? (289)

10. Can you palpate _____? (284)

Learning Objectives

After completing this chapter, students will be able to:

1. Perform a regional exam and differentiate common pathologies of the region

2. Identify and palpate body region bony landmarks, ligaments and muscles

3. Discuss regional kinematics and joint organ biomechanics

4. Demonstrate regional AROM, PROM, goniometry, stretch and strengthen protocols

5. Recognize and execute steps of effective mobilization and joint-play including indications, position, contact, force and relevant clinical notes

6. Perform supine, prone, seated assessment and mobilizations including

   - Pin and stretch
   - Muscle energy technique
   - A-P and P-A Glides
   - Long axis distraction
   - Internal and external rotational motions

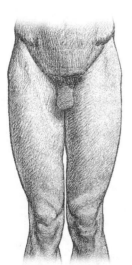
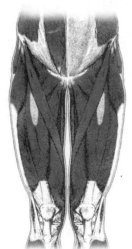
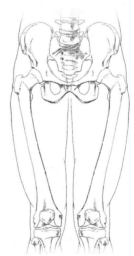

Realize that any mobilization (grade 1-4) can be made into a manipulation (grade 5) with the addition of a high velocity low amplitude (HVLA) thrust & vise versa with the lack of a HVLA thrust

Conversely any technique can be adapted to use IASTM where indicated to save your hands

Hip & Thigh

prohealthsys

> **Follow HIP-MNRS** (see Yellow "Physical Assessment" text for specific details or review)
> History, Inspection, Palpation - Motion, Neurovascular screen, Referred pain, Special tests

Special history questions

- Specific mechanism of injury & forces involved?
- Any numbness, tingling or weakness?
- Any snapping, popping or grinding? (OA)
- Puncture wounds to lower limb? (septic arthritis)
- Type of work, typical posture, sleeping posture?
- Review of systems (GI, urinary, cardiovascular)

Inspection

- Asymmetry, bruising, bumps, color, swelling, iliac crest height
- Posture

Fracture screen (older than 55?)

1. 4 step test, torsion test
2. Bony tenderness on palpation
3. Percussion, tuning fork (128 Hz), ultrasound

Palpation (may be done after ROM assessment)

ASIS/iliac crest	Anterior thigh
TFL/ITB	Iliopsoas
SI joint	Pubic symphysis
Sacrotuberous lig.	Inguinal lig./nodes
Greater trochanter	Femoral triangle
L-spine/sacrum	Greater saph. vein
Hip joint/capsule	Adductor muscles
Gluteus max./med.	Pubic symphysis
Piriformis	Ischial tuberosity
Sciatic nerve	Hamstrings

Functional assessment (ADLs)

- Toe touch or squat & rise

AROM

Flexion .... 80°-90° (straight leg*)
Extension .... 30°
Internal rotation ..... 40°
External rotation .... 50°
Abduction .... 50°
Adduction .... 30°
*Bent knee hip flexion should approach 130°

PROM & Joint Play (if lacking AROM in any motion)

Myotomes (resisted isometric movements)

- Hip flexion (L1-L3, femoral n.)
- Knee extension (L3-L4; femoral n.)

- Knee flexion (L4-S2, sciatic n.)
- Ankle dorsiflexion (**L4**, L5 - deep peroneal),
- Ankle inversion (L5, **S1** - sup. peroneal)
- Ankle eversion (**S1** - sup. peroneal)
- Big toe extension, (L4, **L5**, S1; deep peron.)
- Big toe flexion (L5-S1, tibial nerve)

Leg length measurements

- Greater trochanter to lateral malleolus
- Pubic symphysis to medial malleolus
- Umbilicus to medial malleolus

Neurovascular screen

Sensory: Light touch, sharp/dull or pinwheel
Vibration (DIP, 3rd digit)
UMNL: Babinski (L1 & above)

- **DTR's:** patella (L4), hamstring (L5), Achilles (S1)
- **Pulses:** femoral, tibial, dorsal pedal
- Nail bed blanching
- Buerger's claudication test

Orthopedic tests (if indicated)

Screening
- Heel walk, toe walk
- Trendelenberg
- Anvil test

Hip DJD
- Scour test
- FABERE

Lumbar Radiculopathy
- SLR, Well leg raise (also assess hamstring length)
- Braggard's test

Hip flexor length
- Thomas test
- Gaenslen's test
- Rectus femoris contracture test

Piriformis syndrome
- Sign of the buttock

Instability
- Hip telescoping

 Printable form

Lumbar spine, SI & knee screen

Diagnostic imaging (if indicated)

 youtube: vizniak hip exam brief   prohealthsys.com

Hip & Thigh

Condition	Clinical notes
Avascular necrosis	*Hx:* repetitive hip trauma, corticosteroids, alcohol, diabetes, sickle cell anemia atherosclerosis *SSx:* pain/stiffness in hip joint, pain persists with rest, antalgic limp, limited ROM *DDx:* OA, osteoporosis, hip dislocation, femoral neck fracture
Acetabular labral tear	*Hx:* prior trauma, deep hip/groin pain, worse with fill hip flexion, possible locking *SSx:* audible click with motion, pain with full passive hip flexion (bent knee) *DDx:* internal or external snapping hip, DJD,
Hernia (inguinal or femoral)	*Hx:* M>F (9:1); prior heavy, lifting with valsalva causes more pain *SSx:* palpable protrusion worse with valsalva - **Red flags:** nausea, fever, vomiting, discoloration indicative of strangulated hernia = medical emergency *DDx:* groin strain, testicular torsion
Hip DJD	*Hx:* groin pain worse with weight bearing or cold weather, morning stiffness *SSx:* antalgic gait, (+) scour test, visible on x-ray (sclerosis, ↓ joint space) *DDx:* avascular necrosis

Radiographic Findings

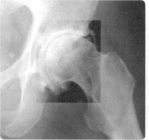

- **Joint space loss** (cartilage thinning)
- **Reactive sclerosis** (subchondral bone remodeling due to abnormal stress)
- **Osteophyte formation** (bone growth around outer margins of joint - bone spur)
- Risk factors include obesity, smoking and repetitive trauma

Muscle strain (hamstring, quads, groin)	*Hx:* sudden onset of pain associated with muscle contraction *SSx:* antalgic gait, local tenderness to palpation, ↓ AROM *DDx:* avulsion fracture
Piriformis syndrome	*Hx:* possible pain down back of leg, worse when sitting on hard surface *SSx:* tender to palpation, (+) SLR, sign of the buttock, (+) piriformis test *DDx:* lumbar radiculopathy, disc herniation, lumbar sprain/strain, stenosis
Septic Arthritis	*Hx:* rapid onset of severe hip pain, prior infection possible (respiratory or other) *SSx:* fever, mincing/painful gait, extremely limited ROM, puncture wound in skin *DDx:* rheumatoid arthritis
Snapping hip	*Hx:* patient may feel a repeatable 'pop' of ITB over greater trochanter *SSx:* tender to palpation over greater trochanter, (+) Ober's test *DDx:* may cause trochanteric bursitis
Trochanteric bursitis	*Hx:* patient may feel 'pop' of ITB or direct trauma to greater trochanter *SSx:* tender to palpation over greater trochanter, (+) Ober's test *DDx:* snapping hip

↑ = increased, ↓ = decreased, Hx = history, SSx = signs & symptoms, DDx = differential diagnosis, SCFE = slipped capital femoral epiphysis
see blue 'Orthopedic Conditions' and yellow 'Physical Assessment' texts for more details

Hip & Thigh

prohealthsys

Joint type: synovial
- Symphysis (pubic symphysis)
- Ball & socket (acetabulofemoral)

Articular surfaces
- **Acetabulofemoral:** *convex* (head of femur) on *concave* (acetabulum)

Hip active range of motion
Flexion (straight leg) ....**90°**
Flexion (bent knee)..............**120°**
Extension ....**30°**
Abduction ....**50°**
Adduction ....**30°**
Lateral (internal) rotation ..**40°**
External (medial) rotation .**50°**

Main muscle actions
- **Flexion:** iliopsoas, rectus femoris, sartorius
- **Extension:** gluteus maximus, hamstrings
- **Abduction:** gluteus medius & minimus, tensor fasciae latae
- **Adduction:** adductor magnus, gracilis, adductor longus & brevis
- **Internal rotation:** tensor fasciae latae, gluteus medius & minimus
- **External rotation:** piriformis, quadratus femoris, superior & inferior gemellus, obturator internus & externus

Resting position
- **Acetabulofemoral:** 30° abduction, 30° flexion & slight external rotation

Close packed position
- **Acetabulofemoral:** full extension, abduction & internal rotation

Capsular pattern of restriction
- **Acetabulofemoral:** internal rotation > extension > abduction

Normal end feel
- **Flexion & adduction:** elastic or tissue approx.
- **Straight leg raise:** elastic
- **Extension & abduction:** elastic / firm
- **Internal/external rotation:** elastic / firm

Abnormal end feel
- **Bony** = osteoarthritis
- **Late myospasm** = instability

Hip arthrokinematics
- **Flexion:** femur rolls superior & glides inferior on acetabulum
- **Extension:** femur rolls inferior & glides superior on acetabulum
- **Abduction:** femur rolls lateral/superior & glides inferior on acetabulum
- **Adduction:** femur rolls medial/inferior & glides superior on acetabulum
- **Internal rotation:** femur rolls medial & glides lateral on acetabulum
- **External rotation:** femur rolls lateral & glides medial on acetabulum

Hip joint forces
- **Standing:** 0.3x body weight
- **Standing one leg:** 2.5x body weight
- **Walking:** 3x body weight
- **Running:** > 4.5x body weight

♂ **<18°**
♀ **<22°**

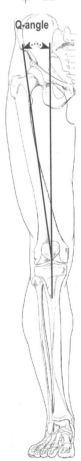

Q angle

"Q" angle
- A line drawn from the anterosuperior iliac spine through the center of the patella & a line drawn from the center of the patella to the center of the tibial tuberosity

- The term 'Q' is used to represent the main pull of the quadriceps muscle group

- The "Q" angle is greater in women as the hips are set wider apart

- **Women:** should be less than 22° with the knee extended and less than 9° with the knee in 90° of flexion

- **Men:** should be less than 18° with the knee extended and less than 8° with the knee in 90° of flexion

- A large "Q" angle may predispose to osteoarthritis of the knee and/or patellar dislocation

Hip & Thigh

prohealthsys

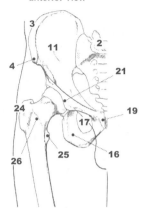
anterior view

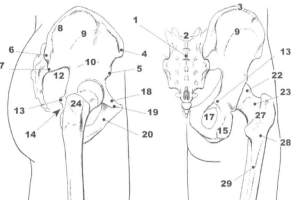
lateral view

posterior view

Sacrum
1. S2 tubercle
2. Sacral base

Os Coxae (ilium, ischium & pubis)
3. Iliac crest
4. Anterior superior iliac spine
5. Anterior inferior iliac spine
6. Posterior superior iliac spine
7. Posterior inferior iliac spine
8. Posterior gluteal line

9. Anterior gluteal line
10. Inferior gluteal line
11. Iliac fossa
12. Greater sciatic notch
13. Ischial spine
14. Lesser sciatic notch
15. Ischial tuberosity
16. Ramus of ischium
17. Obturator foramen
18. Superior pubic ramus
19. Pubic tubercle

20. Inferior pubic ramus
21. Acetabulum

Femur
22. Head
23. Neck
24. Greater trochanter
25. Lesser trochanter
26. Intertrochanteric line
27. Intertrochanteric crest
28. Gluteal tuberosity
29. Linea aspera

Coxa varus & valgus

- During growth it is possible for the femoral neck and acetabulum to have changes in orientations and the deepness of the joint socket

  - **Coxa valgus > 135°**
  - **Coxa varus < 120°**

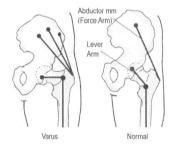
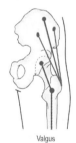

Varus   Normal   Valgus

Anteversion & retroversion

- During growth it is possible for the femur and tibia to have anatomical variation in their long axis causing a rotational variation in alignment

  - **Medial rotation = anteversion**
  - **Lateral rotation = retroversion**

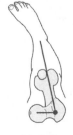
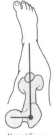
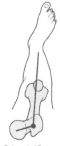

Anteverted Femur (toe in)   Normal Femur   Retroverted Femur (toe out)

Hip & Thigh

anterior view   posterior view

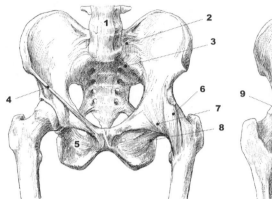

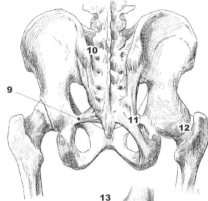

Pelvis & Hip

1. Anterior longitudinal ligament
2. Iliolumbar ligaments
3. Anterior sacroiliac ligaments
4. Inguinal ligament
5. Obturator membrane
6. Iliofemoral ligament
7. Pubofemoral ligament
8. Ischiofemoral ligament
9. Sacrospinous ligament
10. Posterior sacroiliac ligament
11. Sacrotuberus ligament
12. Acetabulofemoral joint capsule
13. Ligamentum teres (to head of femur)

Ligament	Attaches (origin/insertion)	Function
Iliofemoral	AIIS to intertrochanteric line of femur	Supports anterior hip; resists in movements of extension, internal rotation, external rotation
Ischiofemoral	Posterior acetabulum to iliofemoral ligament	Resists adduction & internal rotation
Pubofemoral	Acetabulum, superior rami to intertrochanteric line	Resists in movements of abduction & external rotation
Ligament teres	Acetabular notch to pit on head of femur	Transmits vessels to head of femur; may resist distraction forces of joint
Obturator Membrane	Covers obturator foramen	Attachment point of obturator internus & externus

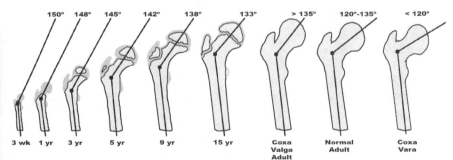

Children are born with ~150° angle, with growth angle usually approaches normal (Normal range 120°-135°)

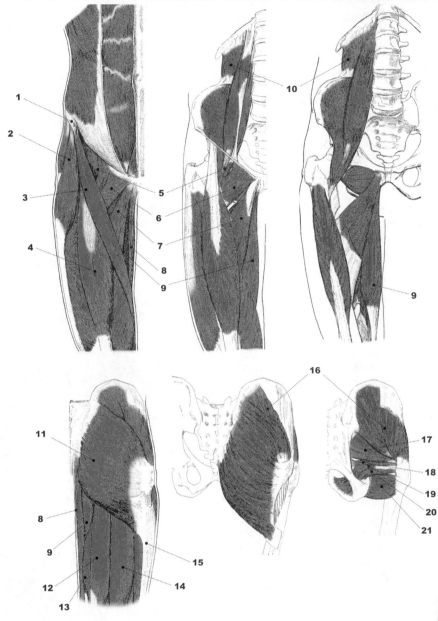

1. ASIS
2. Tensor fascae latae
3. Sartorius
4. Rectus femoris
5. Iliopsoas
6. Pectineus
7. Adductor longus

8. Gracilis
9. Adductor magnus
10. Quadratus lumborum
11. Gluteus maximus
12. Semitendinosus
13. Semimembranosus
14. Biceps femoris (long head)

15. Iliotibial band
16. Gluteus medius
17. Piriformis
18. Superior gemellus
19. Obturator internus
20. Inferior gemellus
21. Quadratus femoris

Hip & Thigh

prohealthsys

Compare bilaterally; prior to ROM examiner should make an introduction statement:
"Try and move as far as possible, if any of the actions or movements are painful or uncomfortable please let me know, do not do any action you feel will cause you further injury."

AROM

Flexion (115°-125° bent knee, 80°-90° straight knee)
Muscles Activated: iliopsoas, rectus femoris, sartorius
Tissue Stretched: gluteus maximus, hamstrings , sciatic nerve
Tissue Compressed: anterior hip muscles, anterior joint capsule, inguinal ligament, femoral artery, femoral nerve

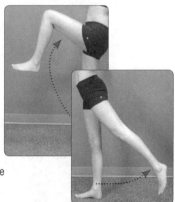

Extension (20°-30°)
Muscles Activated: gluteus maximus, hamstrings
Tissue Stretched: iliopsoas, rectus femoris, sartorius, anterior iliofemoral ligament & joint capsule, femoral nerve
Tissue Compressed: posterior hip muscles, posterior joint capsule

Abduction (40°-50°)
Muscles Activated: gluteus medius & minimus, tensor fasciae latae
Tissue Stretched: adductor magnus, gracilis, adductor longus & brevis, medial hip joint capsule
Tissue Compressed: lateral hip structures (joint capsule, lateral acetabular labrum)

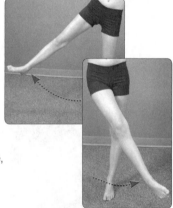

Adduction (15°-30°)
Muscles Activated: adductor magnus, gracilis, adductor longus & brevis
Tissue Stretched: gluteus medius & minimus, tensor fasciae latae, iliotibial band
Tissue Compressed: medial hip structures

Lateral Rotation (25°-50°)
Muscles Activated: piriformis, quadratus femoris, superior & inferior gemellus, obturator internus & externus
Tissue Stretched: tensor fasciae latae, gluteus medius & minimus, anterior joint capsule
Tissue Compressed: posterior hip structures

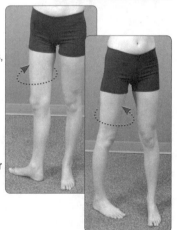

Medial Rotation (35°-50°)
Muscles Activated: tensor fasciae latae, gluteus medius & minimus
Tissue Stretched: piriformis, quadratus femoris, superior & inferior gemellus, obturator internus & externus, posterior joint capsule
Tissue Compressed: anterior joint capsule

Hip & Thigh

prohealthsys

Compare bilaterally; if possible palpate joint during PROM & use the shortest lever possible; apply over pressure at end ROM; introduction statement:
"If any of the actions or movements are painful or uncomfortable please let me know."

Flexion (> 115°-125° bent knee, 80°-90° straight knee)
Tissue Stretched: gluteus maximus, hamstrings , sciatic nerve
Tissue Compressed: anterior hip muscles, anterior joint capsule, inguinal ligament, femoral artery, femoral nerve

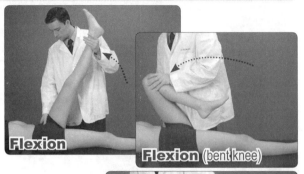

Extension (> 20°-30°)
Tissue Stretched: iliopsoas, rectus femoris, sartorius, anterior iliofemoral ligament & joint capsule, femoral nerve
Tissue Compressed: posterior hip muscles, posterior joint capsule

Abduction (> 40°-50°)
Tissue Stretched: adductor magnus, gracilis, adductor longus & brevis, medial hip joint capsule
Tissue Compressed: lateral hip structures (joint capsule, lateral acetabular labrum)

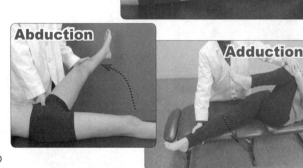

Adduction (> 15°-30°)
Tissue Stretched: gluteus medius & minimus, tensor fasciae latae, iliotibial band
Tissue Compressed: medial hip structures

Medial Rotation (> 35°-50°)
Tissue Stretched: piriformis, quadratus femoris, superior & inferior gemellus, obturator internus & externus, posterior joint capsule
Tissue Compressed: anterior capsule

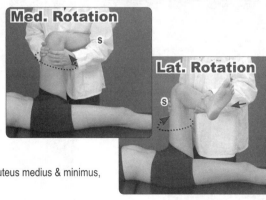

Lateral Rotation (> 25°-50°)
Tissue Stretched: tensor fasciae latae, gluteus medius & minimus, anterior joint capsule

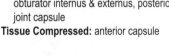

Hip & Thigh

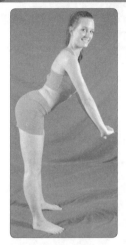

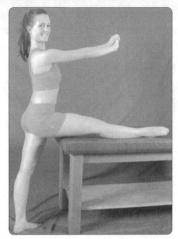

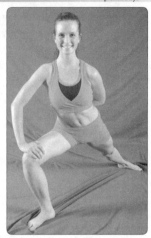

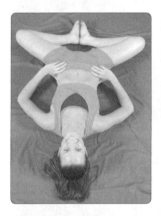

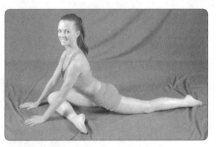

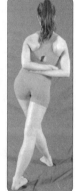

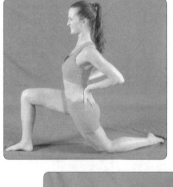

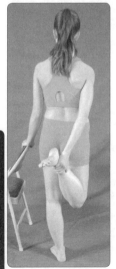

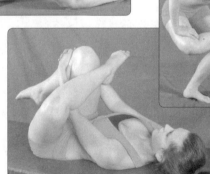

prohealthsys

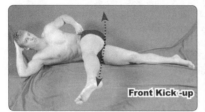
Front Kick-up

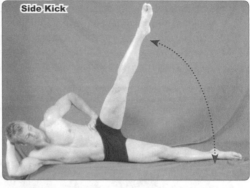
Side Kick

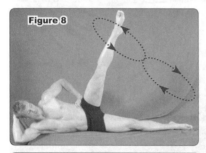
Figure 8

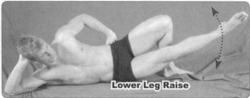
Lower Leg Raise

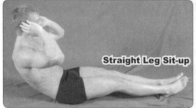
Straight Leg Sit-up

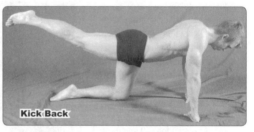
Kick Back

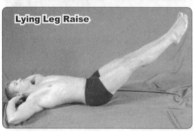
Lying Leg Raise

Printable handouts prohealthsys.com

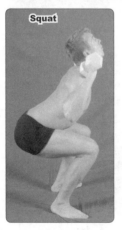
Squat

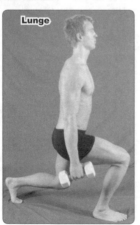
Lunge

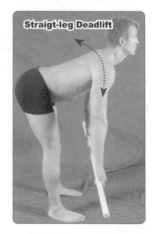
Straigt-leg Deadlift

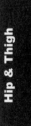
Hip & Thigh

Hip Pin & Stretch

prohealthsys

Pin & Stretch treatments can be adapted & applied to any myofascial structure if the clinician has a detailed understanding of basic anatomy & biomechanics
1. Clinician places muscle in shortened position & pins specific myofascial fibers with other hand
2. Patient is then <u>passively</u> moved to lengthen muscle while pinning force is maintained
3. Hold at tension for ~10 seconds or until myofascial release is felt; repeat & reassess as needed

Gluteus Medius Pin & Stretch

1. Clinician places muscle in shortened position (hip abducted - origin & insertion approximated) & pins specific myofascial fibers with other hand
2. Patient is then passively moved to lengthen muscle (hip adduction - move insertion away from origin) while pinning force is maintained
3. Hold at tension for ~10 sec or until release is felt; repeat as needed

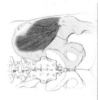 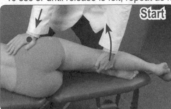 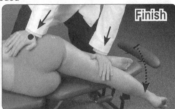

Piriformis Pin & Stretch

1. Clinician places muscle in shortened position (hip neutral or externally rotated - origin & insertion approximated) & pins specific myofascial fibers with other hand
2. Patient is then passively moved to lengthen muscle (hip internal rotation - move insertion away from origin) while pinning force is maintained
3. Hold at tension for ~10 sec or until release is felt; repeat as needed

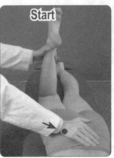 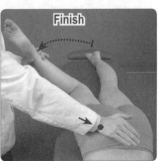

- An **elbow contact or IASTM contact** (proSTM2) may be used to apply more specific pressure through the gluteus maximus to reach piriformis
- Students & clinicians often get confused & must realize that internal rotation of the hip with the knee bent results in the foot going laterally (counter intuitive)

Rectus Femoris Pin & Stretch

1. Clinician places muscle in shortened position (knee extended - origin & insertion approximated) & pins specific myofascial fibers with other hand
2. Patient is then passively moved to lengthen muscle (knee flexion - move insertion away from origin) while pinning force is maintained
3. Hold at tension for ~10 sec or until release is felt; repeat as needed

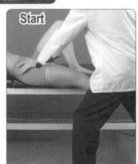 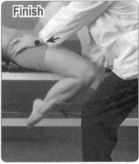

S = stabilization (indifferent hand), ● = contact, ——▶ = examiner force, ·······▶ = patient motion

Hip & Thigh

prohealthsys

With good anatomy & biomechanical understanding, MET can be adapted to any patient
1. Clinician gently stretches patient into direction of restriction or decreased range of motion
2. Patient gently (10% of maximum) contracts in exact opposite motion
3. Clinician resists & patient holds contraction for 3-7 seconds, then patient completely relaxes
4. On relaxation, clinician moves to new resistive barrier; repeat 3-5 times & reassess

Hip Flexion Restriction

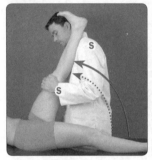

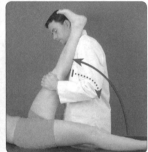

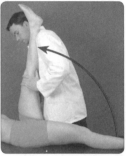

Flexion tissue resistance

Patient contracts ~10% in extension

Clinician finds new end range

Hip Abduction Restriction

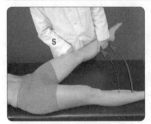

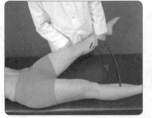

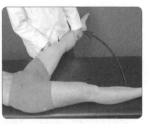

Abduction tissue resistance

Patient contracts ~10% in adduction

Clinician finds new end range

Hip Medial Rotation Restriction

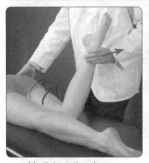

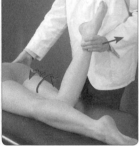

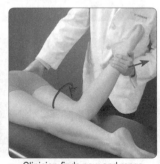

Medial rotation tissue resistance

Patient contracts ~10% in lateral rotation

Clinician finds new end range

Students & clinicians often get confused with medial/internal rotation of the hip when the knee is bent; the ankle actually goes laterally with medial rotation

S = stabilization (indifferent hand),   ● = contact,   ———> = examiner force,   ·········> = patient motion

Hip & Thigh

Mobilization belts are an excellent tool in the toolbox work smarted not harder. By using the mechanical advantage of the belt tied to the clinicians waist or other stronger muscle groups force can be taken off the hands and all body weight to be used to advantage. This is especially true for smaller practitioners and larger/ stronger patients or body regions (hip, spine, ankle)

Use mechanical advantage and good body biomechanics to make your job easier.

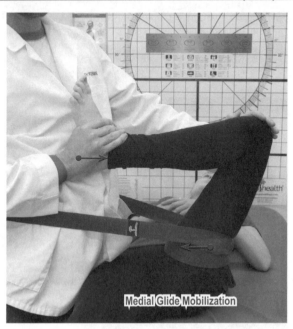

Medial Glide Mobilization

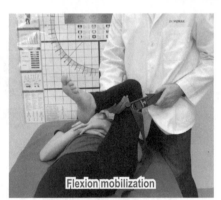

Flexion mobilization

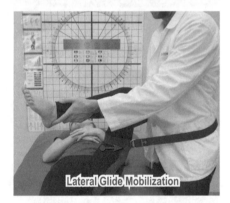

Lateral Glide Mobilization

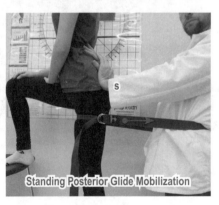

Standing Posterior Glide Mobilization

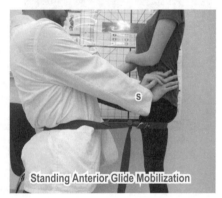

Standing Anterior Glide Mobilization

S = stabilization (indifferent hand),   ● = contact,   ⟶ = examiner force,   ·······▷ = patient motion

Hip & Thigh

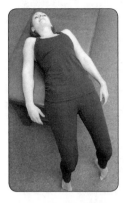

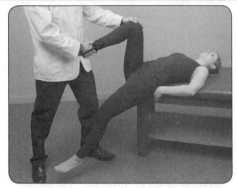

Clinician anchors patient's foot into their pelvis or shoulder (this allow clinician biomechanical advantage of using body weight)

Have patient angled on treatment table to allow for maximum SI joint motion while maintaining balance - sacrum balanced on corner

Clinician leans body toward patient (note left sided hip flexion and knee extension on this patient)

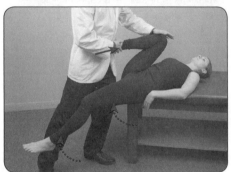

Clinician applies over pressure to the hanging leg to lengthen the left iliopsoas

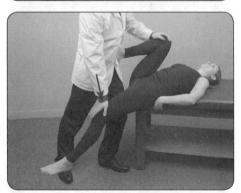

The sequence demonstrated in this page is one of the best SI mobilization techniques this author has used (excellent results, easy on the clinician's body - it just works!)

Clinician also apply over pressure on patient's hand ankle to further stretch (go slow and make sure you have good balance)

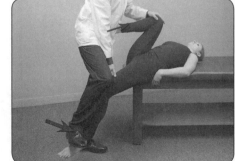

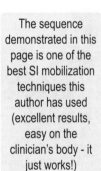

This is also a great position for contract relax or IASTM application

S = stabilization (indifferent hand), ● = contact, ——▶ = examiner force, ·········▶ = patient motion

Hip & Thigh

prohealthsys

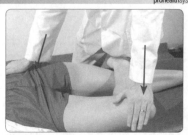

Indications: tight anterior hip

Position: seated or supine, knee bent ~90°

Contact: clinician stabilizes patient's knee & contralateral ASIS

Force: tissue force is P-A; develop tension by gently pushing down;

Clinical notes: slowly progress to increase force & make sure the patient is taking deep relaxing breaths to ensure maximal soft tissue release

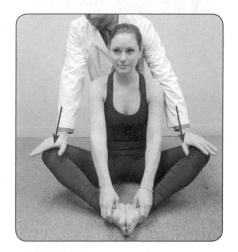

Select Hip IASTM

Supine iliotibial band variation

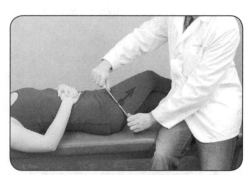

Supine hamstring variation

Long stroking treatments are best done with skin contact and emollient, dark pants were used to better show contrast of instrument - see IASTM text and videos for specific IASTM protocols

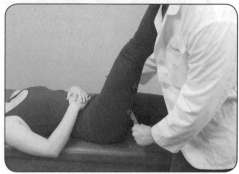

S = stabilization (indifferent hand),　● = contact,　——▶ = examiner force,　·········▶ = patient motion

Hip & Thigh

prohealthsys.com

prohealthsys

Indications: tight short lateral rotators, piriformis syndrome

Position: patient prone knee bent ~90°

Contact: clinician stabilizes patient's ankle & contacts piriformis through gluteus maximus

Force: tissue force is P-A; develop tension by gently pushing into the piriformis; clinician pushes the patients ankle outward & follows by moving the their elbow laterally with the hip rotation

Clinical notes: Clinician should be sure to 'stack' their elbow and shoulder over top of each other to ensure maximum force delivery with the minimum effort and chance of injury

If patient experience numbness or tingling too much pressure is being applied to the sciatic nerve

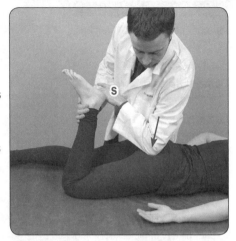

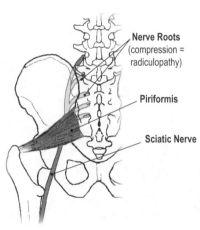

Nerve Roots (compression = radiculopathy)

Piriformis

Sciatic Nerve

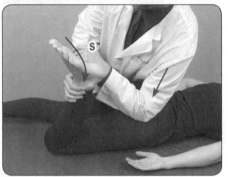

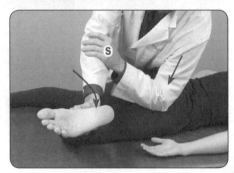

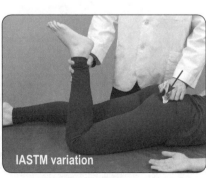

IASTM variation

youtube: IASTM

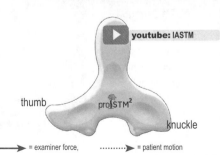

thumb

pro**STM**^{2}

knuckle

S = stabilization (indifferent hand), ● = contact, ——▶ = examiner force, ·········▶ = patient motion

Hip & Thigh

Long Axis Distraction

Indications: hip joint contracture, ↓ ROM, OA

Position: patient supine (or seated)

Contact: clinician stabilizes pelvis & grasps patient's knee

Force: tissue force is S-I; develop tension by gently pulling the knee inferiorly

Clinical notes: maneuver may be performed as a mobilization or manipulation

Contraindicated in patients with prior history of hip dislocation or replacement

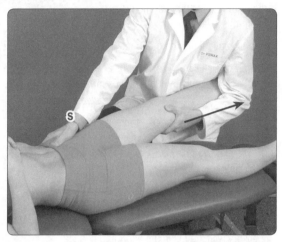

'Bunny hop' mobilization

(clinician's leg are used to help generate long axis distraction)

IASTM variation

(usually done with skin contact - dark pants used to show contrast of instrument)

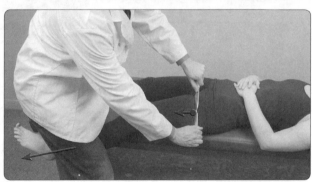

S = stabilization (indifferent hand), ● = contact, ——▶ = examiner force, ·········▶ = patient motion

Hip & Thigh

prohealthsys

A-P Glide

Indications: hip contracture, ↓ ROM, hip pain, scar tissue formation

Position: patient supine

Contact: clinician stabilizes knee & contacts proximal femur

Force: tissue force is A-P; develop tension by gently pushing the proximal femur posteriorly

Clinical notes: maneuver may be performed as a mobilization or manipulation

Two variations shown with knee bent & with knee straight

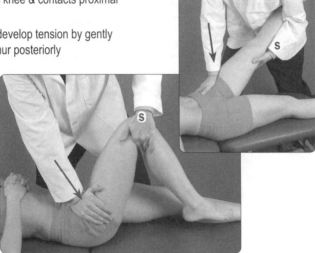

P-A Glide

Indications: hip contracture, ↓ ROM, hip pain, scar tissue formation

Position: patient prone

Contact: clinician stabilizes knee & contacts proximal femur

Force: tissue force is P-A; develop tension by gently pushing the proximal femur anteriorly

Clinical notes: maneuver may be performed as a mobilization or manipulation

Two variations shown with knee bent & with knee straight

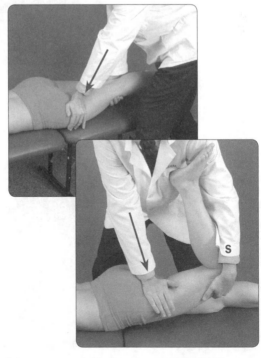

Hip & Thigh

S = stabilization (indifferent hand), ● = contact, ➞ = examiner force, ·········➤ = patient motion

Interanal & External Rotation

Indications: hip contracture, ↓ ROM into rotation, hip pain, scar tissue formation

Position: patient supine with hip & knee flexed 90°

Contact: clinician stabilizes ankle with axilla & contacts mid femur & greater trochanter

Force: tissue force internal or external rotation; develop tension by gently rotating the femur

Clinical notes: maneuver may be performed as a mobilization or manipulation

Main force of motion should be directed through contact hands, try to avoid excessive pressure on the leg that may cause unnecessary torque & tension on the knee

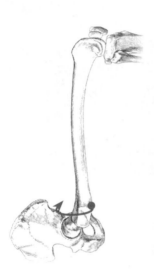
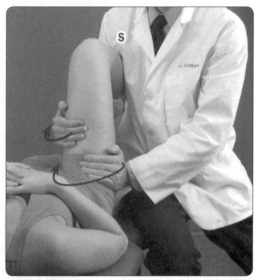

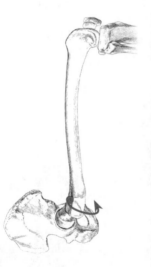
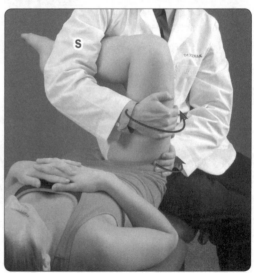

S = stabilization (indifferent hand), ● = contact, ——▶ = examiner force, ·········▶ = patient motion

Hip & Thigh

Inferior Glide in Flexion

Indications: hip contracture, ↓ ROM, hip pain, scar tissue formation

Position: patient prone with hip flexed

Contact: clinician stabilizes patient's ankle over shoulder & contacts proximal femur

Force: tissue force is I-S; develop tension by gently pulling the proximal femur inferiorly

Clinical notes: maneuver may be performed as a mobilization or manipulation

Two variations shown with knee bent & with knee straight (long axis distraction with hip flexion)

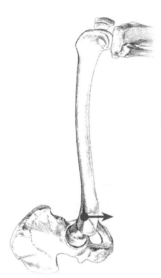

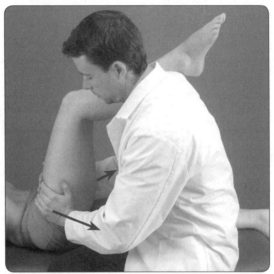

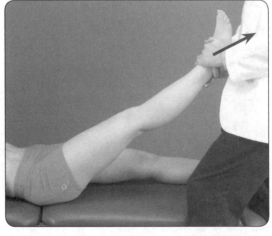

S = stabilization (indifferent hand), = contact, ——————▶ = examiner force, ·········▶ = patient motion

Hip & Thigh

1. Vizniak, NA. Gross Anatomy Human Cadaver Dissections. 1999-2018. McGee S. Evidence-Based Physical Diagnosis. Saunders. 2007.

2. Magee D. Orthopedic Physical Assessment, 5th Edition. Saunders. 2008.

3. Taylor MH, Monroe LG. Physical Rehabilitation: Evidence-Based Examination, Evaluation and Intervention. Saunders. 2007.

4. Warlow C, Hughes R, Uitehaag B, Liberati A. Evidence-Based Neurology. Blackwell Publishing Limited, BMJI Books. 2007.

5. Malanga GA & Nadler. Musculoskeletal Physical Exam, An Evidence-Based Approach. Mosby. 2006.

6. Hoppenfeld S. Physical Examination of the Spine & Extremities. Lippincott Williams & Wilkins. 1976.

7. Hoppenfeld S. Orthopaedic Neurology: A Diagnostic Guide to Neurologic Levels. Lippincott Williams & Wilkins. 1977.

8. Spencer JW, Jacobs JJ. Complementary and Alternative Medicine. An Evidence-Based Approach. Mosby. 2003.

9. Jewell D. Guide to Evidence-Based Physical Therapy Practice. Jones Barlett Publishers Inc. 2007.

10. Iesel SW. Operative Orthopaedics: An Illustrative Approach. Lippincott Williams & Wilkins. 2008.

11. Adams S, Yarnold P. Clinical use of the patellar-pubic percussion sign in hip trauma. Am J Emerg Med. 1 997;15:173-175.

12. Altman R, Alarcon G, Appelrouth D, Bloch D, Borenstein D, Brandt K, Brown C, Cooke TD, Daniel W, Feldman D, et al. The American College of Rheumatology criteria for the classification & reporting of osteoarthritis of the hip. Arthritis Rheum. 1991;34(5):505-51 4.

13. Bache JB, Cross AB. The Barford test: a useful diagnostic sign in fractures of the femoral neck. Practitioner. 1984;228(1 389):305-308.

14. Bird PA, Oakley SP, Shnier R, Kirham BW. Prospective evaluation of magnetic resonance imaging & physical examination findings in patients with greater trochanteric pain syndrome. Arthritis Rheumatism. 2001;44:2138-2145.

15. Birrell F, Croft P, Cooper C, Hosie G, Macfarlane G, Silman A. Predicting radiographic hip Osteoarthritis from range of movement. Rheumatology. 2001 ;40:506-512.

16. Brown M, Gomez-Martin 0, Brookfield K, Stokes P. Differential diagnosis of hip disease versus spine disease. Clin Orthop. 2004;419:280-284.

17. Castelein RM, Korte J. Limited hip abduction in the infant.J Ped Orthoped. 2001;21:668-670.

18. Dorrell JH, Catterall A. The torn acetabular labrum. J Bone Jnt Surg. 1986;68(3):400-403.

19. Jan S, Paton RW, Sninivasan MS. Unilateral limitation of abduction of the hip: a valuable clinical sign for DDH? J Bone Jnt Surg. 2002;84:104-107.

20. Klaue K, Durnin CW, Ganz R. The acetabular rim syndrome: a clinical description of dysplasia of the hip. J Bone Jnt Surg. 1991;73:423-429.

21. Leuning M, Werlen S, Ungersbock A, Ito K, Ganz R. Evaluation of the acetabular labrum by MR arthrography. I Bone Joint Surg Br. 1997;79(2):230-234.

22. Margo K, DreznerJ, Motzkin D. Evaluation and management of hip pain: an algorithmic approach. J Fam Pract. 2003;52(8):607-617.

23. Melchione W, Sullivan S. Reliability of measurements obtained by use of an instrument designed to measure iliotibial band length indirectly. J Orthop Sports Phys Ther. 1993;18:511-515.

24. Misurya RK, Khare A, Mallick A, Sural A, Vishwakarma GK. Use of tuning fork in diagnostic auscultation of fractures. Injury. 1987;18(1):63-64.

25. Mitchell B, McCrory P, Burkner P, O'Donnell J, Colson E, Howells R. Hip joint pathology: clinical presentation & correlation between magnetic resonance arthrography, ultrasound, and arthroscopic findings. Clin J Sport Med. 2003;13:152-156.

26. Narvani A, Tsiridis E, Kendall S, Chaudhuri R, Thomas P. A preliminary report on prevalence of acetabular labrum tears in sports patients with groin pain. Knee Surg TraumatolArthrosc. 2003;11:403-408.

27. Suenaga E, Noguchi Y, Jingushi S, Shuto T, Nakashima Y, Miyanishi K, Iwamoto Y. Relationship between the maximum flexion-internal rotation test & the torn acetabular labrum of a dysplastic hip. J Orthop Sci. 2002;7:26-32.

28. Tiru M, Goh S, Low B. Use of percussion as a screening tool in the diagnosis of occult hip fractures. Singapore Med J. 2002;43:467-469.

29. Woods D, Macnicol M. The flexion-adduction test: an early sign of hip disease. J Ped Orthop. 2001:10:180-185.

30. Akermark C, Johansson C. Tenotomy of the adductor longus tendon in the treatment of chronic groin pain in athletes. Am J Sports Med. Nov-Dec 1992;20(6):640-3.

31. Aksoy B, Oztürk K, Ensenyel CZ, Kara AN. Avulsion of the iliac crest apophysis. Int J Sports Med. Jan 1998;19(1):76-8.

32. Altman RD, Moskowitz R: Intraarticular sodium hyaluronate (Hyalgan) in the treatment of patients with osteoarthritis of the knee: a randomized clinical trial. Hyalgan Study Group [published erratum appears in J Rheumatol 1999 May;26(5):1216]. J Rheumatol 1998 Nov; 25(11): 2203-12

33. American College of Rheumatology: Recommendations for the medical management of osteoarthritis of the hip and knee: 2000 update. American College of Rheumatology Subcommittee on Osteoarthritis Guidelines. Arthritis Rheum 2000 Sep; 43(9): 1905-15

34. Arokoski JP: Physical therapy and rehabilitation programs in the management of hip osteoarthritis. Eura Medicophys 2005 Jun; 41(2): 155-61

35. Azurin DJ, Go LS, Schuricht A, et al. Endoscopic preperitoneal herniorrhaphy in professional athletes with groin pain. J Laparoendosc Adv Surg Tech A. Feb 1997;7(1):7-12.

36. Baber YF, Robinson AH, Villar RN. Is diagnostic arthroscopy of the hip worthwhile? A prospective review of 328 adults investigated for hip pain. J Bone Joint Surg Br. Jul 1999;81(4):600-3.

37. Bijlsma JW, Dekker J: A step forward for exercise in the management of osteoarthritis. Rheumatology (Oxford) 2005 Jan; 44(1): 5-6

38. Blount WP: Don't throw away the cane. J Bone Joint Surg Am 1956 Jun; 38-A(3): 695-708

39. Brandt KD: A pessimistic view of serologic markers for diagnosis and management of osteoarthritis. Biochemical, immunologic and clinicopathologic barriers. J Rheumatol Suppl 1989 Aug; 18: 39-42

40. Browning KH. Hip and pelvis injuries in runners. Phys Sportsmed. 2001;Vol 29:23-34.

41. Brukner P, Bradshaw C, McCory P. Obturator neuropathy. Phys Sportsmed. 1999;27:62-73.

42. Byrd JW. Labral lesions: an elusive source of hip pain case reports and literature review. Arthroscopy. Oct 1996;12(5):603-12.

43. Chan WP, Lang P, Stevens MP: Osteoarthritis of the knee: comparison of radiography, CT, and MR imaging to assess extent and severity. AJR Am J Roentgenol 1991 Oct; 157(4): 799-806

44. Chung CB, Robertson JE, Cho GJ, et al. Gluteus medius tendon tears and avulsive injuries in elderly women: imaging findings in six patients. AJR Am J Roentgenol. Aug 1999;173(2):351-3.

45. Clanton TO, Coupe KJ. Hamstring strains in athletes: diagnosis and treatment. J Am Acad Orthop Surg. Jul-Aug 1998;6(4):237-48.

46. Emery CA, Meeuwisse WH, Powell JW. Groin and abdominal strain injuries in the National Hockey League. Clin J Sport Med. Jul 1999;9(3):151-6.

47. Farjo LA, Glick JM, Sampson TG. Hip arthroscopy for acetabular labral tears. Arthroscopy. Mar 1999;15(2):132-7.

48. Felson DT, Schurman DJ: Risk factors for osteoarthritis: understanding joint vulnerability. Clin Orthop 2004 Oct; S16-21

49. Gilmore J. Groin pain in the soccer athlete: fact, fiction, and treatment. Clin Sports Med. Oct 1998;17(4):787-93.

50. Gray AJ, Villar RN. The ligamentum teres of the hip: an arthroscopic classification of its pathology. Arthroscopy. Oct 1997;13(5):575-8.

51. Jacobson T, Allen WC. Surgical correction of the snapping iliopsoas tendon. Am J Sports Med. Sep-Oct 1990;18(5):470-4.

52. Janzen DL, Partridge E, Logan PM, et al. The snapping hip: clinical and imaging findings in transient subluxation of the iliopsoas tendon. Can Assoc Radiol J. Jun 1996;47(3):202-8.

53. Jones DL, Erhard RE. Diagnosis of trochanteric bursitis versus femoral neck stress fracture. Phys Ther. Jan 1997;77(1):58-67.

54. Kemp S, Batt M. The "sports hernia": A common cause of groin pain. Physician Sportsmed. 1998;26 (1):36-44.

55. Kingzett-Taylor A, Tirman PF, Feller J, et al. Tendinosis and tears of gluteus medius and minimus muscles as a cause of hip pain: MR imaging findings. AJR Am J Roentgenol. Oct 1999;173(4):1123-6.

56. Kujala UM, Orava S, Karpakka J, et al. Ischial tuberosity apophysitis and avulsion among athletes. Int J Sports Med. Feb 1997;18(2):149-55.

57. Lacroix VJ, Kinnear DG, Mulder DS, Brown RA. Lower abdominal pain syndrome in national hockey league players: a report of 11 cases. Clin J Sport Med. Jan 1998;8(1):5-9.

58. Meyers WC, Foley DP, Garrett WE, et al. Management of severe lower abdominal or inguinal pain in high-performance athletes. PAIN (Performing Athletes with Abdominal or Inguinal Neuromuscular Pain Study Group). Am J Sports Med. Jan-Feb 2000;28(1):2-8.

Hip & Thigh Quiz (answer page)

1. What are the joint type classifications for this region? (306) _____

2. What are the joint surface shapes for this region (convex/concave)? (306)

3. What is the normal ROM for _____?
   - Flexion/Ext.: _____, _____
   - Abduction/Add: _____, _____
   - Rotation (ext./int) _____, _____

4. What is the AF resting position? _____

5. What is the AF joint tight packed position?

6. What ligaments resist extension? (308)

   _____

7. What muscles cause flexion to occur? (306)

   _____

8. When running how many ___x body goes through the hip? (306) _____

9. What is the normal femoral neck angle? (306) ___

10. Can you palpate _____ ? (304)

Learning Objectives

After completing this chapter, students will be able to:

1. Perform a regional exam and differentiate common pathologies of the region

2. Identify and palpate body region bony landmarks, ligaments and muscles

3. Discuss regional kinematics and joint organ biomechanics

4. Demonstrate regional AROM, PROM, goniometry, stretch and strengthen protocols

5. Recognize and execute steps of effective mobilization and joint-play including indications, position, contact, force and relevant clinical notes

6. Perform supine, prone, seated assessment and mobilizations including

   • Pin and stretch
   • Muscle energy technique
   • Glides (A-P, P-A, M-L, L-M)
   • Long axis distraction and gapping
   • Internal and external rotational motions

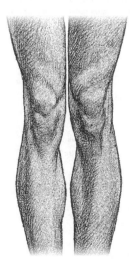
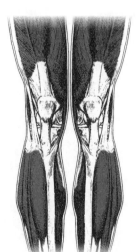
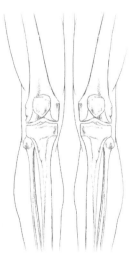

Realize that any mobilization (grade 1-4) can be made into a manipulation (grade 5) with a high velocity low amplitude (HVLA) thrust & vise versa with the lack of a HVLA thrust

Conversely any technique can be adapted to use IASTM where indicated to save your hands

Knee

Follow HIP-MNRS (see Yellow "Physical Assessment" text for specific details or review)
History, Inspection, Palpation - Motion, Neurovascular screen, Referred pain, Special tests

Special history questions
• Specific mechanism of injury & forces involved?
  - did you hear a "popping" sound?
• Age? (teenagers = plica syndrome)
• Do you have pain going up/down stairs?
• Any swelling? (Onset - sudden/slow)
• What type & age of shoes? Running surface?

Inspection
• Asymmetry, bruising, bumps, color, swelling, iliac crest height
• Posture

Fracture screen (older than 55?)
1. 4 step test, torsion test
2. Bony tenderness on palpation
3. Percussion, tuning fork (128 Hz)

Palpation (may be done after ROM assessment)

Quadriceps	Saphenous vein
Patella (facets, bursa)	Popliteal fossa
Patellar ligament	Gastrocnemius heads
Tibial tuberosity	Baker's cyst
Retinaculum/plica	Lateral hamstrings
Adductor canal	Iliotibial band (ITB)
Pes anserine	Popliteus
Med. joint/meniscus	Lateral collateral lig.
Med. femoral condyle	Lateral joint/meniscus
MCL & capsule	Lat. femoral condyle
Medial hamstrings	Lat. tibial condyle

Functional assessment (ADLs) - Squat & rise

AROM
Flexion .... 150°
Extension .... 0° to -5°
Internal rotation* ..... 20-30°
External rotation* .... 30-40°
*Knee must be flexed 90° to assess rotation

PROM & Joint Play (if lacking AROM in any motion)

Myotomes (resisted isometric movements)
• Hip flexion (L1-L3, femoral n.)
• Knee extension (L3-L4; femoral n.)
• Knee flexion (L4-S2, sciatic n.)

• Ankle dorsiflexion (**L4**, L5 - deep peroneal),
• Ankle inversion (L5, **S1** - sup. peroneal)
• Ankle eversion (**S1** - sup. peroneal)
• Big toe extension, (L4, **L5**, S1; deep peron.)
• Big toe flexion (L5-S1, tibial nerve)

Neurovascular screen
Sensory: Light touch, sharp/dull or pinwheel
    Vibration (DIP, 3rd digit)
UMNL: Babinski (L1 & above)
• **DTR's:** patella (L4), hamstring (L5), Achilles (S1)
• **Pulses:** femoral, tibial, dorsal pedal
• Nail bed blanching
• Buerger's claudication test

Orthopedic tests (as indicated)
Screening
• Heel walk, toe walk
• Disco test

Patella
• Ballottement (A-P)
• Bulge/sweep, AP grinding
• Facet (medial/lateral apprehension test)
• Modified Clark's (hold pat, contract quad)
• Step-up test, Rinne (Nobel)

Plica
• Active stutter (sitting active flex)
• Houston's plica test (medial apprehension while passive flex, supine)

Meniscus
• Wilson's, Steinman's, McMurray's
• Apley's compression & hyperflexion
• Apley's distraction
• Bounce home (hand on popliteal fossa)

Ligament stress
• Valgus/varus stress (30° & 0°)
• Wobble test
• Posterior sag sign
• Recurvatum (hyperextension)
• Anterior & posterior drawer
• Lachman's
• Macintosh (pivot-shift) test

Lumbar spine, SI, hip & ankle screen
Diagnostic imaging (if indicated)

Condition	Clinical notes
ACL tear	*Hx:* direct trauma with valgus or hyperextension stress, audible "pop"; playing sport with quick stops or sharp cutting on non-slip surface (b-ball, soccer) *SSx:* severe joint effusion (+) anterior drawer, Lachman's, Lever test *DDx:* often associated with MCL & medial meniscus injury
MCL tear	*Hx:* direct trauma with valgus stress, audible "pop", medial knee pain *SSx:* local tenderness to palpation, (+) valgus stress test *DDx:* often associated with ACL & medial meniscus injury
LCL tear	*Hx:* direct trauma with varus stress, audible "pop", lateral knee pain *SSx:* local tenderness to palpation, (+) varus stress test *DDx:* ITB friction rub
PCL tear	*Hx:* direct trauma with posterior to anterior stress, audible "pop" *SSx:* (+) posterior drawer, reverse Lachman's *DDx:* often associated with ACL & meniscus injury
Chondromalacia patellae	*Hx:* prior trauma, retropatellar pain, worse with prolonged walking, going down stairs, positive Movie/theater sign, crepitus/grinding in knee *SSx:* (+) patellar grind, abnormal tracking *DDx:* condition is effectively patellofemoral DJD, meniscus tear, knee DJD
Menicus tear	*Hx:* painful click or snapping, deep joint line pain, joint locking *SSx:* local tenderness to palpation, (+) McMurray's, Apley's compression/distraction (+) Thessaly test (disco test) *DDx:* MCL & ACL tear (may occur in conjunction)
Osgood-Schlatter's	*Hx:* active pre-teen/teens - insidious onset or after intense activity *SSx:* focal tenderness, swelling, red, pain with RROM, pain brought on by activity, will be able to point to the pain DDx: osteochondroma
ITB friction rub	*Hx:* recent ↑ in running distance, intensity, frequency or duration, lateral knee pain *SSx:* local tenderness, (+) Noble's, Ober's *DDx:* LCL tear, pes planus & genu varum may predispose to condition
Plica syndrome	*Hx:* pain over lateral or medial condyle, snapping sensation *SSx:* tender band or cord from patella to condyle, (+) active stutter, Houston's test *DDx:* ITB friction rub, arthroscopy is the gold standard for diagnosis

↑ = increase, ↓ = decrease, Hx = history, SSx = signs & symptoms, DDx = differential diagnosis, (+) = positive
see blue 'Orthopedic Conditions' and yellow 'Physical Assessment' texts for more details

Knee

Bones

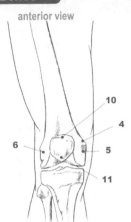

anterior view

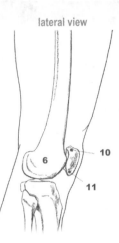

lateral view

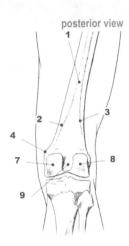

posterior view

1. Linea aspera
2. Medial supracondylar ridge
3. Lateral supracondylar ridge
4. Adductor tubercle
5. Medial epicondyle

6. Lateral epicondyle
7. Medial condyle
8. Lateral condyle
9. Intercondylar fossa

Patella

10. Base
11. Apex

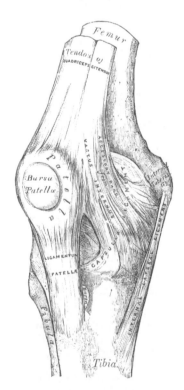

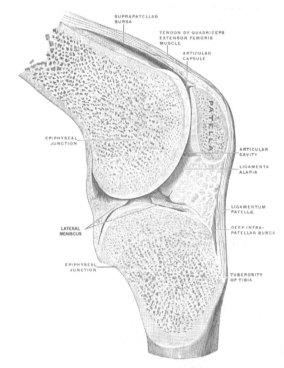

prohealthsys

anterior view

posterior view

Knee

Knee ligaments

1. Lateral (fibular) collateral ligament
2. Medial (tibial) collateral ligament
3. Patellar ligament (infrapatellar tendon)
4. Infrapatellar fat pad
5. Anterior cruciate ligament
6. Posterior cruciate ligament
7. Medial meniscus
8. Lateral meniscus
9. Anterolateral Ligament (ALL)[1]

superior
view right

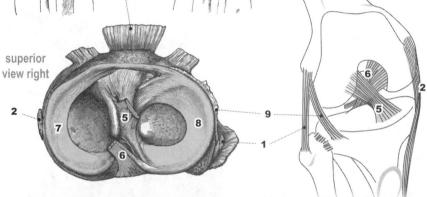

Ligament	Attaches (origin/insertion)	Function
Patellar (infrapatellar tend.)	Interior patella to tibial tuberosity	Transmits force from quadriceps to tibia
Anterior Cruciate	Anterior intercondylar area of tibia to medial surface of lateral femoral condyle	Resists anterior tibial translation & extension, internal rotation, flexion (tight in full extension)
Posterior cruciate	Posterior tibial spine to inner lateral femoral condyle	Resists posterior tibial movement, movements of flexion & rotation (tight in full extension)
Medial (tibial) collateral	Medial epicondyle of femur to medial condyle of tibia & medial meniscus	Resists valgus forces (tight in extension) & internal/external rotation (direct attachment to medial meniscus)
Lateral (fibular) collateral	Lateral epicondyle of femur to head of fibula	Resists varus forces (tight in extension)
Anterolateral lig (ALL)[1]	Lateral femur epicondyle to proximal tibia (attaches to lateral meniscus)	Supports anterolateral stability of the knee (may influence meniscus mobility)
Proximal Tib-Fib	Tibia to fibular head	Holds fibula against tibia, resists superior, anterior and posterior fibular translation (heel strike)

1. Steven Claes, Evie Vereecke, Michael Maes, Jan Victor, Peter Verdonk, Johan Bellemans. Anatomy of the anterolateral ligament of the knee. Journal of Anatomy, 2013; 223 (4): 321 DOI: 10.1111/joa.12087

Coronary ligaments hold the meniscus to the tibia and **transverse ligaments** connect the menisci anteriorly

Knee

Varus/Valgus Stress Test

Valgus Test Procedure (Abduction Stress Test)

Patient supine with legs straight, examiner stabilizes medial ankle & applies a lateral to medial (valgus) force at the knee, procedure is then repeated with the knee slightly flexed (~25°)

Interpretation

(+) Pain → Medial collateral ligament sprain

(+) Increased motion/gapping → Medial collateral ligament rupture

Clinical notes

The term valgus refers to the distal bone moving laterally, Varus stress test is in the opposite direction
Medial collateral ligament injury classification

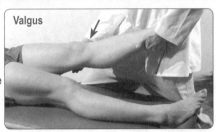

Valgus

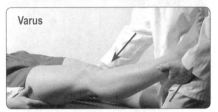

Varus

Anterior/Posterior Drawer Test

Procedure

Patient supine with knee bent 90°, examiner stabilizes foot with hip & places thumbs over the anterior knee joint line & pulls the tibia anteriorly

* Keep index fingers on hamstring tendons - overactive hamstring can stabilize the knee and hide ACL injuries

Interpretation

(+) Pain → Anterior /posterior cruciate ligament sprain

(+) Excessive motion → Anterior or posterior cruciate rupture

Clinical notes

Degrees of knee joint instability

Grade	Description
I	mild, < 5 mm of translation
II	moderate, 5-10 mm of translation
III	severe, > 10 mm translation

This test shows higher sensitivity values when performed on non-acute knee injuries[54]

(SN: 18-95 SP: 86-100 +LR: 1.8-8.3 -LR: 0.1-0.5)[2, 5, 17, 23, 24, 25, 32, 44, 54, 65, 66, 113, 114, 115]

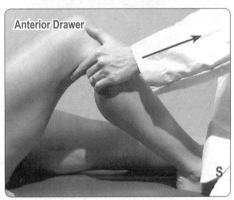

Anterior Drawer

S

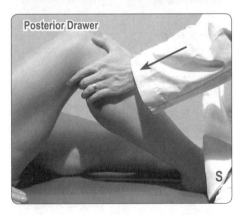

Posterior Drawer

S

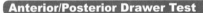

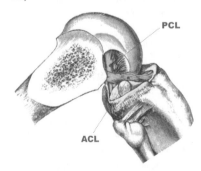

PCL

ACL

Posterior Drawer

Push P-A on the tibia for the posterior drawer test to challange the PCL - watch for overactive quads which can stabilize the knee and hide PCL injuries

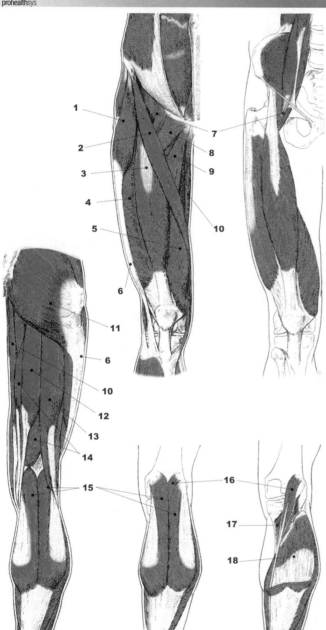

1. Tensor fascae latae
2. Sartorius
3. Rectus femoris
4. Vastus lateralis
5. Vastus medialis
6. Iliotibial band
7. Iliopsoas
8. Pectineus
9. Adductor longus
10. Gracilis
11. Gluteus maximus
12. Semitendinosus
13. Biceps femoris
14. Semimembranosus
15. Gastrocnemius
16. Plantaris
17. Popliteus
18. Soleus
19. Achilles tendon

Knee

Joint type: synovial
- Modified hinge (tibiofemoral) - largest & most complex joint in body
- Gliding (patellofemoral)

Articular surfaces
- **Tibiofemoral:** *concave* (tibial plateau) *on convex* (femoral condyles)

Active range of motion
- Flexion .... 150°
- Extension .... 0° to -5°
- Internal rotation*..... 20-30°
- External rotation*.... 30-40°
- * knee must be flexed 90° to allow rotation

Main muscle actions
- **Flexion:** semitendinosus, semimembranosus, biceps femoris (hamstrings)
- **Extension:** vastus medialis, vastus lateralis, vastus intermedius, rectus femoris (quadriceps)
- **Internal rotation** (tibia): popliteus with pes anserine muscles (knee flexed)
- **External rotation** (tibia): biceps femoris

Resting position
- **Tibiofemoral:** 25° flexion
- **Patellofemoral:** full extension (straight leg)

Close packed position
- **Tibiofemoral:** full extension & external tibial rotation
- **Patellofemoral:** full flexion

Capsular pattern of restriction
- **Tibiofemoral:** flexion > extension

Normal end feel
- **Flexion:** soft tissue or bony approximation
- **Extension:** elastic/firm
- **SLR:** elastic

Abnormal end feel
- **Boggy** = joint effusion; ligamentous pathology
- **Springy block** = loose body (displaced meniscus)

Kinetic chain
- **Tibiofemoral open chain:**
  Flexion: tibia rolls & glides posterior on femur
  Extension: tibia rolls & glides anterior on femur
- **Tibiofemoral closed chain (squat):**
  Flexion: femur rolls posterior & glides ant on tibia
  Extension: femur rolls anterior & glides posterior

- **Patellofemoral** femur moves in relation to patella:
Flexion: glide superior & roll inferior femur on patella
Exten.: glide inferior & roll superior femur on patella

Osteokinematics

- Femoral condyles begin to contact patella at 20° flexion; then progress superior to 90° & medial/lateral at 135° of knee flexion (see image below)

- Medial meniscus is attached to medial collateral ligament & semimembranosus muscle

- Lateral meniscus is attached to posterior cruciate ligament & popliteus muscle

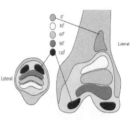

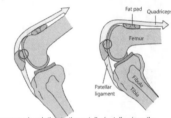

the femur moves in relation to the patella (patella stays the same distance from the tibia due to the patellar ligament)

Patellofemoral loading forces
- **Walking:** 0.3x body weight
- **Up stairs:** 2.5x body weight
- **Down stairs:** 3.5x body weight
- **Squatting:** 7x body weight
- **Deep squat:** ~12x body weight

Genu valgum, varum & recurvatum

- **Genu valgum:** Q angle > 22° (women), 18° (men)
  - Also known as "knocked knees"

- **Genu varum:** Q angle < 0° (distal tibia points medially) - also known as "bow legs"

- **Genu recurvatum:** hyperextension of knee > -5°

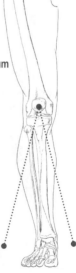

♂ **<18°**   Genu
♀ **<22°**   valgum

During the **last ~15° of knee extension with the foot free, the tibia rotates laterally and "locks" into extension.** When standing as the knee extends the **femur medially rotates** and locks into extension. This "locking" is called the screw home mechanism. ('locks' knee in closed packed position - decreasing the work performed by the quadriceps while standing - low energy state standing)

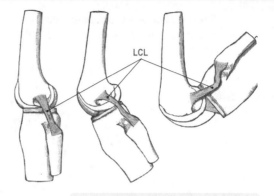

LCL

Clinical note: all knee ligaments are tight in terminal extension and loose with flexion

Screw Home Mechanism

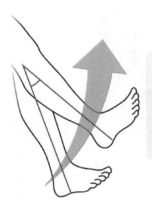

Femur motion (closed chain as in standing)

last 15° of extension femur rotates medial tibia rotates lateral

Tibia motion (open chain as in kicking)

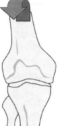
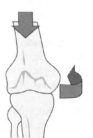
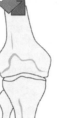
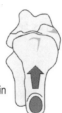
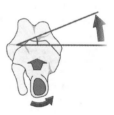

MRI of ACL rupture

- Visible on exam with anterior drawer test (pulls on ACL)

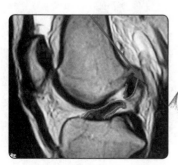

ACL

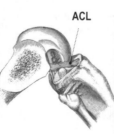

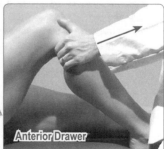

Anterior Drawer

Compare bilaterally, start with unaffected side for PROM & RROM
Prior to assessing ROM the examiner should make an introduction statement:
"Try and move as far as possible, if any of the actions or movements are painful or uncomfortable please let me know, do not do any action you feel will cause you further injury."

AROM

Flexion (130°-150°)
Muscles Activated: semitendinosus, semimembranosus, biceps femoris (hamstrings), popliteus
Tissue Stretched: quadriceps, femoral nerve
Tissue Compressed: popliteal fossa structure (popliteal artery, tibial nerve). patella compressed into femoral condyles

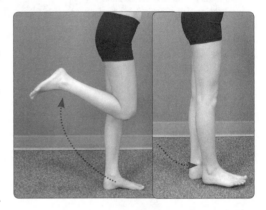

Extension (0° to -5°)
Muscles Activated: vastus medialis, vastus lateralis, vastus intermedius, rectus femoris (quadriceps)
Tissue Stretched: semitendinosus, semimembranosus, biceps femoris (hamstrings), popliteus, gastrocnemius, sciatic nerve
Tissue Compressed: anterior knee structures

Medial Rotation (20-30°)
Muscles Activated: semitendinosus, semimembranosus, sartorius, gracillis

Lateral Rotation (30-40°)
Muscles Activated: biceps femoris
*patient seated, feet flat on floor -knee must be flexed 90°

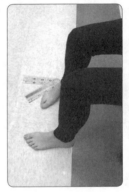
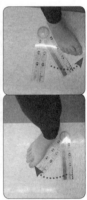

Goniometry

Flexion (normal 130°-150°)
- Patient prone or standing with knees straight (0°)
- Fulcrum aligned with the lateral femoral epicondyle
- Stationary arm in line with greater trochanter; moving arm in line with lateral malleolus
- Ask patient to flex knee

Extension (normal: 0° to -5°)
- Patient prone with a towel under the ankle to assess full extension
- Fulcrum aligned with the lateral femoral epicondyle
- Stationary arm in line with greater trochanter; moving arm in line with lateral malleolus
- Ask patient to extend knee

- If the patient cannot stand on one leg these measurements can also be done in the prone position

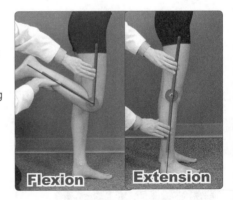

Flexion   Extension

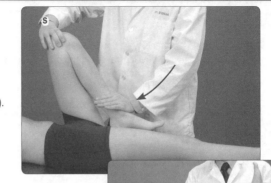

PROM

Flexion (> 130°-150°)
Tissue Stretched: quadriceps, femoral nerve (if done with hip straight)
Tissue Compressed: popliteal fossa structure (popliteal artery, tibial nerve). patella compressed into femoral condyles

Extension (> 0° to -5°)
Tissue Stretched: semitendinosus, semimembranosus, biceps femoris (hamstrings), popliteus, gastrocnemius, sciatic nerve
Tissue Compressed: anterior knee structures

> Knee rotation may also be assessed with AROM, PROM & RROM with the knee bent 90°

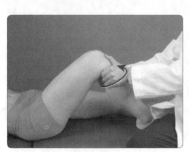
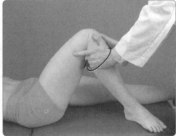

Muscle Testing

Resisted Extension
Muscles Activated: vastus medialis, vastus lateralis, vastus intermedius, rectus femoris (quadriceps)

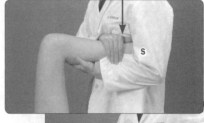

Resisted Flexion
Muscles Activated: semitendinosus, semimembranosus, biceps femoris (hamstrings), popliteus

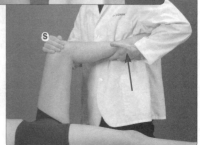

Stretch

Stretch: deliberate lengthening of muscles & fascia, in order to increase muscle flexibility and/or joint range of motion (stretches develop passive tension); **it is crucial to ask patients to demonstrate the stretches they are performing to ensure proper technique & injury avoidance**
Stretches should be held for 15-30 seconds & performed after a mild warm up

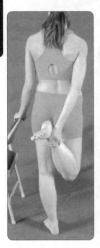
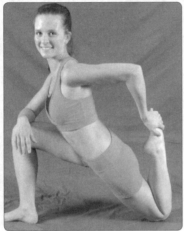
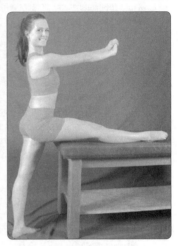

Strengthen

Exercises demonstrated in this text may be performed at home with or without weights, therapy bands, soup cans, pots or any other device that can provide muscle resistance.
KIS - Keep it simple. Exercises & stretches should be easy to do & easy to remember **(show patients how to do it, have them demonstrate it & give handouts with pictures to use at home)**
Keep it short. Time is precious, so keep the home routine to under 15 minutes.
Keep it pain-free. The patient should not work in painful areas; the amount of stretch, weight & reps should be started at below what the practitioner believes the patient's ability is & progress slowly

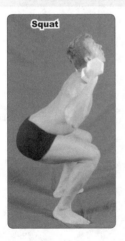
Squat

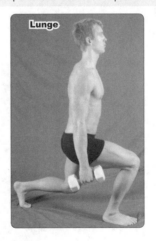
Lunge

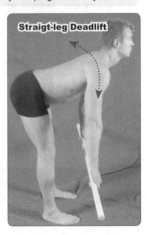
Straigt-leg Deadlift

S = stabilization (indifferent hand),   ● = contact,   ⟶ = examiner force,   ┈┈┈▶ = patient motion

Knee (side tab)

Hamstring pin & stretch

Pin & Stretch treatments can be adapted & applied to any myofascial structure if the clinician has a detailed understanding of basic anatomy & biomechanics

1. Clinician places muscle in shortened position & pins specific myofascial fibers with other hand
2. Patient is then <u>passively</u> moved to lengthen muscle while pinning force is maintained
3. Hold at tension for ~10 seconds or until myofascial release is felt; repeat & reassess as needed

1. Clinician places muscle in shortened position (hip neutral & knee flexed - origin & insertion approximated) & pins specific myofascial fibers with other hand
2. Patient is then passively moved to lengthen muscle (hip flexion - move insertion away from origin) while pinning force is maintained
3. Hold at tension for ~10 sec or until release is felt; repeat as needed

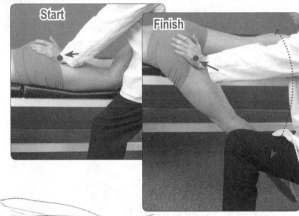

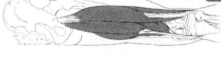

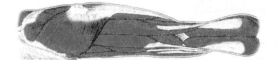

Knee Flexion Restriction

With good anatomy & biomechanical understanding, MET can be adapted to any patient

1. Clinician gently stretches patient into direction of restriction or decreased range of motion
2. Patient gently (10% of maximum) contracts in exact opposite motion
3. Clinician resists & patient holds contraction for 3-7 seconds, then patient completely relaxes
4. On relaxation, clinician moves to new resistive barrier; repeat 3-5 times & reassess

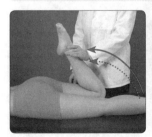

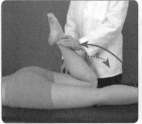

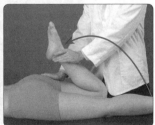

| Flexion tissue resistance | Patient contracts ~10% in extension | Clinician finds new end range |

S = stabilization (indifferent hand),   ● = contact,   ——▶ = examiner force,   ·······▶ = patient motion

Knee

A-P & P-A Glide

Indications: restricted A-P or P-A glide of tibia on femur

Position: patient supine with knee flexed ~90°, clinician stabilizes patients foot with their thigh

Contact: clinician places hands bilaterally with fingers over both gastrocnemius heads, palms over anterior proximal tibia & thumbs on either side of the patellar ligament

Force: tissue force is A-P or P-A; develop tension by gently pulling or pushing the tibia

Clinical notes: essentially an anterior or posterior drawer orthopedic test (lower right picture shows a A-P variation)

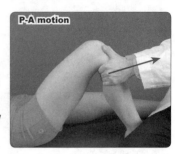

P-A motion

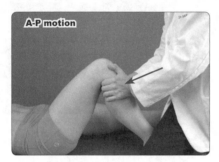

A-P motion

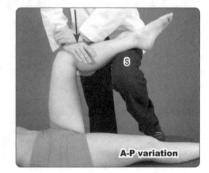

A-P variation

Internal & External Rotation

Indications: restricted A-P or P-A glide of tibia on femur

Position: patient supine with knee flexed ~90°

Contact: clinician places hands bilaterally with fingers over both gastrocnemius heads, palms over anterior proximal tibia & thumbs on either side of the patellar ligament

Force: tissue force is internal or external rotation; clinician develops tension by gently pulling with one hand & pulling with the other hand

Clinical notes: can be performed as a manipulation or mobilization

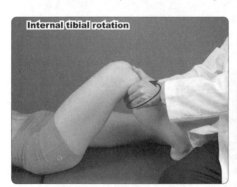

Internal tibial rotation

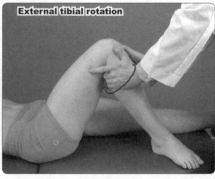

External tibial rotation

S = stabilization (indifferent hand), ● = contact, ──→ = examiner force, ·······▷ = patient motion

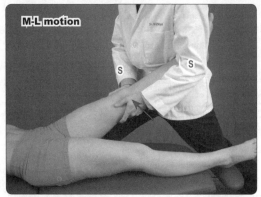

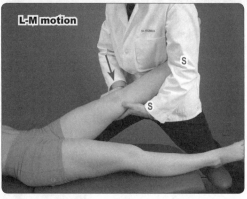

M-L & L-M Glide

Indications: restricted M-L or L-M glide of tibia on femur

Position: patient supine with knee straight

Contact: clinician places hands bilaterally on either side of the knee & the patient's ankle is stabilized between the elbow & hip

Force: tissue force is M-L or L-M; clinician develops tension by gently applying pressure with one hand & stabilizing with the other

Clinical notes: can be performed as a manipulation or mobilization; to improve biomechanical advantage with a M-L glide, consider externally rotating the patient's hip to allow more M-L force to be applied in a downward direction

Grade	Description, ADLs & Healing
Grade I - Mild	• Point tenderness over MCL, no bruising or swelling • Little or no instability with valgus stress test at 30° of knee flexion • Joint space opening < 5 mm • None to very mild limp/loss of function, possible difficulty hopping on one leg • Recovery in 2-14 days
Grade II - Moderate 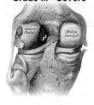	• Possible mild bruising & swelling with point tenderness over MCL • Large spectrum of injury that can include injury to medial meniscus & ACL • Some laxity (5 - 10 mm) with valgus stress test at 30° of knee flexion • Obvious limp, difficulty hopping or running • Recovery in 14-40 days (up to 2 months)
Grade III - Severe	• Complete tear of MCL, marked instability, patient reports a "wobbly knee" • Marked swelling, may or may not cause as much pain as incomplete tears • Significant laxity (> 10 mm) with an empty end feel when valgus stress test 30° • Usually will have concomitant ACL & meniscus damage • Limp with limited ability to bear weight, some loss of ROM • Recovery time 1-3 months (possibly up to 6 months)

S = stabilization (indifferent hand),   ● = contact,   ——▶ = examiner force,   ·········▶ = patient motion

Distraction

Indications: restricted knee ROM, joint contracture or scar tissue formation

Position: patient supine, seated or prone

Contact: see images

Force: clinician develops tension by gently applying pressure with one hand & stabilizing with the other

Clinical notes: can be performed as a manipulation or mobilization, knee distraction is contraindicated in the presence of hypermobility

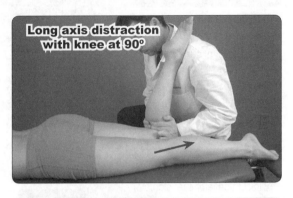

Long axis distraction with knee at 90°

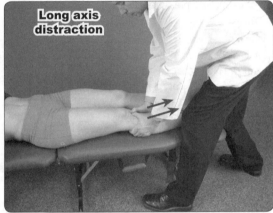

Long axis distraction

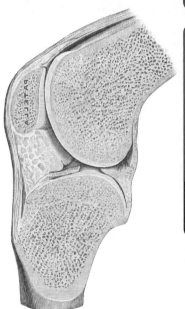

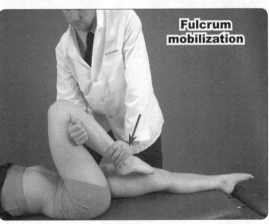

Fulcrum mobilization

S = stabilization (indifferent hand), ● = contact, ——▶ = examiner force, ·········▶ = patient motion

M-L & L-M Patellar Glide

Indications: restricted patellar medial or lateral ROM, patellar tracking abnormalities, joint contracture, surgical rehab or scar tissue formation

Position: patient supine, or seated with knee straight & quadriceps relaxed, clinician at side of table

Contact:

M-L glide - clinician places thumbs over lateral patella

L-M glide - clinician places fingers over medial patella

Force: clinician develops tension by gently pulling (M-L) or pushing (L-M) on patella

Clinical notes: can be performed as a manipulation or mobilization, M-L mobilization is contraindicated in the presence of hypermobility or recent lateral patellar dislocations

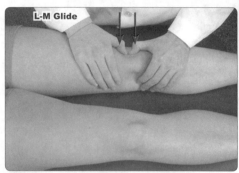

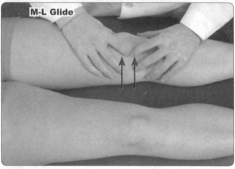

Superior & Inferior Patellar Glide

Indications: restricted patellar ROM, patellar tracking abnormalities, joint contracture, surgical rehab or scar tissue formation

Position: patient supine, or seated with knee straight & quadriceps relaxed, clinician at side of table

Contact:

Superior glide - clinician places hand over inferior patella (patellar apex)

Inferior glide - clinician places hand over superior patella (patellar base)

Force: clinician develops tension by gently pushing the patella superiorly (I-S) or inferiorly (S-I)

Clinical notes: can be performed as a manipulation or mobilization

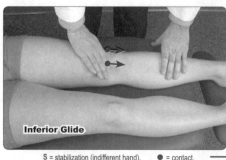

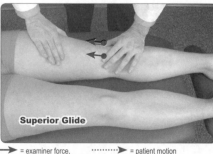

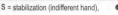
S = stabilization (indifferent hand), ● = contact, ⟶ = examiner force, ┄┄┄▶ = patient motion

prohealthsys

A-P & P-A Fibular Glide

Indications: restricted fibular ROM, joint contracture, or scar tissue formation

Position: patient supine, side-lying, prone or seated with knee flexed at ~90°, clinician at foot of table

Contact:

A-P glide - clinician places palm of hand over anterior lateral fibular head

P-A glide - clinician places fingers over posterior lateral fibular head

Force: clinician develops tension by gently pulling (P-A) or pushing (A-P) on fibula while stabilizing the tibia & knee with the other hand

Clinical notes: can be performed as a manipulation or mobilization

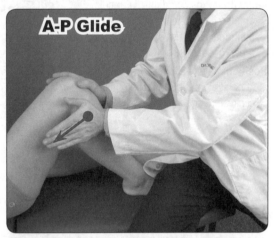

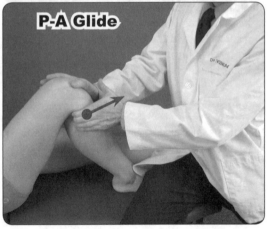

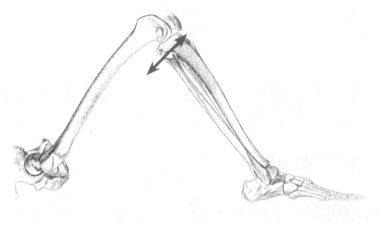

S = stabilization (indifferent hand),　● = contact,　——▶ = examiner force,　·········▶ = patient motion

Superior & Inferior Fibular Glide

Indications: restricted fibular ROM, joint contracture, or scar tissue formation

Position: patient supine, side-lying, prone or seated with knee flexed at ~90°

Contact:

Superior glide - clinician places palm of hand over inferior fibular head

Inferior glide - clinician places palm of hand over superior fibular head

Force: clinician develops tension by gently pushing (S-I or I-S) on fibula while stabilizing the tibia & knee with the other hand

Clinical notes: can be performed as a manipulation or mobilization an alternate variation is shown in the lower pictures by inverting the ankle inferior glide of the fibula may be induced or by everting the ankle superior fibular glide may also be produced

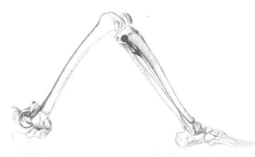

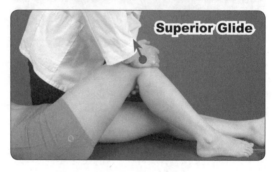

Inferior Glide

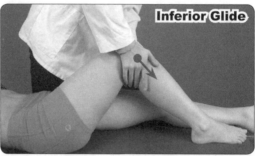

Superior Glide

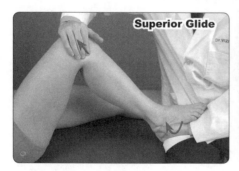

Superior Glide

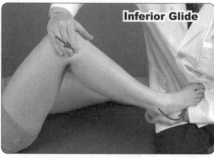

Inferior Glide

S = stabilization (indifferent hand), ● = contact, ——▶ = examiner force, ·········▶ = patient motion

1. Vizniak, NA. Clinical Cadaver Dissections. 1999-2018
2. McGee S. Evidence-Based Physical Diagnosis. Saunders. 2017.
3. Magee D. Orthopedic Physical Assessment, 5th Edition. Saunders. 2008.
4. Taylor MH, Monroe LG. Physical Rehabilitation: Evidence-Based Examination, Evaluation and Intervention. Saunders. 2007.
5. Warlow C, Hughes R, Uitehaag B, Liberati A. Evidence-Based Neurology. Blackwell Publishing Limited, BMJI Books. 2007.
6. Malanga GA & Nadler. Musculoskeletal Physical Exam, An Evidence-Based Approach. Mosby. 2006.
7. Hoppenfield S. Physical Examination of the Spine & Extremities. Lippincott Williams & Wilkins. 1976.
8. Hoppenfield S. Orthopaedic Neurology: A Diagnostic Guide to Neurologic Levels. Lippincott Williams & Wilkins. 1977.
9. Spencer JW, Jacobs JJ. Complementary and Alternative Medicine: An Evidence-Based Approach. Mosby. 2003.
10. Jewell D. Guide to Evidence-Based Physical Therapy Practice. Jones Barlett Publishers Inc. 2007.
11. lesel SW. Operative Orthopaedics: An Illustrative Approach. Lippincott Williams & Wilkins. 2008.
12. Adams S, Yarnold P. Clinical use of the patellar-pubic percussion sign in Abdon P, Lindstrand A, Thorngren KG. Statistical evaluation of the diagnostic criteria for meniscal tears. Int Orthop. 1990;14:341-345.
13. Akseki D, Ozcan 0, Boya H, Pinar H. A new weight-bearing meniscal test and a comparison with McMurray's test and joint line tenderness. Arthroscopy. 2004;20:951 -958.
14. al-Dun Z. Relation of the fibular head sign to other signs of anterior cruciate ligament insufficiency: a follow-up letter to the editor. Clin Orthop Relat Res. 1992:220-225.
15. Allen CR, Kaplan LD, Fluhrne DJ, Harner CD. Posterior cruciate ligament injuries. Curr Opin Rheum. 2002;14:142-149.
16. Amatuzzi MM, Fazzi A, Varella MH. Pathologic synovial plica of the knee: results of conservative treatment. Am J Sports Med. 1990;18:466-469.
17. Anderson AF, Lipscomb AB. Clinical diagnosis of meniscal tears: description of a new manipulative test: Am I Sports Med. 1986;14:291 -293.
18. Anderson AF, Lipscomb AB. Preoperative instrumented testing of anterior and posterior knee laxity. Am I Sports Med. 1 989;17:387-392.
19. Apley, AG. The diagnosis of meniscus injuries. JBJS. 1947;29:78-84.
20. Bach BR, Jr., Warren RF, Wickiewicz TL. The pivot shift phenomenon: results and description of a modified clinical test for anterior cruciate ligament insufficiency. Am J Sports Med. 1988;16:571-576.
21. Baciu CC, Tudor A, Olaru I. Recurrent luxation of the superior tibio-fibular joint in the adult. Acta Orthop Scand. 1974;45:772-777.
22. Barry OC, Smith H, McManus F, MacAuley P. Clinical assessment of suspected meniscal tears. Ir J Med Sci. 1983;152:149-151.
23. Bauer Sj, Hollander JE, Fuchs SH, Thode HC, Jr. A clinical decision rule in the evaluation of acute knee injuries. J Emerg Med. 1995;13:611-615.
24. Boeree NR, Ackroyd CE. Assessment of the menisci and cruciate ligaments: an audit of clinical practice. Injury. 1991;22:291-294.
25. Bomberg BC, McGinty JB. Acute hemarthrosis of the knee: indications for diagnostic arthroscopy. Arthroscopy. 1990;6:221-225.
26. Braunstein EM. Anterior cruciate ligament injuries: a comparison of arthrographic and physical diagnosis. AJR Am J Roent. 1982;1 38:423-425.
27. Clendenin MB, DeLee JC, Heckman ID. Interstitial tears of the posterior cruciate ligament of the knee. Orthopedics. 1 980;3:764-772.
28. Cooperman JM, Riddle DL, Rothstein JM. Reliability and validity of judgments of the integrity of the anterior cruciate ligament of the knee using the Lachman's test. Phys Ther. 1990;70:225-233.
29. Corea JR, Moussa M, al Othman A. McMurray's test tested. Knee Surg Sports Traumatol Arthrosc. 1994;2:70-72.
30. Cross Mi, Schmidt DR, Mackie 1G. A no-touch test for the anterior cruciate ligament. J Bone Joint Surg Br. 1987; 69:300.
31. Daniel DM, Stone ML, Barnett P, Sachs R. Use of the quadriceps active test to diagnose posterior cruciate-ligament disruption and measure posterior laxity of the knee. J Bone Joint Surg Am. 1988;70:386-391.
32. Dervin GF, Stiell IG, Wells GA, Rody K, Grabowski J. Physicians' accuracy and interrater reliability for the diagnosis of unstable meniscal tears in patients having osteoarthritis of the knee. Can] Surg. 2001;44:267-274.
33. Donaldson WF, 3rd, Warren RF, Wickiewicz T. A comparison of acute anterior cruciate ligament examinations: initial versus examination under anesthesia. Am J Sports Med. 1985;13:5-10.
34. Eren OT. The accuracy of joint line tenderness by physical examination in the diagnosis of meniscal tears. Arthroscopy. 2003;19:850-854.
35. Evans P1, Bell GD, Frank C. Prospective evaluation of the McMurray test. Am J Sports Med. 1993;21:604-608.
36. Feltham GT, Albright JP. The diagnosis of PCL injury: literature review and introduction of two novel tests. Iowa OrthopJ. 2001;21:36-42.
37. Ferrari DA, Ferrari JD, Coumas J. Posterolateral instability of the knee. J Bone Joint Surg Br. 1994; 76:187-192.
38. Flanagan JP, Trakru S, Meyer M, Mullaji AB, Krappel F. Arthroscopic excision of symptomatic medial plica: a study of 11 8 knees with 1-4 year follow-up. Acta Orthop Scand. 1994;65:408-411.
39. Fowler PJ, Lubliner JA. The predictive value of five clinical signs in the evaluation of meniscal pathology. Arthroscopy. 1989;5:184-186.
40. Fowler Pj, Messieh SS. Isolated posterior cruciate ligament injuries in athletes. Am J Sports Med. 1987;15:553-557.
41. Galway KR, Macintosh DL. The lateral pivot shift: a symptom and sign of anterior cruciate ligament insufficiency. Clin Orthop Relat Res. 1980:45-50.
42. Greene CC, Edwards TB, Wade MR, Carson EW. Reliability of the quadriceps angle measurement. Am J Knee Surg. 2012;1 4:97-103.
43. Grood ES, Stowers SF, Noyes FR. Limits of movement in the human knee: effect of sectioning the posterior cruciate ligament and posterolateral structures. J Bone Joint Surg Am. 1988;70:88-97.
44. Haim A, Yaniv M, Dekel 5, Amir H. Patellofemoral pain syndrome: validity of clinical and radiological features. Clin Orthop. 2006.
45. Hardaker WT, Jr., Garrett WE, Jr., Bassett FH. Evaluation of acute traumatic hemarthrosis of the knee joint. South Med J. 1990;83:640-644.
46. Hardaker WT, Whipple TL, Bassett FH, 3rd. Diagnosis and treatment of the plica syndrome of the knee. J Bone Joint Surg Am. 1 980;62:221-225.
47. Harilainen A. Evaluation of knee instability in acute ligamentous injuries. Ann Chir Gyn. 1987;76:269-273.
48. Harilainen A, Myllynen P, Rauste J, Silvennoinen E. Diagnosis of acute knee ligament injuries: the value of stress radiography compared with clinical examination, stability, under anaesthesia and arthroscopic or operative findings. Ann Chir Gyn. 1986;75:37-43.
49. Hughston IC, Andrews JR, Cross MJ, Moschi A. Classification of knee ligament instabilities: Part I. The medial compartment and cruciate ligaments. J Bone Joint Surg Am. 1976;58:159-172.
50. Hughston JC, Andrews JR, Cross MJ, Moschi A. Classification of knee ligament instabilities. Part II. The lateral compartment. J Bone Joint Surg Am. 1976;58:173-179.
51. Hughston JC, Norwood LA. The posterolateral drawer test and external rotational recurvatum test for posterolateral rotatory instability of the knee. Clin Orthop. 1980;14 7:82-87.
52. Jackson jL, O'Malley PG, Kroenke K. Evaluation of acute knee pain in primary care. Ann Intern Med. 2003;139:575-588.
53. Jakob RP, Hassler H, Staubli HU. Observations on rotatory instability of the lateral compartment of the knee: experimental studies on the functional anatomy and pathomechanism of the true and reversed pivot shift sign. Acta Orthop Scand. 1981;52:1-32.
54. Jerosch J, Riemer S. CHow good are clinical investigative procedures for diagnosing meniscus lesions? J Sportverletz Sportschaden. 2004;18:59-67.
55. Jonsson T, Althoff B, Peterson L, Renstrom P. Clinical diagnosis of ruptures of the anterior cruciate ligament: a comparative study of the Lachman test and the anterior drawer sign. Am J Sports Med. 1982;10:100-102.
56. Karachalios T, Hantes M, Zibis AH, Zachos V, Karantanas AH, Malizos KN. Diagnostic accuracy of a new clinical test (the Thessaly test) for early detection of meniscal tears. J Bone Joint Surg Am. 2005;87:955-962.
57. Kim SJ, Jeong JH, Cheon YM, Ryu SW. MPP test in the diagnosis of medial patellar plica syndrome. Arthroscopy. 2004;20:1 101-1103.
58. Kocabey Y, Tetik 0, Isbell WM, Atay OA, Johnson DL. The value of clinical examination versus magnetic resonance imaging in the diagnosis of meniscal tears and anterior cruciate ligament rupture. Arthroscopy. 2004;20:696-700.
59. Kocher MS, DiCanzio J, Zurakowski D, Micheli Li. Diagnostic performance of clinical examination and selective magnetic resonance imaging in the evaluation of intraarticular knee disorders in children and adolescents. Am J Sports Med. 2001 ;29:292-296.
60. Koshino T, Okamoto R. Resection of painfulshelf (plica synovialis mediopatellaris) under arthroscopy. Arthroscopy. 1985;1:136-141.
61. Kurosaka M, Yagi M, Yoshiya 5, Muratsu H, Mizuno K. Efficacy of the axially loaded pivot shift test for the diagnosis of a meniscal tear. Int Orthop. 1999;23:271 -274.
62. LaPrade RF, Konowalchuk BK. Popliteomeniscal fascicle tears causing symptomatic lateralcompartment knee pain: diagnosis by the figure-4 test and treatment by open repair. Am J Sports Med. 2005;33:1231-1 236.
63. LaPrade RF, Wentorf F. Diagnosis and treatment of posterolateral knee injuries. Clin Orthop. 2002;402:1 10-121.
64. Larson RL. Physical examination in the diagnosis of rotatory instability. Clin Orthop Relat Res. 1983:38-44.
65. Learmonth DJ. Incidence and diagnosis of anterior cruciate injuries in the accident and emergency department. Injury. 1991;22:287-290.
66. Lee JK, Yao L, Phelps CT, Wirth CR, Czajka J, Lozman I. Anterior cruciate ligament tears: MR imaging compared with arthroscopy and clinical tests. Radiology. 1988;166:861-864.
67. Liu SH, Osti L, Henry M, Bocchi L. The diagnosis of acute complete tears of the anterior cruciate ligament: comparison of MRI, arthrometry and clinical examination. J Bone Joint Surg Br. 1995;77:586-588.
68. Loomer RL. A test for knee posterolateral rotatory instability. Clin Orthop Relat Res. 1 991:235-238.
69. Loomer RL. A test for knee posterolateral rotatory instability. Clin Orthop. 1991;264:235-238.
70. Loos WC, Fox JM, Blazina ME, Del Pizzo W, Friedman MJ. Acute posterior cruciate ligament injuries. Am] Sports Med. 1981;9:86-92.
71. Losee RE. Concepts of the pivot shift. Clin Orthop Relat Res. 1983:45-51.
72. Losee RE. Diagnosis of chronic injury to the anterior cruciate ligament. Orthop Clin North Am. 1985;16:83-97.
73. Loudon JK, Wiesner D, Goist-Foley HL, Asjes C, Loudon KL. Intrarater reliability of functional performance tests for subjects with patellofemoral pain syndrome. J Athl Train. 2002;37:256-261.
74. Malanga GA, Andrus 5, Nadler SF, McLean J. Physical examination of the knee: a review of the original test description and scientific validity of common orthopedic tests. Arch Phys Med Rehabil. 2003;84:592-603.
75. Mariani PP, Adriani E, Maresca G, Mazzola CG. A prospective evaluation of a test for lateral meniscus tears. Knee Surg Sports Traum Arthrosc. 1996;4:22-26.
76. Martens MA, Mulier JC. Anterior subluxation of the lateral tibial plateau: a new clinical test and the morbidity of this type of knee instability. Arch Orthop Trauma Surg. 1981;98:109-111.
77. McClure PW, Rothstein JM, Riddle DL. Intertester reliability of clinical judgments of medial knee ligament integrity. Phys Ther. 1989;69:268-275.
78. McConnell J. The management of chondromalacia patella. Aust J Physiother. 1986;32:21 5-223.
79. Mital MA, Hayden J. Pain in the knee in children: the medial plica shelf syndrome. Orthop Clin North Am. 1979;1 0:71 3-722.
80. Moore HA, Larson RL. Posterior cruciate ligament injuries: results of early surgical repair. Am J Sports Med. 1980;8:68-78.
81. Nijs J, Van Geel C, Van der auwera D, Van de Velde B. Diagnostic value of five clinical tests in patellofemoral pain syndrome. Man Ther. 2006;1 1:69-77.
82. Niskanen RO, Paavilainen Pj, Jaakkola M, Korkala OL. Poor correlation of clinical signs with patellar cartilaginous changes. Arthroscopy. 2001;17:307-310.
83. Nissen CW, Cullen MC, Hewett TE, Noyes FR. Physical and arthroscopic examination techniques of the patellofemoral joint. J

Knee Quiz (answer page)

1. What are the joint type classifications for this region? (332) ________________
2. What are the joint surface shapes for this region (convex/concave)? (332) ____________________________
3. What is the normal ROM for ____________?
   - Flexion/Ext.: ________, ________
   - Rotation (ext./int) ________, ________
4. What is the resting position? __________
5. What is the knee joint tight packed position?
6. What ligaments resist extension? (329) ____________________________
7. What muscles cause flexion to occur? (332) ____________________________
8. With a deep squat, how many times your body weight is placed on the patella? (332) _________________
9. What is the normal Q-angle? (332) ________
10. Can you palpate _______________ ? (326)

Learning Objectives

After completing this chapter, students will be able to:

1. Perform a regional exam and differentiate common pathologies of the region

2. Identify and palpate body region bony landmarks, ligaments and muscles

3. Discuss regional kinematics and joint organ biomechanics

4. Demonstrate regional AROM, PROM, goniometry, stretch and strengthen protocols

5. Recognize and execute steps of effective mobilization and joint-play including indications, position, contact, force and relevant clinical notes

6. Perform supine, prone, seated assessment and mobilizations including

   • Pin and stretch
   • Muscle energy technique
   • Tibiotalar, subtalar, tarsal, phalangeal glides (A-P, P-A, M-L, L-M)
   • Long axis distraction and gapping
   • Internal and external rotational motions

Leg, Ankle & Foot

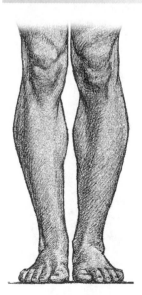
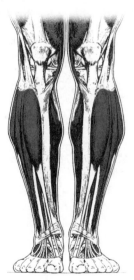
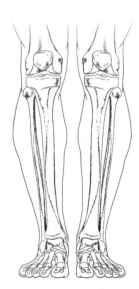

Realize that any mobilization (grade 1-4) can be made into a manipulation (grade 5) with a high velocity low amplitude (HVLA) thrust & vise versa with the lack of a HVLA thrust

Conversely any technique can be adapted to use IASTM where indicated to save your hands

Special history questions
- Specific mechanism of injury & forces involved?
  - did you hear a "popping" sound?
- Any swelling?
- What type & age of shoes? Running surface?
- Wear pattern on shoes? Possible fracture?

Inspection
- Asymmetry, bruising, bumps, color, swelling
- Posture (pes planus, cavus)

Fracture screen (older than 55?)
1. 4 step test, torsion test
2. Bony tenderness on palpation
3. Percussion, tuning fork (128 Hz)

Palpation (may be done after ROM assessment)

Tibial tub./fibular head	Subtalar joint
Tibial crest	Midtarsal joint
Lateral malleolus	Tarsometatarsal joints
Medial malleolus	MP joints
Navicular	PIP joints
Cuboid	DIP joints
Cuneiforms	Gastrocnemius/soleus
Talus (head, neck, trochlea)	Lateral leg muscles
Calcaneus	Anterior leg muscles
Sustentaculum tali	Achilles tendon
Metatarsals	Fibularis tendons
Phalanges	TDH muscles
Sinus tarsi	Tarsal tunnel
Ant. talofibular lig.	Tibialis anterior
Calcaneofibular lig.	Calcaneal bursa
Post. talofibular lig.	Plantar fascia
Spring ligament	Plantar muscles
Deltoid ligament	Saphenous vein

TDH = Tom Dick & Harry - Tibialis posterior, Flexor
Digitorum Longus & Flexor hallicus longus

Functional assessment (ADLs)
- Squat & rise, heel walk, toe walk

AROM
Talocrural
Plantar flexion .... 40°
Dorsiflexion .... 20°
Subtalar
Inversion .... 20°
Eversion .... 10°

PROM & Joint Play (if lacking AROM in any motion)

Myotomes (resisted isometric movements)
- Hip flexion (L1-L3, femoral n.)
- Knee extension (L3-L4; femoral n.)
- Knee flexion (L4-S2, sciatic n.)
- Ankle dorsiflexion (**L4**, L5 - deep peroneal),
- Ankle inversion (L5, **S1** - sup. peroneal)
- Ankle eversion (**S1** - sup. peroneal)
- Big toe extension, (L4, **L5**, S1; deep peron.)
- Big toe flexion (L5-S1, tibial nerve)

Neurovascular screen
Sensory: Light touch, sharp/dull or pinwheel
Vibration (DIP, 3rd digit)
UMNL: Babinski (L1 & above)
- **DTR's:** patella (L4), hamstring (L5), Achilles (S1)
- **Pulses:** femoral, tibial, dorsal pedal
- Nail bed blanching
- Buerger's claudication test

Orthopedic tests (as indicated)

Screening
- Heel walk, toe walk

Instability/Ligament stress
- Anterior drawer/plantar flexed
- Posterior drawer/neutral ankle
- Inversion talar tilt (neutral)
- Inversion talar tilt (plantar flex)
- Eversion talar tilt
- Subtalar glide test
- Rotational stress

Vascular
- Claudication test
- Buerger's claudication test
- Tourniquet test
- Homan's test

Stress fracture
- Calcaneal squeeze test
- Morton's squeeze test

Achilles tendonitis/rupture
- Achilles tap test
- Achilles squeeze test
- Hoffa's/Simmond's test

Nerve compression
- Tinel's test

Lumbar, SI, hip & knee screen

Diagnostic imaging (if indicated)

youtube: vizniak ankle exam brief

Condition	Clinical notes
Achilles tendinitis	*Hx:* painful tendon, worse with running, jumping & stairs, better with rest *SSx:* tender to palpation, (+) Achilles squeeze test, Thompson test *DDx:* Achilles strain
Plantar fascitis	*Hx:* pain in morning worse with first few steps *SSx:* tender to palpation, (+) calcaneal squeeze *DDx:* calcaneal stress fracture 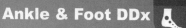
Stress fractures	*Hx:* insidious onset of pain, better with rest, overuse injury (repetitive stress) *SSx:* tender to palpation (common locations: tibia, calcaneus, metatarsals) **Tibial Stress Fracture** - most common stress fracture of body; usually involves dominant or long leg; repetitive trauma (long distance running/walking/marching, military recruits, ballet dancers); usually proximal posterior diaphysis region which is usually stable; less common in mid-shaft where the "dreaded black line" may be observed indicating more significant injury **Metatarsals Stress Fracture** (March fracture) - common usually involve 2nd & 3rd (1st and 5th rarely); secondary to repetitive stress (more often long leg, distance running, sprinting, pronation syndrome); tenderness with metatarsal squeeze test **Calcaneus Stress Fracture** – common stable fracture; secondary to repetitive trauma (distance running, military recruits, dancers, gymnasts, & jumpers); heel pain that may mimic plantar fasciitis or retrocalcaneal bursitis/achilles tendonitis; tenderness with calcaneal side squeeze & calcaneal percussion; may be painful with heal strike during gait – patient will often have altered gait (soft heel strike)
Compartment syndrome	*Hx:* symptoms exercise induced, better with rest, muscle weakness *SSx:* local swelling & tightness, (+) calf circumference test, muscle weakness *DDx:* tibial stress fracture, tibialis anterior strain
Ankle sprain	*Hx:* significant trauma, mild-moderate pain *SSx:* local swelling (+) talar tilt tests, anterior/posterior drawer, rotational stress test *DDx:* avulsion fracture
Tarsal tunnel syndrome	*Hx:* medial or plantar foot pain of paresthesia *SSx:* tenderness around tarsal tunnel, (+) Tinel's test *DDx:* lumbar radiculopathy
Morton's neuroma	*Hx:* burning pain between metatarsals *SSx:* local tenderness, (+) Morton's neuroma test (metatarsal squeeze) *DDx:* lumbar radiculopathy, metatarsal stress fracture

↑ = increase, ↓ = decrease, Hx = history, SSx = signs & symptoms, DDx = differential diagnosis, (+) = positive
see blue 'Orthopedic Conditions' and yellow 'Physical Assessment' texts for more details

Leg, Ankle & Foot

Joint type: synovial
  Hinge (talocrural, metatarsophalangeal &
    interphalangeal)
  Gliding (subtalar, midtarsal joints)

AROM
Talocrural (talotibial)
  Plantar flexion .... 40°
  Dorsiflexion .... 20°
Subtalar
  Inversion .... 30°
  Eversion .... 15°
Metatarsophalangeal
  Flexion .... 75°
  Extension .... 35°
Interphalangeal
  Flexion .... ~60°
  Extension .... ~20°

Normal joint end feels
  Talocrural: firm ligamentous
  Subtalar: firm ligamentous
  TMT: elastic firm
  MTP extension: elastic / ligamentous

MTP flexion: firm / ligamentous
MTP big toe: firm / bony
PIP flexion: firm / bony
PIP extension: firm / ligamentous
DIP flexion: firm / ligamentous / elastic
DIP extension: firm / ligamentous / elastic

Main muscle actions
  Plantar flexion: soleus, gastrocnemius, tibialis
    posterior, flexor digitorum longus, flexor hallucis
    longus
  Dorsiflexion: tibialis anterior, extensor digitorum
    longus
  Inversion: tibialis anterior, tibialis posterior
  Eversion: fibularis longus, brevis & tertius

  1st toe flexion: flexor hallucis longus & brevis
  Toe 2-5 flexion: flexor digitorum longus & brevis,
    lumbricals
  1st toe extension: extensor hallicus l. & brevis
  Toe extension: extensor digitorum longus & brevis
  Abduction: dorsal interossei
  Adduction: palmar interossei

Joint		Resting Position	Tight Packed	Capsular Pattern
Talocrural		~10° plantar flexion	Full dorsiflexion	Plantar flex. > dorsiflex.
Subtalar		Mid ROM	Full supination	Varus, valgus
Midtarsal		Mid ROM	Supination	Dorsiflexion > plantarflex
TMT	1st toe	Mid ROM	Supination	None
	2-5 toes	Mid flexion & extension.		
1st MTP		5° extension	Full extension	Flexion > extension
2-5 MTP		2° flexion	Full extension	Variable
IP		2° flexion	Full extension	Flexion > extension

MTP = metatarsal phalangeal, TMT = tarsometatarsal, MTP = metatarsophalangeal, IP = interphalangeal

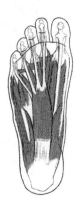
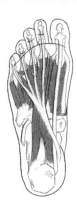
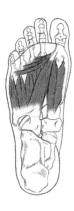
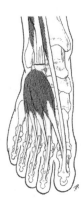

prohealthsys

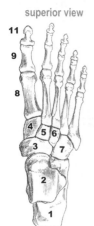

superior view   inferior view

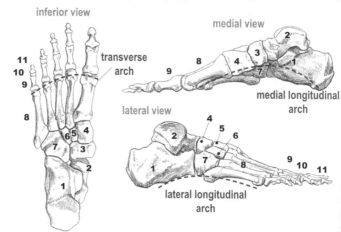

medial view

transverse arch

medial longitudinal arch

lateral view

lateral longitudinal arch

Leg, Ankle & Foot

1. Calcaneus
2. Talus
3. Navicular
4. Medial (1st) Cuneiform

5. Intermediate (2nd) Cuneiform
6. Lateral (3rd) Cuneiform
7. Cuboid
8. Metatarsals (5)

9. Proximal phalanges (5)
10. Middle phalanges (4)
11. Distal phalanges (5)

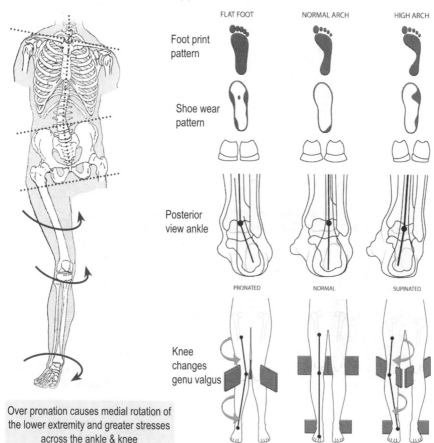

FLAT FOOT   NORMAL ARCH   HIGH ARCH

Foot print pattern

Shoe wear pattern

Posterior view ankle

PRONATED   NORMAL   SUPINATED

Knee changes genu valgus

Over pronation causes medial rotation of the lower extremity and greater stresses across the ankle & knee

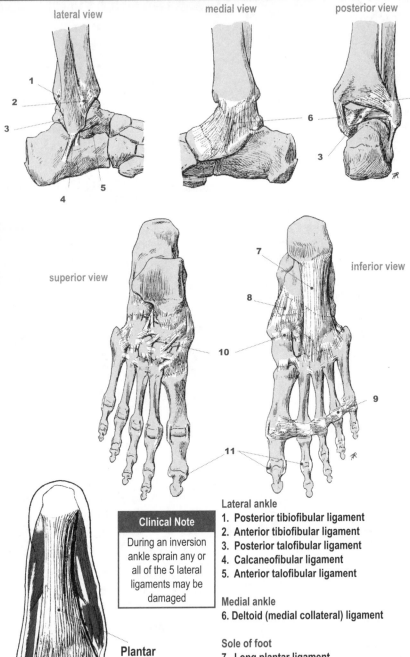

lateral view

medial view

posterior view

superior view

inferior view

Plantar
fascia

Clinical Note

During an inversion
ankle sprain any or
all of the 5 lateral
ligaments may be
damaged

Lateral ankle
1. Posterior tibiofibular ligament
2. Anterior tibiofibular ligament
3. Posterior talofibular ligament
4. Calcaneofibular ligament
5. Anterior talofibular ligament

Medial ankle
6. Deltoid (medial collateral) ligament

Sole of foot
7. Long plantar ligament
8. Spring (plantar calcaneonavicular) ligament
9. Transverse metatarsal ligament

10. Intertarsal ligaments
11. Interphalangeal collateral ligaments

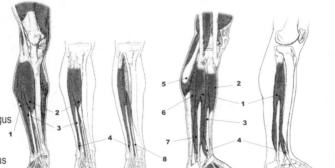

1. Fibularis (peroneus) longus
2. Tibialis anterior
3. Extensor digitorum longus
4. Fibularis (peroneus) tertius
5. Gastrocnemius
6. Soleus
7. Fibularis (peroneus) brevis
8. Extensor hallucis longus
9. Plantaris
10. Popliteus
11. Tibialis posterior
12. Flexor hallucis longus
13. Flexor digitorum longus
14. Achilles tendon

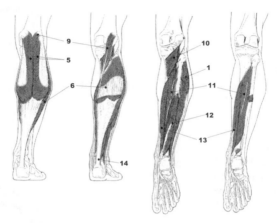

Leg, Ankle & Foot

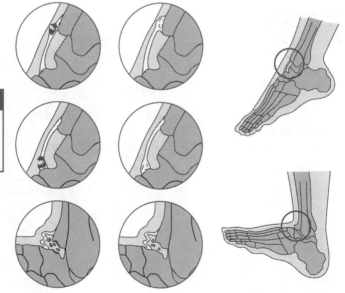

Clinical Note

During forced dorsiflexion or plantar flexion specific injuries may occur

Compare bilaterally, start with unaffected side for PROM & Muscle Testing
Prior to assessing ROM the examiner should make an introduction statement:
"Try and move as far as possible, if any of the actions or movements are painful or uncomfortable please let me know, do not do any action you feel will cause you further injury."

Leg, Ankle & Foot

AROM

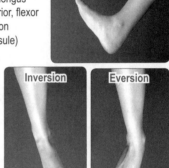

Plantar flexion

Plantar Flexion (20°-40°)
Muscles Activated: soleus, gastrocnemius, tibialis posterior, flexor digitorum longus, flexor hallicus longus, plantaris
Tissue Stretched: tibialis anterior, extensor digitorum longus, anterior ankle joint capsule & ligaments
Tissue Compressed: posterior ankle structures

Dorsiflexion (0°-20°)
Muscles Activated: tibialis anterior, extensor digitorum longus
Tissue Stretched: soleus, gastrocnemius, tibialis posterior, flexor digitorum longus, flexor hallicus longus, Achilles tendon
Tissue Compressed: anterior ankle structure (joint capsule)

Inversion (adduction) (20°-35°)
Muscles Activated: tibialis anterior, tibialis posterior
Tissue Stretched: fibularis longus, brevis & tertius, lateral ankle ligaments (anterior talofibular, calcaneofibular & posterior talofibular)
Tissue Compressed: medial ankle structures

Inversion   Eversion

Eversion (abduction) (5°-15°)
Muscles Activated: fibularis longus, brevis & tertius
Tissue Stretched: tibialis anterior, tibialis posterior, medial collateral (deltoid) ligament of ankle
Tissue Compressed: lateral ankle structures

PROM

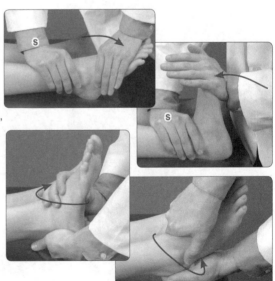

Plantar Flexion (> 20°-40°)
Tissue Stretched: tibialis anterior, extensor digitorum longus, anterior ankle joint capsule & ligaments

Dorsiflexion (> 0°-20°)
Tissue Stretched: soleus, gastrocnemius, tibialis posterior, flexor digitorum longus, flexor hallicus longus, Achilles tendon

Eversion (abduction) (> 5°-15°)
Tissue Stretched: tibialis anterior, tibialis posterior, medial collateral (deltoid) ligament of ankle

Inversion (adduction) (> 20°-35°)
Tissue Stretched: fibularis longus, brevis & tertius, lateral ankle ligaments (anterior talofibular, calcaneofibular & posterior talofibular)

Muscle Testing

Plantar Flexion
Muscles Activated: soleus, gastrocnemius, tibialis posterior, flexor digitorum longus, flexor hallucis longus, plantaris

Dorsiflexion
Muscles Activated: tibialis anterior, extensor digitorum longus, extensor hallucis longus

Eversion (abduction)
Muscles Activated: fibularis longus, brevis & tertius

Inversion (adduction)
Muscles Activated: tibialis anterior, tibialis posterior

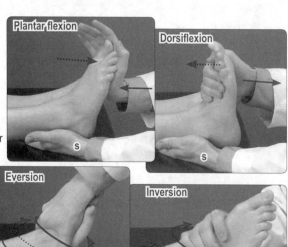

Plantar flexion

Dorsiflexion

Eversion

Inversion

Goniometry

Procedure
- Patient seated with legs off the table, ankle in neutral position (~90°)

Plantar Flexion (normal: 20°-40°)
- Fulcrum aligned with the medial malleolus
- Stationary arm in line tibia; moving arm is parallel to the 1st metatarsal
- Ask patient to plantar flex ankle

Dorsiflexion (normal 0°-20°)
- Fulcrum aligned with the medial malleolus
- Stationary arm in line tibia; moving arm is parallel to the first metatarsal
- Ask patient to dorsiflex ankle

Inversion (20°-35°)
- Fulcrum aligned between malleoli
- Stationary arm in midline tibia; moving arm is parallel to the 2nd metatarsal
- Ask patient to invert ankle

Eversion (5°-15°)
- Fulcrum aligned between malleoli
- Stationary arm in midline tibia; moving arm is parallel to the 2nd metatarsal
- Ask patient to evert ankle

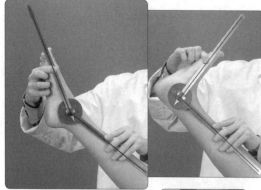
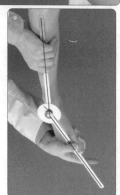
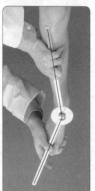

prohealthsys

Leg, Ankle & Foot

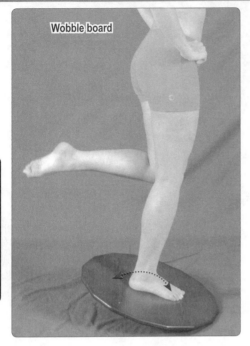

Wobble board

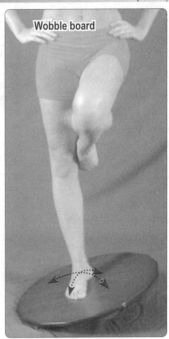

Wobble board

Strengthen
- Dorsiflxion with rubber band
- Walking/running on sand
- Wobble board
- Resistance elastic bands

Short Toe

Short Foot

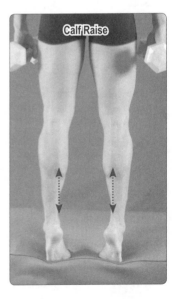

Calf Raise

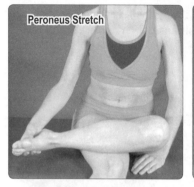

Peroneus Stretch

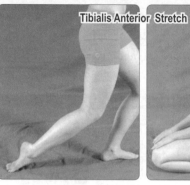

Tibialis Anterior Stretch

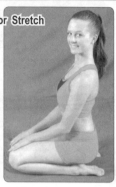

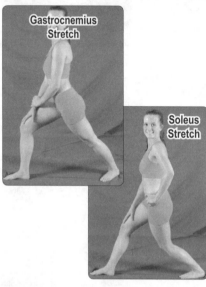

Gastrocnemius Stretch

Soleus Stretch

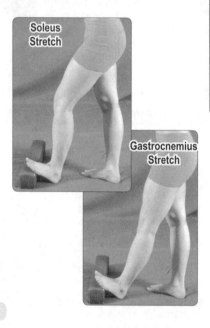

Soleus Stretch

Gastrocnemius Stretch

Printable patient handouts

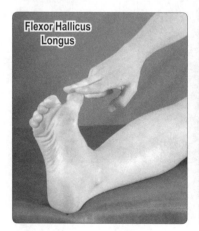

Flexor Hallicus Longus

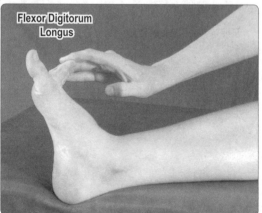

Flexor Digitorum Longus

Leg, Ankle & Foot

Pin & Stretch treatments can be adapted & applied to any myofascial structure if the clinician has a detailed understanding of basic anatomy & biomechanics

1. Clinician places muscle in shortened position & pins specific myofascial fibers with other hand
2. Patient is then _passively_ moved to lengthen muscle while pinning force is maintained
3. Hold at tension for ~10 seconds or until myofascial release is felt; repeat & reassess as needed

Plantar Fascia Pin & Stretch

1. Clinician places muscle in shortened position (toes in neutral or flexed - origin & insertion approximated) & pins origin of plantar fascia with other hand
2. Patient is then passively moved to lengthen muscle (toe extension - move insertion away from origin) while pinning force is maintained
3. Hold at tension for ~10 sec or until release is felt; repeat as needed

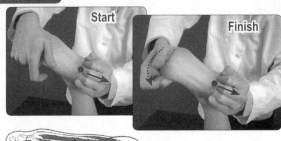

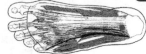

Gastrocnemius Lateral Head

1. Clinician places muscle in shortened position (ankle plantar flexed - origin & insertion approximated) & pins specific myofascial fibers with other hand
2. Patient is then passively moved to lengthen muscle (ankle dorsiflexion - move insertion away from origin) while pinning force is maintained
3. Hold at tension for ~10 sec or until release is felt; repeat as needed

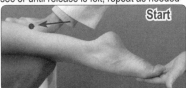

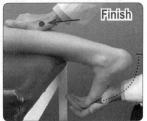

Tibialis Anterior Pin & Stretch

1. Clinician places muscle in shortened position (ankle dorsiflexed & inverted - origin & insertion approximated) & pins specific myofascial fibers with other hand
2. Patient is then passively moved to lengthen muscle (ankle plantar flexion & eversion - move insertion away from origin) while pinning force is maintained
3. Hold at tension for ~10 sec or until release is felt; repeat as needed

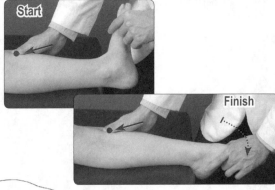

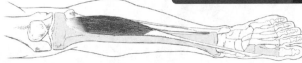

With good anatomy & biomechanical understanding, MET can be adapted to any patient
1. Clinician gently stretches patient into direction of restriction or decreased range of motion
2. Patient gently (10% of maximum) contracts in exact opposite motion
3. Clinician resists & patient holds contraction for 3-7 seconds, then patient completely relaxes
4. On relaxation, clinician moves to new resistive barrier; repeat 3-5 times & reassess

Dorsiflexion Restriction

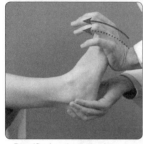
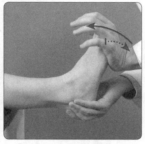
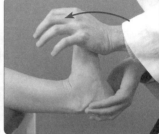

| Dorsiflexion tissue resistance | Patient contracts ~10% into plantar flexion | Clinician finds new end range |

Ankle Plantar Flexion Restriction

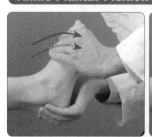
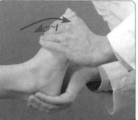
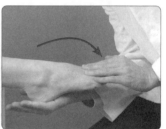

| Plantar flexion tissue resistance | Patient contracts ~10% into dorsiflexion | Clinician finds new end range |

Ankle Eversion Restriction

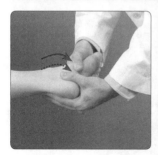
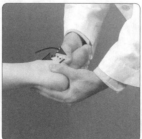
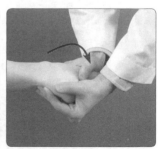

| Eversion tissue resistance | Patient contracts ~10% into inversion | Clinician finds new end range |

S = stabilization (indifferent hand),   ● = contact,   ⟶ = examiner force,   ·········▷ = patient motion

Leg, Ankle & Foot

Long Axis Distraction

Indications: ankle joint contracture, scar tissue formation, ↓ ROM

Position: patient supine (or seated) with ankle in neutral position; clinician at foot of table

Contact: clinician grasps patient foot over both the calcaneus & talus

Force: tissue force is S-I; develop tension by gently pulling or pushing the foot inferiorly

Clinical notes: maneuver may be performed as mobilization or manipulation (HVLA thrust)

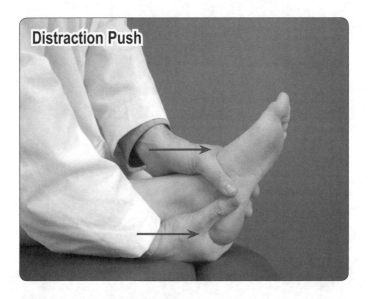

Distraction Push

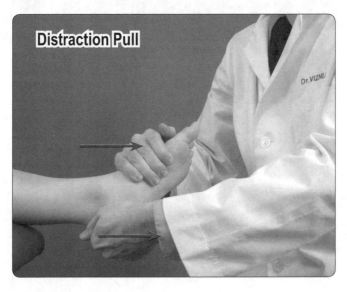

Distraction Pull

S = stabilization (indifferent hand),   ● = contact,   ──────▶ = examiner force,   ·········▶ = patient motion

Leg, Ankle & Foot

prohealthsys

Tibiotalar A-P Glide

Indications: ankle joint contracture, scar tissue formation, ↓ ROM

Position: patient supine (or seated); clinician at foot of table

Contact:

A-P Talus push: clinician grasps patient's foot over talus & stabilizes plantar surface of foot

Tibial pull: clinician grasps patient's foot over talus & stabilizes distal tibia/fibula with other hand

Force: tissue force is A-P with hand over the talus; develop tension by gently pushing the talus posteriorly

Clinical notes: maneuver may be performed as mobilization or manipulation (HVLA thrust)

Even though both methods look different they can be used to create the same motion in the joint

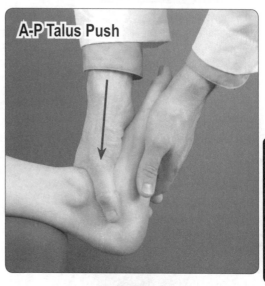

A-P Talus Push

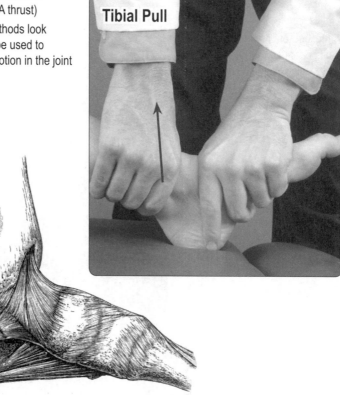

Tibial Pull

S = stabilization (indifferent hand), ● = contact, ⟶ = examiner force, ┈┈┈▸ = patient motion

Talotibular P-A Glide

Indications: ankle joint contracture, scar tissue formation, ↓ ROM

Position: patient prone or supine (or seated); clinician at foot of table

Contact:

Tibial push: clinician grasps patient's foot over talus & stabilizes plantar surface of foot

Talocalcaneal push: clinician grasps patient's foot over talus & stabilizes distal tibia/fibula with other hand

Force: tissue force is P-A with hand over the talus; develop tension by gently pushing the talus anteriorly

Clinical notes: maneuver may be performed as mobilization or manipulation (HVLA thrust)

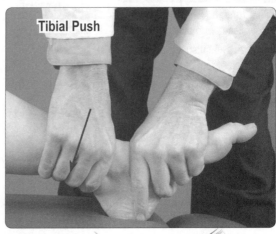

Tibial Push

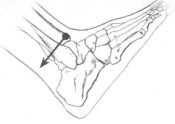

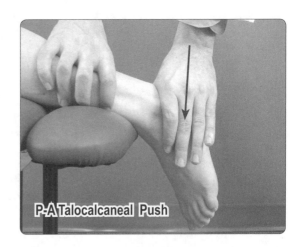

P-A Talocalcaneal Push

S = stabilization (indifferent hand), ● = contact, ⟶ = examiner force, ·········▷ = patient motion

Leg, Ankle & Foot

Talotibular M-L & L-M Glide

Indications: ankle joint contracture, scar tissue formation, ↓ ROM

Position: patient supine; clinician at foot of table

Contact:

Web push: clinician grasps patient's foot over talus with web of thumb & stabilizes over metatarsals with other hand

Reinforced digital pull: clinician grasps patient's foot over talus with a reinforced digital contact

Force: tissue force is S-I with L-M or M-L (depending upon the specific motion required) with hand over the talus; develop tension by gently pushing or pulling the talus with a medial or lateral force

Clinical notes: maneuver may be performed as mobilization or manipulation (HVLA thrust)

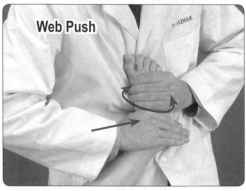

Web Push

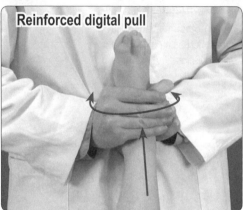

Reinforced digital pull

Leg, Ankle & Foot

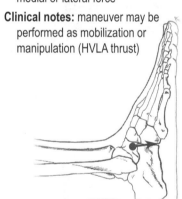

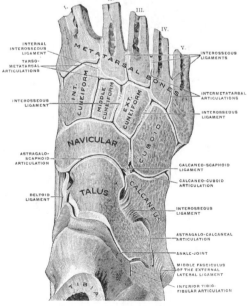

S = stabilization (indifferent hand), ● = contact, ➝ = examiner force, ┈┈➤ = patient motion

Leg, Ankle & Foot

Subtalar M-L & L-M Glide

Indications: subtalar joint contracture, scar tissue formation, ↓ medial or lateral glide ROM

Position: patient supine (or seated) with ankle in neutral position; clinician at foot of table

Contact: clinician contacts navicular and/or cuboid (depending on specific subtalar issue)

Force: tissue force is M-L or L-M; develop tension by gently pulling or pushing in required direction

Clinical notes: maneuver may be performed as mobilization or manipulation (HVLA thrust)

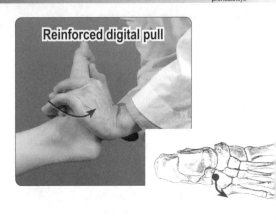

Reinforced digital pull

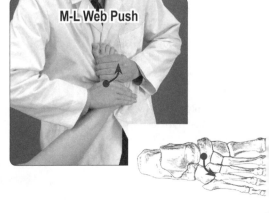

M-L Web Push

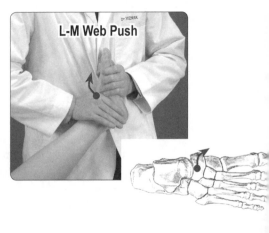

L-M Web Push

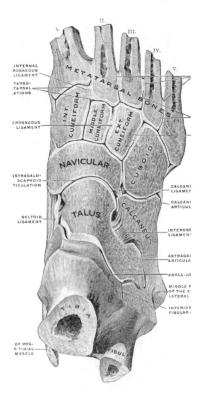

S = stabilization (indifferent hand), ● = contact, ⟶ = examiner force, ┈┈┈▶ = patient motion

Subtalar Distraction

Indications: subtalar joint contracture, scar tissue formation, ↓ ROM

Position: patient supine (or seated) with ankle in neutral position; clinician at foot of table

Contact: clinician contacts navicular &/or cuboid (depending on specific subtalar issue) with a reinforced digital contact & uses thumbs to stabilize the metatarsals

Force: tissue force is S-I; develop tension by gently pulling the navicular or cuboid inferiorly

Clinical notes: maneuver may be performed as mobilization or manipulation (HVLA thrust)

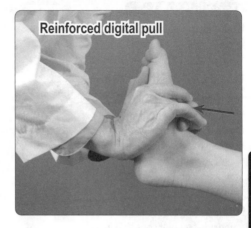

Reinforced digital pull

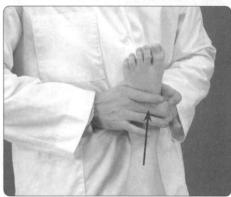

Leg, Ankle & Foot

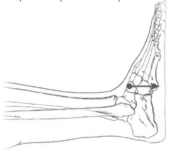

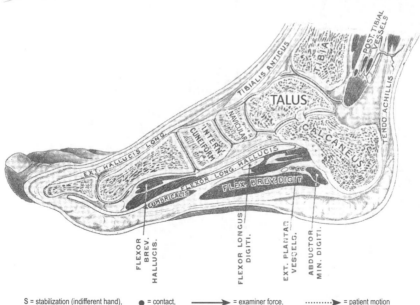

S = stabilization (indifferent hand), ● = contact, ——▶ = examiner force, ·······▶ = patient motion

Tarsal I-S Glide

Indications: tarsal joint contracture, scar tissue formation, ↓ ROM

Position: patient prone with ankle in neutral position & knee bent 90º; clinician at foot of table

Contact: clinician contacts specific tarsal (navicular, cuboid, cuneiforms) with thumb or palm of hand & stabilizes metatarsals distally

Force: tissue force is I-S; develop tension by gently pushing in desired direction

Clinical notes: maneuver may be performed as mobilization or manipulation (HVLA thrust)

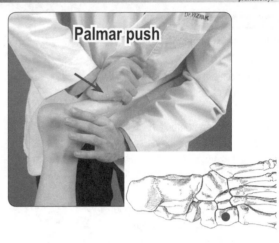
Palmar push

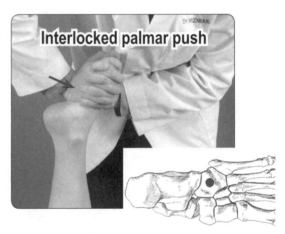
Interlocked palmar push

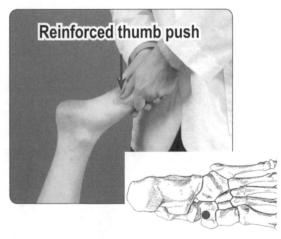
Reinforced thumb push

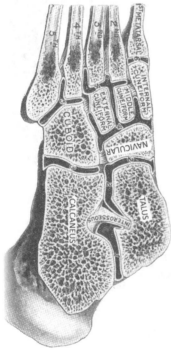

S = stabilization (indifferent hand),   ● = contact,   ⟶ = examiner force,   ⋯⋯▶ = patient motion

prohealthsys

Tarsal S-I Glide

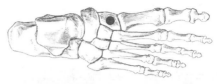

Indications: tarsal joint contracture, scar tissue formation, ↓ ROM

Position: patient supine or seated with ankle in neutral position; clinician at foot of table

Contact: clinician contacts specific tarsal (navicular, cuboid, cuneiforms) with reinforced digital or palmar contact & stabilizes metatarsals distally

Force: tissue force is S-I; develop tension by gently pushing or pulling in desired direction

Clinical notes: maneuver may be performed as mobilization or manipulation (HVLA thrust)

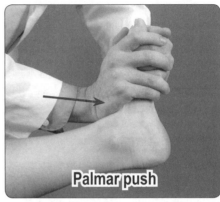

Palmar push

Leg, Ankle & Foot

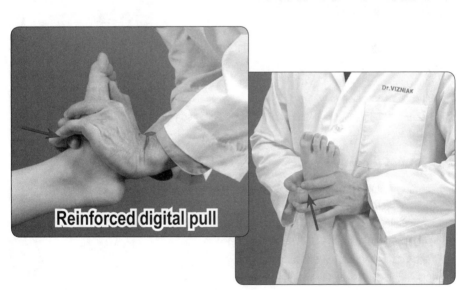

Reinforced digital pull

Dr. VIZNIAK

S = stabilization (indifferent hand),   ● = contact,   ——————▶ = examiner force,   ·········▶ = patient motion

Metatarsal I-S Glide

Indications: metatarsal joint contracture, scar tissue formation, ↓ ROM

Position: patient prone with ankle in neutral position; clinician at foot of table

Contact: clinician contacts metatarsal with reinforced thumb or palmar contact & stabilizes metatarsals distally

Force: tissue force is I-S; develop tension by gently pushing in desired direction over the specific area of restriction or malposition

Clinical notes: maneuver may be performed as mobilization or manipulation

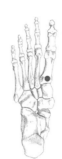

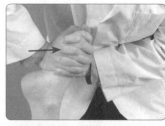

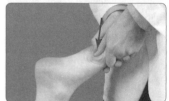

Metatarsal S-I Glide

Indications: metatarsal joint contracture, scar tissue formation, ↓ ROM

Position: patient supine or seated with ankle in neutral position; clinician at foot of table

Contact: clinician contacts metatarsal with reinforced digital or palmar contact & stabilizes metatarsals distally

Force: tissue force is I-S; develop tension by gently pushing or pulling in desired direction over the specific area of restriction/malposition

Clinical notes: maneuver may be performed as mobilization or manipulation

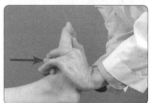

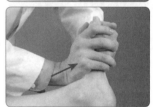

Metatarsal Head Glide

Indications: distal metatarsal joint contracture, scar tissue formation, ↓ ROM

Position: patient supine or seated with ankle in neutral position; clinician at foot of table

Contact: clinician contacts metatarsal superiorly with palm of hands & inferiorly with fingers

Force: tissue force is I-S or S-I or in a spreading action (M-L & L-M); develop tension by gently tractioning in desired direction over the specific area of restriction or malposition

Clinical notes: maneuver may be performed as mobilization or manipulation

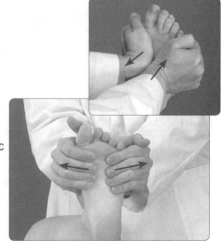

S = stabilization (indifferent hand), ● = contact, ──────► = examiner force, ·········► = patient motion

MTP & Digital Mobes

Indications: metatarsal phalangeal or interphalangeal joint contracture, scar tissue formation, ↓ ROM, pain, motion restriction

Position: patient supine or seated with ankle relaxed; clinician at foot of table

Contact: clinician contacts specific digit (proximal, middle or distal) with finger, thumb or pincer contact & stabilizes the proximal bone

Force: tissue force is into the direction of restriction; develop tension by gently pushing or pulling in desired direction

Clinical notes: maneuver may be performed as mobilization or manipulation (HVLA thrust)

There are numerous variations that will work equally well for a variety of given digital joint dysfunctions (see images below)

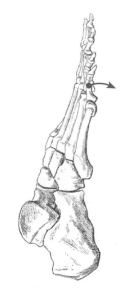

Leg, Ankle & Foot

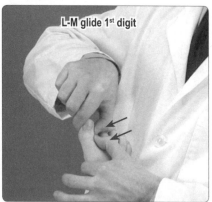

L-M glide 1st digit

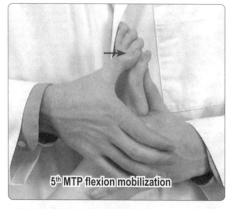

5th MTP flexion mobilization

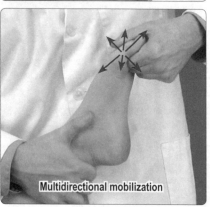

Multidirectional mobilization

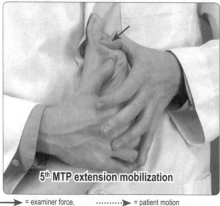

5th MTP extension mobilization

S = stabilization (indifferent hand),　● = contact,　━━━▶ = examiner force,　┈┈┈▶ = patient motion

1. Vizniak, NA. Clinical Cadaver Dissections. 1999-2018.
2. McGee S. Evidence-Based Physical Diagnosis. Saunders. 2017.
3. Magee D. Orthopedic Physical Assessment, 5th Edition. Saunders. 2008.
4. Taylor MH, Monroe LG. Physical Rehabilitation: Evidence-Based Examination, Evaluation and Intervention. Saunders. 2007.
5. Warlow C, Hughes R, Uitehaag B, Liberati A. Evidence-Based Neurology. Blackwell Publishing Limited, BMJI Books. 2007.
6. Malanga GA & Nadler. Musculoskeletal Physical Exam, An Evidence-Based Approach. Mosby. 2006.
7. Hoppenfield S. Physical Examination of the Spine & Extremities. Lippincott Williams & Wilkins. 1976.
8. Hoppenfield S. Orthopaedic Neurology: A Diagnostic Guide to Neurologic Levels. Lippincott Williams & Wilkins. 1977.
9. Spencer JW, Jacobs JJ. Complementary and Alternative Medicine: An Evidence-Based Approach. Mosby. 2003.
10. Jewell D. Guide to Evidence-Based Physical Therapy Practice. Jones Barlett Publishers Inc. 2007.
11. Iesel SW. Operative Orthopaedics: An Illustrative Approach. Lippincott Williams & Wilkins. 2008.
12. Alonso A, Khoury L, Adams R. Clinical tests for ankle syndesmosis injury: reliability and prediction of return to function. J Orthop Sports Phys Ther. 1998;27(4):276-284.
13. Bachmann LM, Kolb E, Koller MT, Steurer. Accuracy of Ottawa ankle rules to exclude fractures of the ankle and mid-foot: systematic review. BMJ. 2003;32:417.
14. Beumer A, Swierstra BA, Mulder PG. Clinical diagnosis of syndesmotic ankle instability: evaluation of stress tests behind the curtains. Acta Orthop Scand. 2002;73(6):667-669.
15. Beumer A, van Hemert WL, Swierstra BA, Jasper LE, Belkoff SM. A biomechanical evaluation of clinical stress tests for syndesmotic ankle instability. Foot Ankle. 2003;24(4):358-363.
16. Cranley JJ, Canos AJ, Sull WJ. The diagnosis of deep venous thrombosis: fallibility of clinical symptoms and signs. Arch Surg. 1976;1 11(1):34-36.
17. Egol KA, Amirtharajah M, Tejwani NC, Capla EL, Koval KJ. Ankle stress test for predicting the need for surgical fixation of isolated fibular fractures. J Bone Joint Surg Am. 2004;86(11):2393-2398.
18. Glasoe WM, Allen MK, Saltzman CL, Ludewig PM, Sublett SH. Comparison of two methods used to assess first-ray mobility. Foot Ankle. 2002;23(3):248-252.
19. Glasoe WM, Grebing BR, Beck S, Coughlin MJ, Saltzman CL. A comparison of device measures of dorsal first ray mobility. Foot Ankle Int. 2005;26(1 1):957-961.
20. Hertel J, Denegar CR, Monroe MM, Stokes WL. Talocrural and subtalar joint instability after lateral ankle sprain. Med Sd Sports Exerc. 1 999;31(11):1501-1508.

21. Knox FW. The clinical diagnosis of deep vein thrombophelbitis. Practitioner. 1965;1 95:214-216.
22. Liu SH, Nuccion SL, Finerman G. Diagnosis of anterolateral ankle impingement: comparison between magnetic resonance imaging and clinical examination. Am J Sports Med. 1 997;25(3):389-393.
23. Loudon JK, Bell SL. The foot and ankle: an overview of arthrokinematics and selectedjoint techniques. J Athi Train. 1996;31(2):173-178.
24. Molloy S, Solan MC, Bendall SP. Synovial impingement in the ankle: a new physical sign. J Bone Joint Surg Br. 2003;85(3):330-333.
25. Oloff LM, Schulhofer SD. Flexor hallucis longus dysfunction. J Foot Ankle Surg. 1998;37(2);101 -109.
26. Petersen EJ, Irish SM, Lyons CL, Miklaski SF, Bryan JM, Henderson NE, Masullo LN. Reliability of water volumetry and the figure eight method on patients with ankle joint swelling. J Orthop Sports Phys Ther. 1999;29(10):609-615.
27. Picciano AM, Rowlands MS, Worrell T. Reliability of open and closed kinetic chain subtalar joint neutral positions and navicular drop test. J Orthop Sports Phys Ther. 1993;18(4):553-558.
28. Sell KE, Verity TM, Worrell TW, Pease BJ, Wigglesworth J. Two measurement techniques for assessing subtalar joint position: a reliability study. J Orthop Sports Phys Ther. 1 994;1 9(3):162-167.
29. Shafer N, Duboff S. Physical signs in the early diagnosis of thrombophlebitis. Angiology. 1971 ;22(1):18-30.
30. Smith J, Szczerba JE, Arnold BL, Perrin DH, Martin DE. Role of hyperpronation as a possible risk factor for anterior cruciate ligament injuries. J Athl Train. 1997;32(1):25-28.
31. Tatro-Adams D, McGann SF, Carbone W. Reliability of the figure-of-eight method of ankle measurement. J Orthop Sports Phys Ther. 1995;22(4):161-163.
32. Thompson TC, Doherty JH. Spontaneous rupture of tendon of Achilles: a new clinical diagnostic test. J Trauma. 1962;2:126-129.
33. Vinicombe A, Raspovic A, Menz HB. Reliability of navicular displacement measurement as a clinical indicator of foot posture. J Am Podiatr Med Assoc. 2001;91 (5):262-268.
34. Wells PS, Hirsh I, Anderson DR, Lensing AW, Foster C, Kearon C, Weitz I, D'Ovidio R, Cogo A, Prandoni P. Accuracy of clinical assessment of deep-vein thrombosis. Lancet. 1995;345:1326-1330.
35. Anderson DL, Sanderson DJ, Hennig EM. The role of external nonrigid ankle bracing in limiting ankle inversion. Clin J Sport Med. 1995;5(1):18-24.
36. Balduini FC, Tetzlaff J. Historical perspectives on injuries of the ligaments of the ankle. Clin Sports Med. Mar 1982;1(1):3-12.
37. Bosien WR, Staples OS, Russell SW. Residual disability following acute ankle sprains. J Bone Joint Surg Am. Dec 1955;37-A(6):1237-43.
38. DeLee JC, Drez D: Orthopaedic Sports Medicine: Principles and Practice. Vol 2. WB Saunders Co; 1994:1718-1724.

39. Foster AP, Thompson NW, Crone MD: Rupture of the tibialis posterior tendon: an important differential in the assessment of ankle injuries. Emerg Med J. 2005; 22: 915-6.
40. Gerber JP, Williams GN, Scoville CR, et al. Persistent disability associated with ankle sprains: a prospective examination of an athletic population. Foot Ankle Int. Oct 1998;19(10):653-60.
41. Hubbard TJ, Denegar CR: Does Cryotherapy Improve Outcomes With Soft Tissue Injury? J Athl Train 2004 9; 39(3): 278-279
42. Kibler WB: Rehabilitation of the ankle and foot. Functional Rehabilitation of Sports and Musculoskeletal Injuries. Aspen Publishers Inc; 1998:273-279
43. LeBlanc KE: Ankle problems masquerading as sprains. Prim Care 2004 Dec; 31(4): 1055-67
44. Leddy JJ, Smolinski RJ, Lawrence J, et al. Prospective evaluation of the Ottawa Ankle Rules in a university sports medicine center. With a modification to increase specificity for identifying malleolar fractures. Am J Sports Med. Mar-Apr 1998;26(2):158-65.
45. Lephart SM, Pincivero DM, Giraldo JL, Fu FH. The role of proprioception in the management and rehabilitation of athletic injuries. Am J Sports Med. Jan-Feb 1997;25(1):130-7.
46. Lephart SM, Pincivero DM, Rozzi SL. Proprioception of the ankle and knee. Sports Med. Mar 1998;25(3):149-55.
47. Liu SH, Nguyen TM. Ankle sprains and other soft tissue injuries. Curr Opin Rheumatol. Mar 1999;11(2):132-7.
48. Löfvenberg R, Kärrholm J, Sundelin G, Ahlgren O. Prolonged reaction time in patients with chronic lateral instability of the ankle. Am J Sports Med. Jul-Aug 1995;23(4):414-7.
49. Lohrer H, Alt W, Gollhofer A. Neuromuscular properties and functional aspects of taped ankles. Am J Sports Med. Jan-Feb 1999;27(1):69-75.
50. Man IO, Morrissey MC: Relationship between ankle-foot swelling and self-assessed function after ankle sprain. Med Sci Sports Exerc 2005 Mar; 37(3): 360-3
51. Manfroy PP, Ashton-Miller JA, Wojtys EM. The effect of exercise, prewrap, and athletic tape on the maximal active and passive ankle resistance of ankle inversion. Am J Sports Med. Mar-Apr 1997;25(2):156-63.
52. McCarthy D. Nonsteroidal anti-inflammatory drug-related gastrointestinal definitions and epidemiology. Am J Med. Nov 2 1998;105(5A):3S-9S.
53. Osborne MD, Rizzo TD Jr. Prevention and treatment of ankle sprain in athletes. Sports Med. 2003;33(15):1145-50.
54. Pfeffer G, Claim MR, Frey C. Foot and ankle. In: Essentials of musculoskeletal care. ed. 1997:366-489.
55. Plint AC, Bulloch B, Osmond MH, et al. Validation of the Ottawa Ankle Rules in children with ankle injuries. Acad Emerg Med. Oct 1999;6(10):1005-9.
56. Renstrom PAFH, Kannus P. Injuries to the foot and ankle. Orthop Sports Med. 1994;1705-67.
57. Stiell IG, McKnight RD, Greenberg GH, et al. Implementation of the Ottawa ankle rules. JAMA. Mar 16 1994;271(11):872-3.

Leg, Ankle & Foot

Ankle & Foot Quiz (answer page)

1. What are the joint type classifications for this region? (348) _____

2. What are the joint surface shapes for this region (convex/concave)? (332)

_____

3. What is the normal ROM for _____?
   - Plantar/dorsi flexion._____, _____
   - Inversion/eversion _____, _____

4. What is the resting position? _____

5. What is the ankle joint tight packed position?

6. What ligaments support foot arches? (350)

_____

7. What some good ankle strengthening exercises? (354) _____

8. Over pronation causes what change at the knee? (349) _____

9. Stress fractures of the foot are caused by _____? (347) _____

10. Can you palpate _____ ? (346)

Clinical Rehabilitation Goals

Phase	~Time Course	Clinical Objective
1 Acute*	2-3 days (up to ~7 days)	• **Reduce pain; PRICE or METH as needed** • Prevent excess swelling & possible ischemia • Basic PFROM, IASTM & activity as tolerated
2 Post Acute	2 days - 6 weeks	• Pain reduction, prevent early scar tissue adhesions • Begin orienting repair tissue along line of tension (IASTM) • Basic stretch, strength, functional & proprioceptive retraining
3 Chronic*	3 weeks - 12 month or more	• Proper alignment of repair collagen & myofascial tissue • Increase elasticity of scar tissue (↑ ROM & strength) • Advanced stretch, strength, functional & proprioceptive retraining

*Chronic recurrent episodes may be treated as acute during a flare-up; PFROM = Pain Free Range of Motion

Functional Rehab

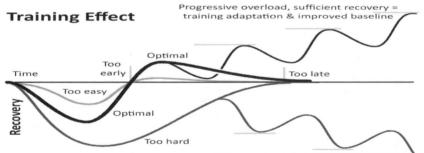

Training Effect

Progressive overload, sufficient recovery = training adaptation & improved baseline

Time — Too early — Optimal — Too late

Recovery — Too easy — Optimal — Too hard

High overload, insufficient recovery = no training adaptation & risk of injury (sprain, strain, stress fracture)

There are many expert-based strategies for rehab. to target inhibited/weak muscles, relax/stretch overactive tissues.

- **Remove mechanical blockage** (tight tissues, joint dysfunction - massage, stretch, pin & stretch, IASTM, joint mobilization)

- To restore functional motor control, endurance and strength, **follow the ACE protocol** during rehab.

A = **A**ctivate muscles with **verbal & tactile cues** to make the patient consciously aware of the neuromuscular pathway that needs training

C = **C**ontrol motor function by repeating the motion with good form, avoiding recruitment

E = **E**ndurance increases by adding resistance or difficulty to build strength and further augment control and activation

prohealthsys

Gauging Intensity using Heart Rate (HR)

The basic way to calculate maximum heart rate is to **subtract age from 220**.

220 - 40 yrs old = 180 beats/min max
- **Moderate intensity: 50-70% max HR**
- **Vigorous intensity: 70-85% max HR**
- If patient is not fit or just beginning an exercise program, aim for the lower end of your target zone (50 percent). Then, gradually build up the intensity. If patient is healthy and wants a vigorous intensity, opt for the higher end of the zone.

Exercise prescription must include F I T T

Frequency: __ x wk - find a balance between enough stress for body adaptation & allow enough rest to heal.

Intensity: effort during exercise (% of max). Balance intensity hard enough to overload the body but not so difficult that it results in overtraining, injury or burnout.

Time: how long each session should last. Varies based on the intensity and type.

Type: cardiovascular, strength and flexibility training. Based on goals & specific exercises performed

Cardiovascular training
3-5 x week, 60-85% 1 rep max, 20-60 min

Strength training
2-3x wk, 70-90% 1 rep max, 8-10 reps, 1-3 sets

Flexibility training
2-3x wk, 10-30 sec holds, 2-4 reps (yoga)

adapted from ACSM (American College of Sport Medicine)

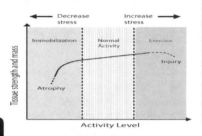

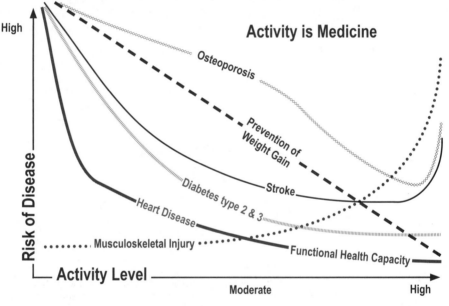

Activity is Medicine. For most conditions, activity reduces risk factors and improves functional health capacity. At extremes of activity, the risk of stroke, osteoporosis and musculoskeletal injury increases.

(Type 2 diabetes is insulin resistant form associated with obesity, type 3 diabetes is Alzheimer's Disease)

"Those who do not find the time for exercise will have to find time for illness"

all good health care providers

Definitions
- **Rep (repetition)** = 1 complete movement (concentric & eccentric)
- **Set** = number of times a group of reps is done
- **1 RM** = 1 Repetition Maximum (the most weight that can be done for one rep)

- **Total volume** = reps x sets x weight
  - 3 sets of 10 reps with 100 lbs = 3,000
  - 10 sets of 3 reps with 100 lbs = 3,000.
  - Research suggests for hypertrophy **even though the number of sets and reps are different, the gains in muscle hypertrophy are very close to the same using the same total volume**
  - **For strength, studies show that the most important factor is the intensity.** The heavier you lift, the stronger you become.

Optimal Sets & Reps

Two meta-analyses measured difference in strength gains & muscle hypertrophy. comparing single vs multi set sessions. In both, **multiple set training came out on top.** (Krieger, J. W. (2009) Single versus multiple sets of resistance exercise: a meta-regression. Journal of Strength and Conditioning Research. 23.6: 1890 – 1901.; Krieger, J.W. (2010) Single vs. multiple sets of resistance exercise for muscle hypertrophy: a meta-analysis. Journal of Strength and Conditioning Research. 24.4: 1150 – 1159.)

> **Train the motion, not the muscle**

Eccentric contractions (lowering phase) are ~10% stronger, thus increase total work volume
- Eccentric-focused sets (*'negatives'*) can serve as a finishing set to slightly increase gains
- Lifting a slower eccentric phase, assures control of the weight down, keeping more tension in muscle-tendon units
- Generally a slower rep scheme is good for beginners to work on form and prevent injury
- **Studies consistently show greater total work volume = greater muscle growth**

HIIT - High Intensity Interval Training

Alternating periods of short, high intensity activity with periods of low intensity recovery
- Eg: alternate walk/sprint (walk 5 – 30 sec, sprint 5 -10 sec,), total session length: 5 – 20 min; 3 d/wk - ratios (eg. 2:1, 4:1 rest : exercise)
- Body goes through intense activity, it needs to be able to keep up with energy demand
- Drawback - extremely strenuous, may cause joint pain due to high impact and may lead to serious injuries & longer recovery time

> HIIT training more accurately represents human evolutionary needs - when there would have been times of brief maximum effort during fight or flight for survival

Functional Rehab

Reps	< 2	3	4	5	6	7	8	9	10	11	12	13	14	15	16	17	18	19	> 20

Training goal

Power

STRENGTH (3-5 sets, 3-5 reps)

HYPERTROPHY (3-4 sets, 8-12 reps)

ENDURANCE (1-2 sets, 15+ reps)

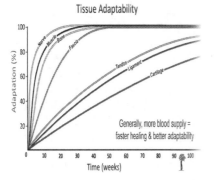

Tissue Adaptability

Generally, more blood supply = faster healing & better adaptability

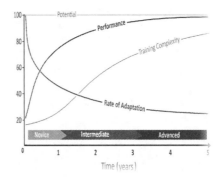

Nutrition & Feeding Window

- "Feeding window" = within 1 hr after workout

- Research shows, immediately after workout insulin levels spike rapidly for a few hours priming the body for synthesizing new muscle, limiting exercise-induced muscle loss, and restoring energy levels (evolutionary this would correspond to meal time following a hunt or work from a harvest - you eat when the work to get the meal is done)

  - Research shows consuming **20-40g of protein within 2 hrs following workout significantly increases muscle growth** compared to consuming more than 4 hrs later (feeding window may extend out up to 24 hrs)

1. Stark M, Lukaszuk J, Prawitz A, Salacinski A. Protein timing and its effects on muscular hypertrophy and strength in individuals engaged in weight-training. Journal of the International Society of Sports Nutrition. 2012;9:54. doi:10.1186/1550-2783-9-54.
2. Kerksick C, Harvey T, Stout J, Campbell B, Wilborn C, Kreider R, Kalman D, Ziegenfuss T, Lopez H, Landis J, Ivy JL, Antonio J: International Society of Sports Nutrition position stand: nutrient timing. J Int Soc Sports Nutr. 2008, 5: 17-10.1186/1550-2783-5-17.

> **Basic physiology and evolutionary anatomy support that to heal damaged or stressed tissue you need the building blocks of that tissue** (protein, carbohydrates, fats, DNA, collagen, fascia and cartilage); **and the sooner after the stress you get those building blocks into the bloodstream the better the outcome**

Soreness & Recovery

DOMS - delayed onset muscle soreness is theorized to be due to very small tears happen in the muscle at a cellular level. Pain receptors in muscles then send pain signals to brain and calcium builds up in muscle causing low level inflammation

- Be aware that mild DOMS is a good thing! - it shows good workout intensity - the best way to alleviate DOMS long term is to progress slowly into a new exercise program, giving muscles enough time to adapt to new stress being placed

- Rest, light motion, sleep and nutrition improve recovery (creatine, fish oil, taurine, branched chain amino acids, caffeine, citrulline malate)

- Studies show that massage, foam rolling and other manual therapies can alleviate DOMS

- Be aware that increased performance and lowered recovery time is possible with performance enhancing substances (anabolic steroids)

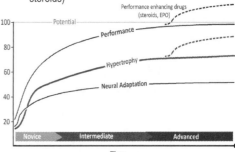

Performance increase occur fastest during initial training as neural adaptation develops appropriate muscle firing patterns and biomechanics, then muscle hypertrophy continues as activity intensity is increased with skill. Performance enhancing substance can take athletes beyond natural genetic potential.

Detraining Effect - injury, illness, lack of motivation cause loss in performance after...

- **1-2 week for cardio** (stroke volume, work capacity, cardiac output - VO$_2$ max can drop by ~20% in 2 weeks - beginners lose more easily, trained athletes lose more slowly)

- **2-3 weeks for strength** and **muscle size**

- Also influenced by age, injury, overall activity level, nutrition, prior training ability

Theodorou, A. et al. (2016). Aerobic, resistance and combined training and detraining on body composition, muscle strength, lipid profile and inflammation in coronary artery disease patients. Research in Sports Medicine Vol. 24:3

Coetsee, C. Terblance, E. (2015). The time course of changes induced by resistance training and detraining on muscular and physical function in older adults. Eur Rev Aging Phys Act. 2015; 12: 7

Mujika, I.; Padilla, S.(2000). Detraining: loss of training-induced physiological and performance adaptations. Part I: short term insufficient training stimulus. Journal of Sports Med. (2), 79 – 87.

Contralateral Training Effect

- Evidence suggests by training the uninjured side, there is ↑ **gene expression** and up to a **35% strength** transfer to the injured limb

- Molecular responses to acute exercise are not confined to exercising muscles but also extend to contralateral resting muscles

- Mechanisms include motor pathway projecting & neuroplasticity to contralateral muscles to enhance performance

Catoire, M., Mensink, M., Boekschoten, M. V., Hangelbroek, R., Müller, M., Schrauwen, P., & Kersten, S. (2012). Pronounced Effects of Acute Endurance Exercise on Gene Expression in Resting and Exercising Human Skeletal Muscle. Plos ONE, 7(11), 1-10. doi:10.1371/journal

Lee, M., & Carroll, T. J. (2007). Cross Education: Possible Mechanisms for the Contralateral Effects of Unilateral Resistance Training. Sports Medicine, 37(1), 1-14. doi:10.2165/00007256-200737010-00001

Basic Principles

1. **Keep objects that you are lifting or carrying close to your body**

   - The farther the object is from your body, the greater the strain will be - slide objects close to you or step toward them before lifting

2. **Work with your upper body as close to upright as possible & minimize twisting of your upper body**

   - Work with loads between waist and shoulder height; keep loads off of the floor if possible

   - For low level work, bend your knees, squat or kneel or consider a longer handled tool

3. **Maintain the natural inward (lordosis) curve of your low back -** this curve has a tendency to flatten when you bend or sit, increasing the strain on the low back

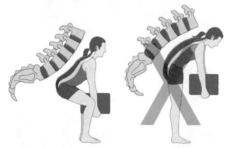

4. **Unexpected movements are more likely to cause injuries than deliberate movements**

   - Keep walking surfaces clear and take care to avoid slips, trips or falls

   - Make sure objects you are moving do not shift during transport. Proper storage will minimize injuries related to sudden movements to catch falling objects

5. **Use a footrest for prolonged standing** (~8 inches high can be used to help avoid static postures)

   - Vary standing postures by shifting body weight from both to one or the other leg.

Work Organization

1. **Frequent short breaks are better than infrequent long breaks**

   - The most important determinant of risk of injury is how long the activity is performed

continuously without interruption not the total time spent performing the activity

   - Performing an activity for 2 hours all at once has a higher risk of injury than performing the 2 hours of activity in shorter segments, alternated with less fatiguing activities. Strained muscles heal if given time to heal and the healing time required depends on how long the muscles are strained.

2. **Rest break doesn't mean that no work can be performed**

   - Switching to a task that puts less strain on that muscle group. Alternating sitting and standing tasks, or performing some stretches

   - Alternating tasks that involve a lot of bending with those that utilize more upright postures. Performing the task using different muscle groups (e.g., use your right hand instead of your left)

3. **Take extra care & warm-up at high risk times**

   - After a day off, first thing in the morning or just after waking up, after breaks or long periods of inactivity.

4. **Physical fitness (diet, exercise & rest)**

   - Higher physical fitness reduces the risk of back injury; Exercise - most forms of physical activity will strengthen the back, as the back is central to any whole body movement

   - Rest - proper rest enhances physical fitness. In addition, when we are well rested we are less likely to make mistakes that can lead to injuries.

5. **Pain is not always bad**

   - **Pain can tell us if what we are doing is causing body damage; however, you must remain active after a back injury even if it mildly hurts; inactivity can lead to further tissue weakening and long term disability. Some tissue challenge & pain is necessary for proper, normal healing**

   - Characteristics of pain that may not be associated with harm:
     - You bring it on yourself purposefully & can control the intensity
     - Mild discomfort can lead to stronger muscles and more flexible joints
     - Pain is less as you continue to repeat the activity over the course of a few days

Pin & Stretch treatments can be adapted & applied to any myofascial structure if the clinician has a detailed understanding of basic anatomy & biomechanics

1. Clinician places **muscle in shortened position** & pins specific myofascial fibers with other hand
2. Patient is then **passively** moved to lengthen muscle while pinning force is maintained
3. Hold at tension for ~10 seconds or until myofascial release is felt; repeat & reassess as needed

Note: some protocols involve having the patient actively move to lengthen muscle while the pinning force is maintained; also consider 'resetting' the tissue afterwards with AROM after treatment

Middle Deltoid Example

1. Clinician places muscle in shortened position (shoulder abducted - origin & insertion approximated) & pins specific myofascial fibers with other hand
2. Patient is then passively moved to lengthen muscle (shoulder adduction - move insertion away from origin) while pinning force is maintained
3. Hold at tension for ~10 sec or until release is felt; repeat as needed

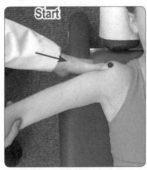
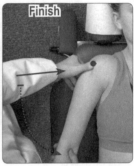

Pectoralis Major Example

1. Clinician places muscle in shortened position (origin & insertion approximated) & pins specific myofascial fibers with other hand
2. Patient is then passively moved to lengthen muscle (shoulder abduction - move insertion away from origin) while pinning force is maintained
3. Hold at tension for ~10 sec or until release is felt; repeat as needed

Note: any region of pectoralis major may be stretched by altering the specific pinning contact

This is an especially useful method to apply to patients with rounded shoulders secondary to poor posture or tight pectoralis muscles

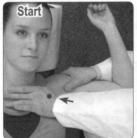
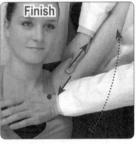

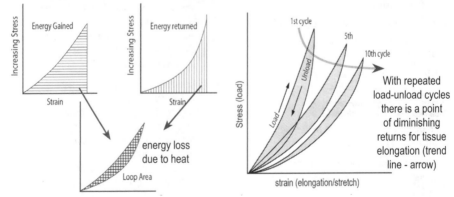

energy loss due to heat

With repeated load-unload cycles there is a point of diminishing returns for tissue elongation (trend line - arrow)

Functional Rehab

Flexibility/ROM Resistance by Tissue Type
Muscle/Fascia............ ~40%
Tendons.....................~10%
Skin............................~2%
Ligaments/Capsule....~48%

the percentages above will vary somewhat based on
the joint and person specific variations

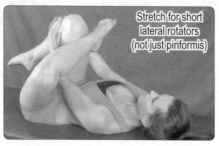

Stretch for short
lateral rotators
(not just piriformis)

Stretching is a fundamental way to improve your overall health & fitness. Possible effects include:

- **Increased flexibility & circulation; muscle relaxation**
- **Reduced risk for injury, reduced muscle or ROM imbalance**
- **Decreased anxiety & stress; can give patients an overall feeling of well being**

Warm-up - do a large muscle warm-up such as brisk walking for 5-10 minutes before stretching

Basic technique - simply move the origin & insertion of a muscle away from each other until tension is felt in the muscle (this can be applied to every muscle in the body)

Perform balanced stretching - always stretch the muscles on both sides of your body evenly; do not stretch one side more than the other side

Avoid over stretching - never stretch to severe pain or discomfort - 'joyful discomfort' is the goal (over-stretching can cause a muscle strain or even ligament sprain). Recent studies have shown that over-stretching before physical activity may actually increase the chance of injury and lower performance in ballistic/power events

Go slow - stretch slowly & hold the stretch for about ~30 seconds & release slowly as well

Breathe - flexibility exercises should be relaxing; deep, easy, even **breathing is key to relaxation** (never hold your breath while you stretch - **consider breathing or exhaling into the stretch to find more length**)

Stretching Types

Passive stretching - static stretching where external force exerts upon the limb to move it into the new position. Passive stretching resistance is normally achieved through the force of gravity on the limb, or on the body weighing down on it.

Active stretching involves the use of muscle contraction to facilitate increased stretching & is usually based around the two main principles of reciprocal inhibition & autogenic inhibition (See PNF section)

Static stretching is used to stretch muscles while the body is at rest. Muscles are gradually lengthened to an elongated position (to the point of mild discomfort) & held 10-30 secs. Static stretching slightly lessens the sensitivity of tension receptors, which allows the muscle to relax & to be stretched to greater length – this may predispose to injury if long stretches are held prior to vigorous physical activity.

Dynamic stretching similar to what is done when waking from sleep; the body is moving through range of motion. Dynamic stretches are useful in developing neuromuscular coordination for movements such as leg lifts, dance movements, kicks, & development of speed & power.

Ballistic stretching (or bouncing stretches) forces the limb into an extended range of motion when the muscle has not relaxed enough to enter it. This may cause injury if not controlled properly or without adequate preparation/warming-up. Some believe that controlled ballistic stretching in the form of bouncing can increase flexibility. This is true to a certain extent, but this could cause injury & is not the safest method of stretching (though it may lead to quick gains). Can lead to higher levels of flexibility not normally attainable.

Evidence suggests, stretching does not appear to reduce muscle soreness (DOMS); also if muscles are is stretched and you don't build strength at these new ranges of motion, it will simply revert back to its normal length -

Yoga is one of the best options for stretching flexibility with proprioceptive motor control and strength

Functional Rehab

prohealthsys

Definition IASTM: **Instrument-assisted Soft Tissue Manipulation** use of a tool or instrument for the treatment of disease or discomfort; a therapeutic modality and manual therapy technique that when combined with rehabilitative exercises improves musculoskeletal function - **given the potential for over dosing and injury, special training is highly recommended for this technique**

Indications	Specific Conditions
• Sub-acute & chronic soft tissue injuries • Loss of ROM or scar tissue (contracture) • Fascial restriction or adhesions • Post surgical rehabilitation (later stages) • Unsuccessful treatment with traditional cross-fiber therapeutic massage • Fluid movement to minimize stasis (edema reduction) • **Practitioner looking to minimize wear and tear on their own body** (decreases clinician fatigue)	**Scar tissue adhesions (contracture)** • Post surgical or traumatic (sprain/strains) **Ligament sprains -** MCL/LCL, AC sprain **Tendinopathy -** Lateral & medial epicondylosis • Supraspinatus tendinopathy, DeQuervain's • Achilles or patellar tendinopathy **Fascial syndromes** • Plantar fascitis, ITB syndromes • Compartment syndromes, Dupuytren's **Nerve Entrapment syndromes** • Carpal Tunnel, Thoracic outlet syndrome

Basic Application

Warm-up (5-10 min)
• Light massage (assess by hand 1st), hot pack, or light exercise as needed

Instrument application (5-7 minutes)
• Apply emollient (gel)
• **Scan of area** to find 'adhesions' or MFTPs - challenge tissue in multiple directions to locate maximum 'resistance' & treat in that direction
• Broad strokes over region using a **concave** instrument (more general)
• Precise, intense strokes using **convex** instrument
• Limit total stroke count to 20-30 max
• Finish with broad strokes back toward heart or basic hand massage techniques

Stretching, mobes or manip

Rehabilitative exercise:
• Posture or proprioceptive training
• Stabilization exercises
• High rep, low weight exercise

Functional Rehab

proSTM¹

Do NOT over treat

Excessive treatment may exacerbate the patient's condition if using too much pressure or time spent in one location

Specialized training is highly recommended for this technique

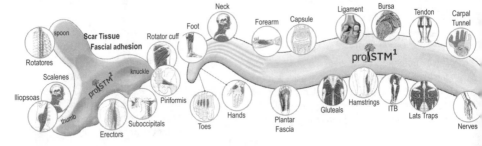

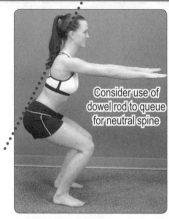

Consider use of dowel rod to queue for neutral spine

Squat & Rise

Procedure

Standing patient is instructed to squat down & then return to a standing position, examiner observes motion

Interpretation

(+) Inability to perform motion → SI/lumbar/hip/knee/ankle pathology (depends on the region the patient reports pain)

(+) Heels lifting off of ground → Tight gastrosoleus muscles

Clinical notes

Useful as a general screen & functional assessment procedure, however the examiner must be aware of certain patient limitations (elderly patients & patients with known pathologies that may limit their ability to perform task)

Examiner should be available to provide support to the patient should they lose their balance

The **ability to squat and rise in patients has been correlated with life expectancy** - test is scored between 1 and 10 (5 points for sitting, 5 more points for standing back up). Each time you use an arm or knee for help in balancing during the test, you subtract one point from 10 possible points. Half a point is subtracted each time you lose balance, or when the fluidity of the feat becomes clumsy. Patients aged 51 to 80, and found that people who scored less than 8 points on the test were twice as likely to die within the next six years (sample size was 2000+ people) - Brito, LB, et. al. Ability to sit and rise from the floor as a predictor of all-cause mortality - European Journal of Preventive Cardiology 2047487312471759, December 13, 2012

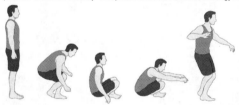

Minus 1 point each if...

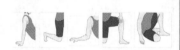

As nature intended, this author recommends deep body weight squats daily for most people

Do not squat deep or dead lift with heavy weight once lumbar neutrality is lost ('butt wink') - body weight is OK, but heavy weights will predispose to injury as proper biomechanics are lost

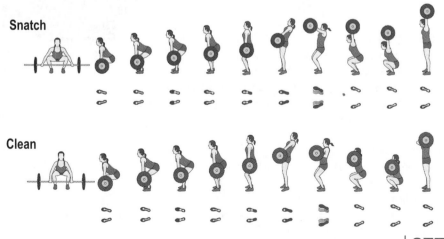

Snatch

Clean

Functional Rehab

Indication
- First step in most lumbar stabilization/core body strength programs
- Good for improving proper biomechanical motion & pelvic stability

Application
1. Patient supine, seated or standing – rock pelvis back & forth ("pelvic clocking")
2. Patient finds pain free area ("neutral pelvis"); if there is no pain free area – patient finds area where they feel most stable
3. Patient "locks" pelvis by contracting abdominal musculature ("abdominal bracing")
4. Patient performs motions (sitting/bending/twisting & eventually tracts) with abdominal bracing

Note: only progress to more difficult tasks as endurance & strength increase

Standing   **Seated**

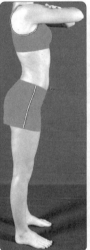
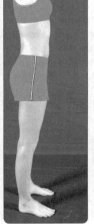

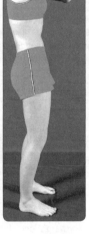
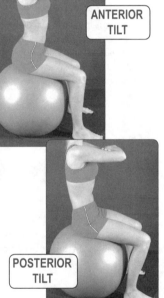

ANTERIOR TILT

POSTERIOR TILT

ANTERIOR TILT   NEUTRAL   POSTERIOR TILT

Functional Rehab

Proper Technique
- Breath & focus on muscles you are working
- Maintain neutral pelvis & do not arch back
- Do movements slowly, if shaking occurs step down a level

Warning: if back pain is aggravated STOP, muscle 'burn' is OK, muscle soreness over the next few days is common & normal

Outcome Measure
- Patient should be able to do 10 contractions with 10 sec holds before moving on to next track

Prescription
_____ reps,   _____ sets,   _____ seconds to hold,   _____ times/day or week

Indication

- Lumbar stabilization/core body strength & aerobic conditioning
- Weak/inhibited gluteals, hip flexors, abdominals

Application

1. Patient supine, with knees bent – attempts to raise pelvis & holds for 1 minute (or as long as possible)
2. As endurance increases – patient lifts one heel off table & holds for 1 minute, then alternates legs
3. As endurance increases – patient lifts one straight leg off table & hold for 1 minute, then alternates legs

Note: only progress to next level of difficulty as endurance & strength increase

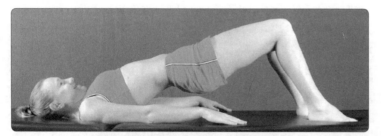

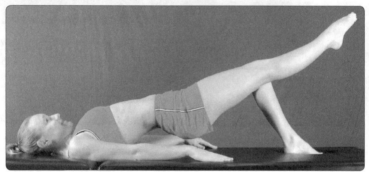

Functional Rehab

Proper Technique

- Breath & focus on muscles you are working
- Maintain neutral pelvis & do not arch back
- Do movements slowly, if shaking occurs step down a level

Warning: if back pain is aggravated STOP, muscle 'burn' is OK, muscle soreness over the next few days is common & normal

Outcome Measure

 Patient handout see website

- Increased endurance & difficulty of activity
- Patient work up to maintaining activity for up to 2 minutes

Prescription

_____ reps, _____ sets, _____ seconds to hold, _____ times/day or week

prohealthsys

Indication

- Lumbar stabilization & aerobic conditioning
- Good for patients that cannot do abdominal curls due to pain or other pathologies
- Weak abdominal musculature

Application

1. Patient supine, with knees bent – raise arm over head
2. Lift one foot off table, then alternate
3. Lift one straight leg off table
4. Lift one straight leg off table & raise opposite arm over head
5. Lift both legs off table & perform alternating kicks ("bicycling") & alternate arms overhead

Note: only progress to next level of difficulty as endurance & strength increase

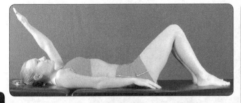
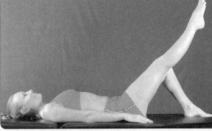
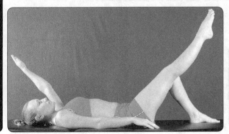
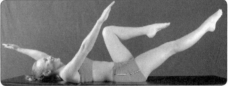

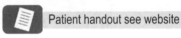 Patient handout see website

Proper Technique

- Breath & focus on muscles you are working
- Maintain neutral pelvis & do not arch back
- Do movements slowly, if shaking occurs step down a level

Warning: if back pain is aggravated STOP, muscle 'burn' is OK, muscle soreness over the next few days is common & normal

Outcome Measure

- Increased endurance & difficulty of activity
- Patient work up to maintaining activity for up to 2 minutes

Prescription

_____ reps, _____ sets, _____ seconds to hold, _____ times/day or week

Functional Rehab

Indication

- May be used in place of quadriped track
- Contraindicated in spinal stenosis & acute phase disc herniation

Application

1. Patient prone (may be performed on floor, table, or Swiss-ball)
2. Patient raise one arm, then alternate
3. Patient raise one leg, then alternate
4. Patient raise opposite arm & leg simultaneously, then alternate

Note: only progress to more difficult tasks as endurance & strength increase

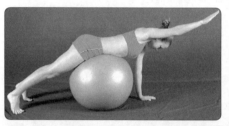
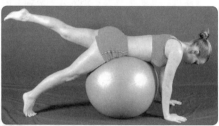
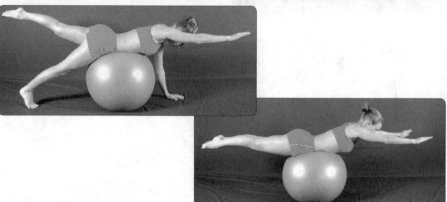

Functional Rehab

Proper Technique

- Breath & focus on muscles you are working
- Maintain neutral pelvis & do not arch back
- Do movements slowly, if shaking occurs step down a level

Warning: if back pain is aggravated STOP, muscle 'burn' is OK, muscle soreness over the next few days is common & normal

Patient handout see website

Outcome Measure

- Patient should be working toward maintaining 2 minutes of activity

Prescription

_____ reps, _____ sets, _____ seconds to hold, _____ times/day or week

Indication
- Weak abdominal obliques, erector spinae, multifidi, quadratus lumborum
- Contraindicated in spinal stenosis, acute phase disc herniation, acute low back strain/sprain

Application
1. Patient side lying (may be performed on floor, table, or Swiss-ball)
2. Patient resting on elbow straightens (raises) torso & pelvis off the ground
3. Patient repeats procedure repeated on opposite side
4. Decrease difficulty by having knees bent, increase difficulty by straightening leg, moving more slowly, supporting on hand (not elbow), placing a Swiss-ball under feet (very advanced)

Note: only progress to more difficult tasks as endurance & strength increase

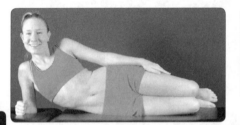
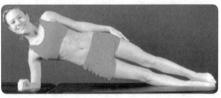
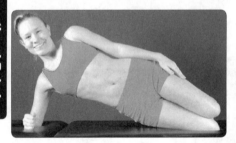
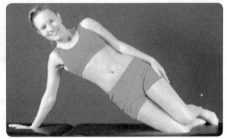

Functional Rehab

Proper Technique
- Breath & focus on muscles you are working
- Maintain neutral pelvis & do not arch back
- Do movements slowly, if shaking occurs step down a level

Warning: if back pain is aggravated STOP, muscle 'burn' is OK, muscle soreness over the next few days is common & normal

📄 Patient handout see website

Outcome Measure
- Patient should be working toward maintaining 2 minutes of activity

Prescription
_____ reps,   _____ sets,   _____ seconds to hold,   _____ times/day or week

Indication

- Weak gluts & multifidi
- Track places minimal load on spine (usually safe for most patients)

Application

1. Patient prone on hands & knees (on floor or table)
2. Patient raise one arm, then alternate
3. Patient raise one leg, then alternate
4. Patient raise opposite arm & leg simultaneously, then alternate

Note: only progress to more difficult tasks as endurance & strength increase

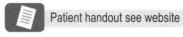
Patient handout see website

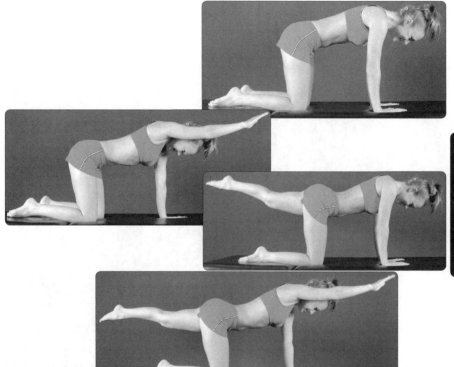

Functional Rehab

Proper Technique

- Breath & focus on muscles you are working
- Maintain neutral pelvis & do not arch back
- Do movements slowly, if shaking occurs step down a level

Warning: if back pain is aggravated STOP, muscle 'burn' is OK, muscle soreness over the next few days is common & normal

Outcome Measure

- Patient should be working toward maintaining 3 minutes of activity or hold positions for 5 seconds

Prescription

_____ reps, _____ sets, _____ seconds to hold, _____ times/day or week

Indication

- Weak core body strength (abdominal obliques, erector spinae, multifidi, quadratus lumborum)
- Contraindicated in spinal stenosis, acute phase disc herniation, acute low back strain/sprain

Application

1. Patient supine (may be performed on floor, table, or Swiss-ball)
2. Patient slowly rotate arms to one side
3. Patient repeats procedure repeated on opposite side
4. Decrease difficulty by lowering weight or bringing arms closer to body, increase difficulty by increasing weight moving more slowly

Note: only progress to more difficult tasks as endurance & strength increase

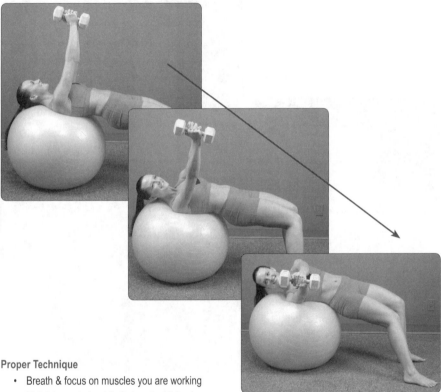

Functional Rehab

Proper Technique

- Breath & focus on muscles you are working
- Maintain neutral pelvis & do not arch back
- Do movements slowly, if shaking occurs step down a level

Warning: if back pain is aggravated STOP, muscle 'burn' is OK, muscle soreness over the next few days is common & normal

Outcome Measure

- Patient should be working toward maintaining 2 minutes of activity

Prescription

_____ reps,   _____ sets,   _____ seconds to hold,   _____ times/day or week

Indication

- Weak core body strength (abdominal obliques, erector spinae, multifidi)
- Contraindicated in spinal stenosis, acute phase disc herniation, acute low back strain/sprain

Application

1. Patient supine with feet on Swiss-ball
2. Patient flexes knees
3. Increase difficulty by moving more slowly or lifting arms off floor

Note: only progress to more difficult tasks as endurance & strength increase

📄 Patient handout see website

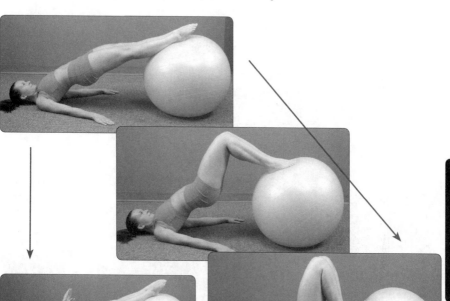

Functional Rehab

Proper Technique

- Breath & focus on muscles you are working
- Maintain neutral pelvis & do not arch back
- Do movements slowly, if shaking occurs step down a level

Warning: if back pain is aggravated STOP, muscle 'burn' is OK, muscle soreness over the next few days is common & normal

Outcome Measure

- Patient should be working toward maintaining 2 minutes of activity

Prescription

_____ reps, _____ sets, _____ seconds to hold, _____ times/day or week

Indication

- Poor balance or jobs that require lots of walking or standing
- Rehabilitation of recurrent ankle sprains & proprioception & muscle endurance improvement

Application

1. Patient stands on two legs with eyes open/closed
2. Patient stands on one leg with eyes open/closed
3. Change foot angle on board to focus on lateral muscles
4. Toss ball from hand to hand or back & forth with clinician
5. Walk from rocker board to rocker board (advanced)
6. Try #1 thru #5 on wobble board (advanced)

Note: clinician should be ready to support patient or catch them if they fall or lose balance

Functional Rehab

Eyes closed   One leg

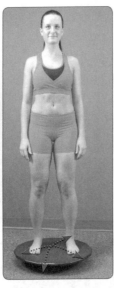
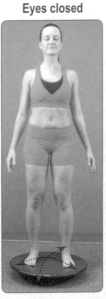
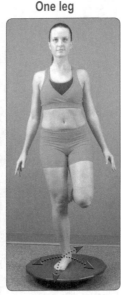

Wobble board

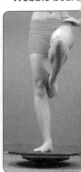

Proper Technique

- Barefoot, try on carpet near wall or corner, thicker carpet is easier
- Breath & focus on muscles you are working
- Maintain neutral pelvis & knee slightly bent, good posture
- Do movements slowly, if shaking occurs step down a level

Warning: if ankle, leg or back pain is aggravated STOP, muscle 'burn' is OK, muscle soreness over the next few days is common & normal

Outcome Measure

- Patient should be working toward maintaining 3 minutes of activity

ROCKER BOARD   **WOBBLE BOARD**

Prescription

_____ reps, _____ sets, _____ seconds to hold, _____ times/day or week

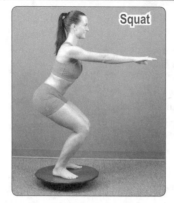

The exercises below are variations designed to provide multidirectional forces to improve proprioceptive ability and strength and are often quite enjoyable for the patient as they provide variety on basic routines

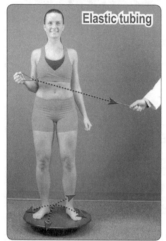

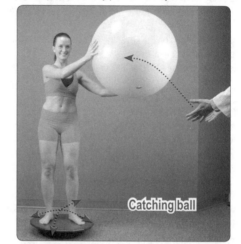

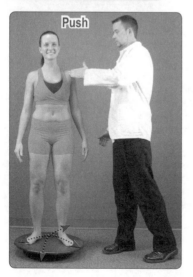

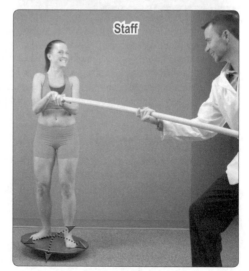

Functional Rehab

prohealthsys

Chair

- Your chair should allow you to sit straight, with your arms relaxed at your side and your hands/wrists at a 90° angle to your keyboard/desktop (chair should have short and adjustable armrests)
- Height of your chair should have your thighs horizontal to the floor, with your feet resting flat (if your feet don't reach the floor, use a footrest)

The most important thing is to regularly change your posture and work positions - use a standing desk!

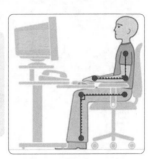

Keyboard & Mouse

- Shoulders should be in a relaxed position, arms horizontally in front of you, and the mouse within easy reach
- Keep your wrists straight and flat, NOT bent up or down
- Your keyboard should be fairly flat, or on a negative slant
- Consider a keyboard tray to help keep your hands and arms in a neutral position
- Use a light touch on the keys; try not to pound, even with a deadline just moments away
- Keep your mouse as close to your keyboard as possible

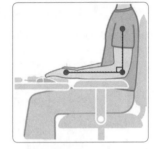

Monitor & Work Station

- Your workstation should be positioned to avoid glare from windows or overhead lighting
- Your monitor should be perpendicular to any window
- Line up your eyes with the upper third of the screen, and about 55 cm to 65 cm (22-26 inches) or an arms length away
- Adjust the brightness of your screen according to your comfort level on a regular basis
- Keep ambient lighting low and add task lighting as needed
- Keep your screen and eyeglasses clean

Telephone & Gagets

- Your phone and any other gadget (calculator, stapler) you use regularly should be within 25 cm (10 inches) away from you.
- Don't cradle your phone on your shoulder while using the computer; when multi-tasking, hold the phone in one hand and the mouse in the other, use a headset or speaker phone
- If you're referring to documents as you work on the computer, use a document holder, set close to the monitor

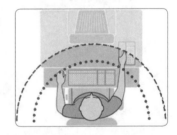

Laptops & Road Trips

- If you're packing more than 10 pounds, use a wheeled carrying case or try a backpack with padded straps
- Try to get a bulkhead or exit row seat (more room), and you'll be more comfortable working on your laptop
- Avoid screen reflection by lowering the window shade and overhead light
- Adjust your chair height and laptop in your hotel room or while working in a conference room. Your arms should remain at a 90° angle to your laptop
- Use a phone book or briefcase to act as a footrest.
- Avoid any position that means you're straining your neck

Reference: Canadian Centre for Occupational Health & Safety - http://www.ccohs.ca/oshanswers/ergonomics/office/

Functional Rehab

Learning Objectives

After completing this chapter, students will be able to:

1. Discuss scar tissue healing by tissue type (muscle, ligament, cartilage, bone)

2. Summarize muscle, ligament and bone injury severity grading and healing cascades

3. Recognize the indications, contraindications and application of orthotics

4. Explain and demonstrate the practical testing outcomes for joint assessment and mobilization

5. Recognize the high value of prohealthsys content in text, online and in person CE seminars

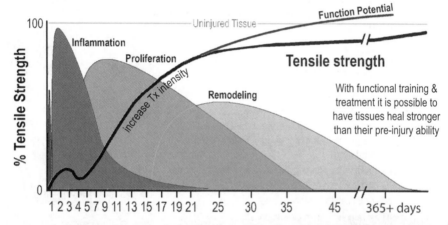

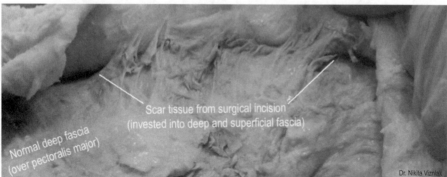

Image: surgical scar tissue following a mastectomy on the left the upper deep fascia is intact, the right side ~lower 2/3 of the pectoralis muscle and associated fascia have the typical random fiber direction and investing adhesions. Upon palpation, the superficial fascia and be separated from the deep fascia/muscle layer easily by hand; at the scar fibers are extremely strong and next to impossible to break by hand - the use of an instrument is required to get through this tissue. Through longer term lever stretching and IASTM techniques it is possible to improve mobility of scar tissue contracture. Larger scars tend to cause more pain.

Early accurate assessment & treatment results in better long-term outcomes.

prohealthsys

Fascia: (Latin for 'band' or 'bandage') flat bands of dense irregular connective tissue below skin that covers the underlying tissues & separates layers of tissue. Fascia encloses muscles, organs, nerves, blood vessels, ligaments & bones; found throughout the entire body.

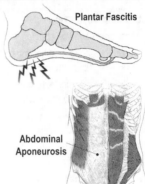
Plantar Fascitis

- Inflammation of the fascia is referred to as *fascitis* (e.g. plantar fascitis)
- Increased blood pressure can sometimes occur in body regions enclosed with fascia resulting in a *compartment syndrome* (e.g. anterior compartment syndrome of the leg)

- *Superficial fascia:* located directly deep to skin & surrounds the entire body. It is filled with fat, nerves, blood vessels & other connective tissue

Abdominal Aponeurosis

- *Deep fascia:* dense fibrous connective tissue that interpenetrates & surrounds the muscles, bones, nerves & blood vessels of the body; **many** muscles directly attach to fascia **to generate force (*e.g. TFL, tib. anterior, glut. max, biceps brachii, plamaris longus*)**

  - *Aponeurosis* - a sheet-like fibrous membrane that binds muscles together or to connect muscle to bone or other fascia (*e.g. abdominal aponeurosis*)

Example of Fascial Connection
(posterior kinetic chain)

- *Visceral fascia:* suspends organs within their cavities (e.g. pericardium, pleura, peritoneum, mesentery)

Functions of Fascia:

- Fascia contains soft tissues & transmits mechanical tension generated by muscular activities or external forces throughout the body (**fascia glides & sticks together; failure of this basic principle = pathology**)

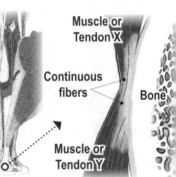
Muscle or Tendon X
Continuous fibers
Bone
Muscle or Tendon Y

  - Provides a sliding & gliding environment for muscles (creates bursae) origin/insertion point of many muscles
  - Suspends organs in their proper place
  - Transmit movement from muscle to bones
  - Provide a supportive & movable wrapping for nerves & blood vessels as they pass through & between muscles
  - Superficial (subcutaneous) **fascia contains many nerve endings**, blood vessels & adipocytes (fat & vitamin storage)
    - Some sources suggest superficial fascia with skin as a human sex organ (a common source of pleasure is rubbing our skin/fascia against each other)

Muscles, fascia, ligaments, and joint capsules attach to each other, creating myofascial connections & kinetic chains through the entire body!

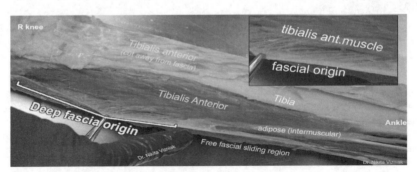
R knee
Tibialis anterior *(cut away from fascia)*
tibialis ant. muscle
fascial origin
Tibialis Anterior
Tibia
Deep fascial origin
adipose (intermuscular)
Ankle
Free fascial sliding region
Dr. Nikita Vizniak

390 | Joint Mobilization

Appendix

Muscles, fascia, ligaments, and joint capsules attach to each other, creating myofascial connections & kinetic chains through the entire body!

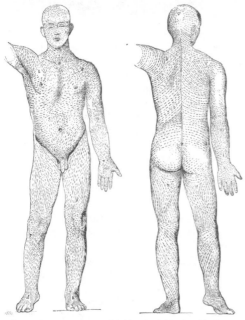

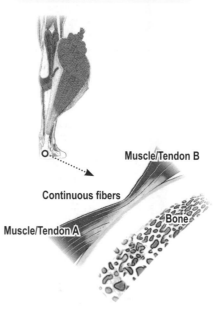

Muscle/Tendon B

Continuous fibers

Bone

Muscle/Tendon A

General course of superficial fascia determined by linear cleft made in skin with a round awl

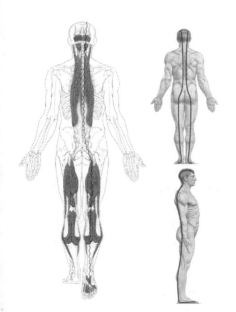

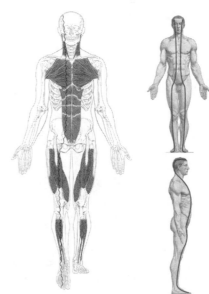

Example of posterior myofascial chain

Example of anterior myofascial chain

Appendix

Grade	Description, ADLs & Healing

Grade I - Mild

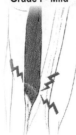

Minimal 'stretch' of fibers (< 10% fibers damaged)
- Common findings: mild pain with activity, muscle guarding, mild myofascial trigger points & local mild compensatory joint motion restrictions
- No bruising or loss of function (minimal or no loss of ROM)
- Minimal pain with motion, mild pain with palpation over damaged site
- Slight weakness may be noted with strong muscle contraction (AROM/RROM)
- Delayed onset muscle soreness (DOMS) is classified as grade 1
- Usually self limiting unless there is repeat trauma to an area which can progress into grade II & III (chronic injury)
- Functional healing time: 2-7 days (structural healing time: 4-14 days)

Grade II - Moderate

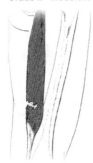

Moderate to severe tearing of fibers (11%-99% fibers torn) - some sources suggest a 2+ or 2- scale to further distinguish severity within range
- Common findings: moderate to severe pain, guarding, loss of function, bruising & edema, decreased range of motion, moderate joint motion restriction
- Antalgic limp, muscle weakness
- Significant pain with AROM & PROM stretch of damaged tissue
- Moderate to severe pain with palpation tissue challenge
- Defect is likely palpable at higher end of range
- Significant loss of strength (3/5 or 4/5) with resisted muscle testing
- Consider referral for diagnostic imaging & surgical evaluation - large partial tears can progress to full tears with repeated trauma
- Functional healing time: 1-10 weeks (structural healing: 3-12+ wks)

Grade III - Severe

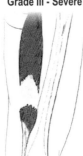

Complete tearing (100% fibers torn = full thickness tear)
- Common findings: severe pain at time of injury then minimal or no pain afterward, significant muscle guarding, severe bruising, loss of function
- Can usually visualize - ruptured muscle balls up under skin, palpable defect
- Complete loss of muscle strength an function (0/5 or 1/5)
- Usually requires surgical intervention (surgical gap closure)
- May be associated with avulsion fracture
- Return to full function is not expected, often with chronic sequelae
- If left untreated there is massive scar tissue formation, loss of function & increased risk of future injury developing into a chronic condition
- Functional healing time: 10 weeks - 6 months (muscle may heal in lengthened position there by changing function) - (structural healing time: 12+ months)

Key Principles for Myofascial Healing

Acute phase (~1-5 days)
- PRICE or METH, avoid aggravating activities & pain control - ↑ protein, Zn, Mg, Mn, Ca & water intake
- Avoid re-injury of damaged tissue & development of chronic condition - COMPLETE FULL REHAB.

Post-acute phase (~2 days - 6 wks)
- As tolerated, begin pain-free ROM ASAP; switch to heat to improve local blood flow
- Soft tissue mobilization & manipulation to improve ROM & reduce contracture (regular stretching)

Remodelling phase (1 wk - 12+ months)
- Work toward functional recovery, proprioception improvement, proper warm-up before activity; address technique issues or biomechanical imbalances that may predispose to injury
- Strengthen exercises, work hardening, or activity specific actions - stretch after exercise for flexibility

1. Injury & Inflammation

- **Initial rupture & necrosis of myofibers** (muscle cell) - within hours necrosis stops
- **Hematoma formation** occurs between ruptured stumps of myofibers
- Torn blood vessels release inflammatory cells & local hormones

2. Proliferation (post-acute repair)

- **Phagocytosis of necrotized tissue** - within first days macrophages phagocytose necrotic tissue
- **Regeneration of myofibers & neurons**
  - Satellite stem cells (present since fetal development) proliferate in response to injury, differentiate into myoblasts & join together to form multinucleated myotubes (these myotubes then fuse with injured myofiber that survived the trauma)
  - Regeneration of intramuscular nerves is also occurs (lack of innervation causes atrophy)
- **Production of a connective tissue scar**
  - Initial injury results in a hematoma; within the first day is invaded by inflammatory cells
  - Fibroblasts then synthesize proteins to restore integrity of the fascial connective tissue framework
  - Hematoma is replaced with Type 3 collagen and then Type 1 collagen (scar/granulation tissue)
- **Capillary in-growth into injured area**
  - Vascularization is the first sign of regeneration & required for subsequent recovery process
  - Regeneration does not progress beyond the newly formed thin myotube/scar tissue stage unless a sufficient capillary in-growth has ensured the required supply of oxygen for aerobic metabolism

3. Remodelling (recovery & fibrosis)

- **Maturation of regenerated myofibers**
- **Contraction & reorganization of scar tissue fibrosis**
  - Myofibers form branches & try to pierce through the scar and adhere to the connective tissue (scar); reinforced lateral adhesions (branches) also form to reduce the movement of the stumps & reduce the pull on the fragile scar; lateral adhesions are formed as a result of intentional mechanical stress (Pain free ROM, massage, stretching & muscle use without tearing)
  - Overtime the scar progressively diminishes bringing the stumps closer together – until the myofibers become interlaced (though likely not reunited - there is usually some remaining fibrosis)
- **Recovery of the functional capacity of the muscle**
  - Depends on severity of injury, prevention of re-injury, appropriate nutrition & rehabilitation

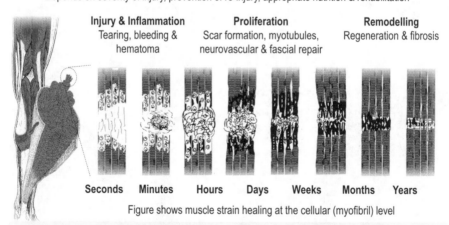

| Injury & Inflammation | Proliferation | Remodelling |
| Tearing, bleeding & hematoma | Scar formation, myotubules, neurovascular & fascial repair | Regeneration & fibrosis |

Seconds   Minutes   Hours   Days   Weeks   Months   Years

Figure shows muscle strain healing at the cellular (myofibril) level

Muscle strain healing occurs in 3 overlapping phases

Duration varies depending on injury severity & general health, activity, nutrition & age of the individual involved. Early return to full activity increases the likelihood of re-injury & the development of chronic pain, repetitive injury results in a increased scar tissue/fibrosis formation & loss of function

Dermatome - region of **skin supplied by neurons from a single spinal root**
(note there is an exception where the dermatomes of the face are supplied by the trigeminal nerve CN-V)

Myotome - region of **muscle supplied by neurons from a single spinal root** (note there are exception where cranial nerves supply muscles - see cranial nerve exam)

Sclerotome - area of **bone supplied by neurons from a single spinal root** (most programs do not even mention or teach sclerotome distribution)

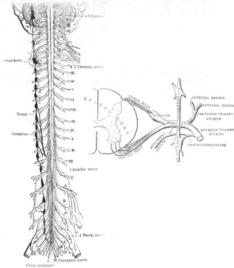

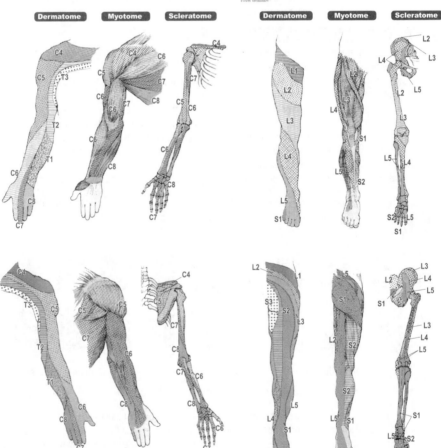

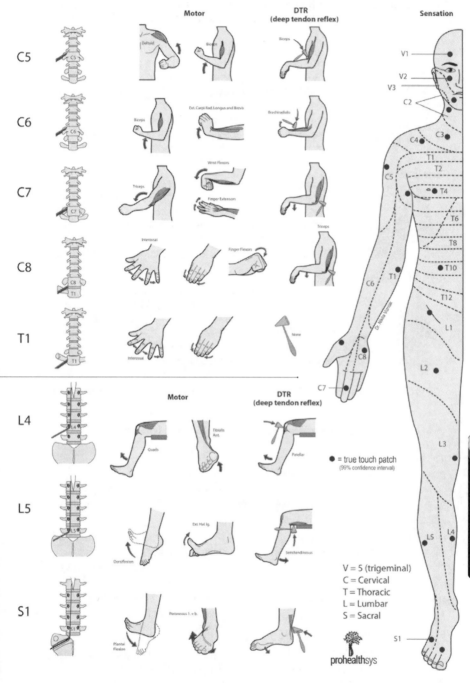

remember there is overlap and anatomical variation in specific nerve innervation look for multiple levels of evidence to support findings (DTRs, motor pathways, dermatomes, myotomes and sclerotomes)

Ligament sprains occur when ligaments surrounding joint are forced beyond their normal ROM; because of a lower blood supply, ligaments usually take longer to heal than muscles

Description, ADLs & Healing

Grade I - Mild

- Mild swelling & point tenderness over ligament, no bruising
- Estimated > 10% fiber damage
- Single ligament, mild stretch, no instability
- (-) stress tests, mild pain at extreme end ROM (PROM w/ over pressure)
- No or mild limp/loss of function, mild difficulty hopping on one leg
- Functional recovery in 2-14 days (structural healing 6-30 days)

Grade II - Moderate

- Bruising is common, mild to moderate swelling
- Large spectrum of injury that can include partial tearing of many ligaments
- Estimated 11-99% fiber damage (2+/- can be used to further grade severity)
- Mild to moderate instability demonstrated on stress tests
- Obvious limp, unable to hop or run
- Functional recovery in 14 days - 2 months (structural healing 1-3 months)

Grade III - Severe

- Severe bruising & swelling - fracture must be ruled out!
- Difficult to visualize structures due to swelling & tenderness
- Complete tearing of multiple ligament & joint capsule may also be involved
- Marked instability (+) stress tests
- Unable to bear weight, almost complete loss of ROM
- Functional recovery time 1-3 months (structural healing 6 month+)

Given the huge range of a Grade 2 sprain, 2+ or 2- can be used to denote the upper or lower range

Key Principles for Ligament Healing

Acute phase (~1-5 days)

- PRICE or METH, avoid aggravating activities/ positions & pain control
- Short-term immobilization (tensor bandage with ice), NSAIDS for short term pain reduction
- Avoid re-injury of damaged tissue & development of chronic instability - COMPLETE FULL REHAB.

Post-acute phase (~2 days - 6 wks)

- As tolerated, begin pain-free ROM ASAP
- Switch to heat to improve blood flow (METH)
- Consider IFC, TENS or MENS
- Gentle mobilization & manipulation to improve ROM & reduce contracture
- Consider prolotherapy if unstable

Remodelling phase (1 wk - 12+ months)

- Work toward function recovery, proper warm-up before activity
- Address biomechanical imbalances that may predispose to injury
- SLOWLY as tolerated by patients move from simple isometric activities to eccentric & then activity specific or work hardening activities
- Surgical consultation is warranted with failure to respond to conservative care, marked joint instability or severe cases which may have multifactoral causes (occult fracture of surrounding bone or cartilage)

Appendix

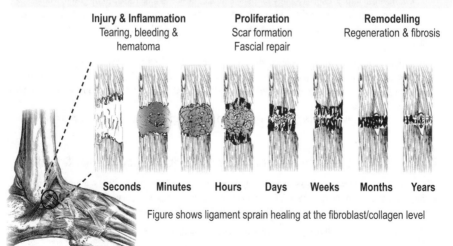

1. Injury & Inflammation

- **Initial rupture, hematoma formation** occurs between ruptured stumps of collagen & fibroblasts
- Torn blood vessels release inflammatory cells & local hormones

2. Proliferation (post-acute repair)

- **Phagocytosis of necrotized tissue** - within first few days macrophages phagocytose necrotic tissue
- **Production of a connective tissue scar**
  - Initial injury results in a hematoma; within the first day is invaded by inflammatory cells
  - Fibroblasts then synthesize proteins to restore integrity of the fascial connective tissue framework
  - Hematoma is replaced with Type 3 collagen & then Type 1 collagen (scar/granulation tissue)
- **Capillary in-growth into injured area**
  - Vascularization is somewhat limited in ligaments, which results in a longer healing time than more vascular tissue (muscle). Vascularization is the first sign of regeneration & required for subsequent recovery process

3. Remodelling (recovery & fibrosis)

- **Contraction & reorganization of scar tissue fibrosis**
  - Can last for up to a year plus
  - Maturation of collagen tissue from Type 3 to Type 1 & realignment of collagen tissue
    - When it is first laid down, the collagen tissue is haphazard & does not have a lot of tensile strength; ligaments gradually become stronger through controlled stress & loading in a functional pattern, which aligns the fibres in a longitudinal fashion (pain free ROM, massage, stretch, mobilization & exercise use without tearing)
  - Because remodelling phase lasts a year plus, there is a potential for weakness in the ligament & a risk of re-injury; risk is reduced by increasing the strength of muscles which also provide support to the joint & by doing proprioceptive exercises to increase the patient's sense of joint positioning
- **Recovery of the functional capacity of the muscle**
  - Depends on severity of injury, prevention of re-injury, appropriate nutrition & rehabilitation

Ligament sprain healing occurs in 3 overlapping phases
Duration varies depending on injury severity & general health, activity, nutrition & age of the individual involved. Early return to full activity increases the likelihood of re-injury & the development of chronic pain, repetitive injury results in increased scar tissue/fibrosis formation & loss of function

Injury & Inflammation	Proliferation	Remodelling
Tearing, bleeding & hematoma	Scar formation Fascial repair	Regeneration & fibrosis

Seconds   Minutes   Hours   Days   Weeks   Months   Years

Figure shows ligament sprain healing at the fibroblast/collagen level

Appendix

The leading cause of cartilage damage is osteoarthritis (degenerative joint disease); three processes:

1. A progressive loss of cartilage (either direct damage or slow wear & tear)
2. The body's attempt to repair cartilage (usually very slow scar tissue formation)
3. Finally, destruction of bone underneath the articular cartilage

Lifelong moderate use of normal joints does not appear to increase the risk. Factors such as high-impact, twisting injuries; abnormal joint anatomy & biomechanics; joint instability; inadequate muscle strength, balance or endurance, nutritional deficiency & medical or genetic factors can contribute to osteoarthritis

Progression of Osteoarthritis (OA) Joint Degeneration

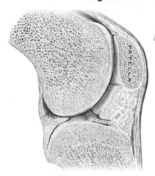 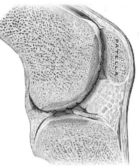 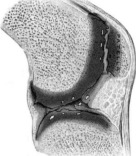

Grade I - OA	**Grade II-III - Moderate OA**	**Grade IV - Late OA**
Mild cartilage damage (tears); very mild subchondral reactive sclerosis (bone remodeling due to abnormal stress)	Irregular joint space due to loss of cartilage; cartilage fragmentation ('joint mice'); reactive sclerosis	Osteophytes, periarticular fibrosis, cartilage calcification; subchondral cysts (geodes); sever cases may include ankylosis (fusion)

Cartilage Healing

- Articular cartilage is avascular which prevents it from mounting a vascular response to injury (no direct blood supply which imposes limits on healing potential (some traumatic defects in cartilage never heal)

Mechanisms of repair (type of cartilage healing is influenced by the <u>depth</u> of the injury)

- With **subchondral injury**, capillary injury forms a fibrin clot, which is then replaced by granulation tissue & fibrocartilage; if defect is limited to cartilage, no blood vessels are disrupted & inflammatory response is less intense than if injury extends through cartilage into subchondral bone, as occurs in intra-articular fracture

- Injury **isolated only to cartilage** is dependent on chondrocytes to synthesize a new matrix
  - Since cartilage is largely avascular, healing is dependent on diffusion of nutrients from synovial fluid
  - Regeneration of cartilage is slow & highest potential for growth occurs in the perichondrium (periphery regions of articular cartilage)
  - Isolated injuries to cartilage (which do not extend to subchondral bone) heal slowly & incompletely

Regular motion & activity are crucial to ensure optimal joint health & healing

During normal movements, the synovial fluid held within the cartilage is squeezed out mechanically (weeping lubrication) to maintain a layer of fluid on the cartilage surface & circulate nutrients - synovial fluid that bathes cartilage provides adequate nutrition diffusion through several millimeters of matrix

Research suggests that prolonged joint immobilization results in cartilage thinning & degradation

Grade	Description, ADLs & Healing
Grade I Cartilage softening & swelling	• Estimated > 5% fiber damage, no radiographic changes visible • (-) scour tests, no or very mild pain after extreme activity • No or mild limp/loss of function, respond well to conservative care • Functional recovery in 2-14 days (structural healing 6-30 days)
Grade II Partial-thickness defect with fissures on the surface that do not reach subchondral bone or exceed 1.5 cm in diameter	• Estimated 5-50% fiber damage • Mild swelling is possible after activity, crepitus with ROM or scour test • Possible limp, may or may not respond to conservative care • Mild reactive sclerosis & joint space due to loss of cartilage visible on x-ray • Functional recovery time 1-3 months (structural healing 6 month+)
Grade III Fissuring to the level of subchondral bone in an area with a diameter more than 1.5 cm	• Estimated 50-99% fiber damage, swelling is common after activity • Crepitus will be noted with ROM or scour test, possible mild instability • Possible limp or altered gait • Irregular joint space & reactive subchondral sclerosis visible on x-ray • Will likely result in a permanent & progressive defect
Grade IV Exposed subchondral bone	• 100% cartilage loss! Bone is directly exposed & remodels under stress • Marked crepitus & instability (+) stress & scour tests • Reactive sclerosis, osteophytes, subchondral cysts visible on x-ray • Permanent defect that often requires surgical consultation

Based on Outerbridge classification system for cartilage damage (note: grade 0/4 = normal cartilage)

Key Principles for Joint Cartilage Healing

Acute phase (~1-5 day)

• PRICE or METH as indicated, avoid aggravating activities, positions & pain

• Short-term immobilization (1-2 days maximum)

   • **Pain free ROM is good for fluid movement & synovial fluid nutrient exchange!**

• Medications for short term pain reduction: aspirin, ibuprophen & naproxen

   • Glucocorticoid injection (initially relieve pain but increase cartilage degeneration with long term use)

Post-acute phase (~2 days - 6 wks)

• As tolerated begin pain-free ROM ASAP

• Switch to heat to improve blood flow & nutrient exchange

• Consider IFC, TENS or MENS

• Gentle mobilization & manipulation to improve ROM, reduce contracture & increase synovial fluid movement

Post-acute phase (continued)

• Improve diet & weight control

• **Glucosamine Sulfate & GAG supplementation** (variable effectiveness but very few side effects)

• Consider platelet rich plasma (PRP) injections

Remodelling phase (3 wks - 12+ months)

• Work toward function recovery - improve aerobic & cardiovascular fitness

• Address biomechanical imbalances

• SLOWLY as tolerated by patients move from simple isometric activities to eccentric & then activity specific or work hardening activities

• Surgical consultation is warranted with failure to respond to conservative care or in severe cases

• Consider microfracture surgery (drill tiny holes into bone/cartilage; allows blood & stem cells from bone marrow to leak out & patch the injury - variable effectiveness)

Appendix

- **Fracture** - cracking or breaking of a hard object or material (bone)
- **Bone bruise:** can be described as a stage before the fracture (includes: sub-periosteal hematoma, inter-osseous bruising & sub-chondral lesion); fracture means that all bone trabeculae of that specific place are fractured, in a bone bruise only a few of the trabeculae are broken (visible on MRI)
- **Pathologic fracture** - bone breaks in an area weakened by another disease process (tumors, infection, osteoporosis & certain inherited bone disorders)
- **Stress (fatigue) fracture** - microfracture caused by repetitive stress, as may occur in sports, strenuous exercise, or heavy physical labor (bone does not heal sufficiently from each repetitive trauma event); if the forces on the bone continue with inadequate healing may progress to a full fracture
- **Closed fracture** - fracture does not penetrate skin
- **Open (compound) fracture** - fracture penetrates skin (a spike of bone sticks out or object penetrates skin)
- **Avulsion fracture** - separated bone fragment from a muscle, tendon or ligament attachment site
- **Comminuted fracture** - more than 2 bony fragments
- **Compression** (impaction) **fracture** - decreased bone size from trabecular compression (common in osteoporosis)
- **Greenstick fracture** - buckled trabeculae (not completely broken bone - occurs in children)
- **Oblique fracture** - fracture at 45° to long axis of bone
- **Occult fracture** - non-visualized fracture, often diagnosed through soft tissue swelling (fat pad signs) or advanced imaging (MRI/CT)
- **Spiral fracture** - fracture circumferential & longitudinal to long axis of bone
- **Torus fracture** - buckled trabeculae & cortical bulge
- **Transverse fracture** - fracture ~90° to long axis of bone
- **Salter-Harris fracture** - fractures involving growth plates (see below)

Avulsion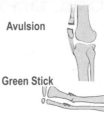

Green Stick

Transverse

Angulated

Oblique

Spiral

Comminuted

Impaction

Compression

Fracture Dislocation

Salter-Harris Fracture Types

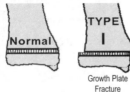

Normal	TYPE I	TYPE II	TYPE III	TYPE IV	TYPE V
	Growth Plate Fracture	Growth Plate & Metaphysis Fracture	Growth Plate & Epiphysis Fracture	Growth Plate, Metaphysis & Epiphysis Fracture	Growth Plate Compression Fracture

Fracture Complications

Immediate concerns	Short-term concerns	Long-term concerns
• Neurovascular damage • Compartment syndrome • Fat embolism • Thrombus formation • Gas gangrene (infection)	• Refracture • Synostosis • Delayed union • Osteomyelitis • Reflex sympathetic dystrophy • Myositis ossificans	• Osteonecrosis • Nonunion • Malunion • DJD • Osteoporosis

Fractures heal through physiological processes; the healing process is mainly determined by the periosteum
- Periosteum is the primary source of precursor cells which develop into chondroblasts & osteoblasts
- Bone marrow, endosteum, small blood vessels & fibroblasts are secondary sources of precursor cells
- Immobilization protects & surgery can help realign to facilitate healing (excessive immobilization can have negative effects including muscle & bone atrophy - osteoporosis)

Phases of fracture healing

Inflammation/Reactive Phase (0 to ~3 days)
- *Fracture & inflammatory phase* - following break blood cells fill adjacent tissue, blood vessels constrict, stopping any further bleeding & a blood clot (hematoma) forms
- *Granulation tissue formation* - fibroblasts replicate & form a loose aggregate of cells, interspersed with small blood vessels (granulation tissue)

Proliferation/Reparative Phase (~3 days to 6 wks)
- *Soft callus formation* - cells of the periosteum replicate & blood vessels start to regrow
  - Fibroblasts within granulation tissue also develop into chondroblasts & form hyaline cartilage
  - Periosteal cells around the fracture gap develop into osteoblasts & form woven bone
  - Eventually, fracture gap is bridged by hyaline cartilage & woven bone, restoring some of its original strength
- *Hard callus formation* - hyaline cartilage & woven bone is replaced with lamellar bone through endochondral ossification

Remodeling Phase (4-6+ weeks)
- *Remodeling to original bone contour* - process substitutes trabecular bone with compact bone
  - Trabecular bone is resorbed by *osteoclasts*; then *osteoblasts* deposit compact bone
  - Eventually, the fracture callus is remodelled into a new shape which closely duplicates the bone's original shape & strength

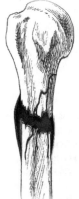
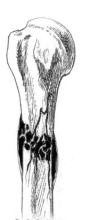
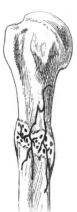
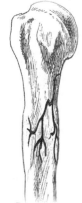

Reactive Phase	**Soft Callus**	**Hard Callus**	**Remodeling**
inflammation granulation	blood vessel & cartilage growth	endochondral ossification	compact bone remodelling

Key Principles for Fracture Healing

- **Protection from re-injury** (soft cast with appropriate bone orientation) - avoid re-injury!
- **Age:** younger individuals heal more rapidly
- **Nutrition:** adequate metabolic products (Ca, Mg, Zn, phosphate, carbohydrates & protein)
- **Systemic Diseases:** osteoporosis, diabetes & other conditions slow healing (smoking)
- **Hormones:** thyroid hormone, growth hormone, calcitonin, estrogen & others play significant roles in bone healing (corticosteroids slow healing)

A custom orthotic is device designed to **align the foot and ankle into the most anatomically efficient position**. They look similar to insoles but are more structurally sound and have medical applications based on the custom specifications your body needs. Orthotics help correct various lower body kinetic chain & foot imbalances. Custom orthotics work to correct how your foot and ankle work similar to the way glasses help your eyes focus and see clear.

Orthotics help reduce the strain and stress on your body by properly aligning your feet and supporting your transverse and longitudinal arches. The orthotic device helps realign the foot and assists in redirecting and reducing certain motion patterns that appear during the gait cycle. Custom orthotics fit into the various shoes you wear day to day as easily as most over the counter insoles do. The major advantage here is that these custom orthotic devices are fit exactly to each of your feet and establish proper foot, ankle, knee, hip and low back biomechanics that restore proper function from the ground up. This helps you eliminate pain and reduce overall wear and tear.

Who might need a custom orthotic?

If you have any of the following symptoms or pain patterns you will benefit from a thorough lower body assessment, gait analysis and potentially a custom orthotic prescription.

- Localized foot pain (heel, sole of foot, burning pain in the toes, ankle pain)
- Bunions or hammer toes
- Leg/calf, knee pain
- Hip or low back pain
- Those who are on their feet all day everyday
- Anyone working or standing on hard surfaces for several hours a day

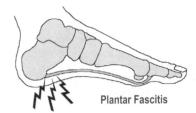
Plantar Fascitis

Indications

Custom orthotics are designed to improve joint position, motion and efficacy of the lower body. Any time orthotics are prescribed the following goals need to be kept in mind:

- Enhance the patient's functional capabilities
- Redistribute weight more evenly across joints of the lower body
- Reduce or eliminate pain
- Improve the patient's day to day performance and activities of daily living

Specific conditions indicated for orthotics
- Over pronation syndrome
- 'Shin splints' when DDx correctly
- Patellofemoral syndrome
- Posterior tibial syndrome
- Iliotibial band syndrome
- Limb length discrepancy
- Plantar fascitis

Conservative care must always be attempted prior to initiating custom orthotic devices. For example, the 27 bones of the foot need to be free and moving congruently with one another prior to stepping into an orthotic device. Failing to do this is akin to casting a broken limb before the bone has been realigned or set. You must first ensure the bones are in place and working throughout the foot. You must also determine if the pain in the foot is from a stress fracture or hairline fracture in which case the orthotic would be unlikely to help.

Conservative care includes: **soft tissue and myofascial release of the foot and leg. Manipulation of key bones of the foot such as the talus and navicular may also be indicated to help support joint motion and aid with pain relief**. Corrective exercises to maintain and develop a strong arch. Barefoot exercises and sand walking for example.

Once conservative care and a proper gait analysis has been conducted a patient may be a good candidate for custom orthotics in any of the following instances:

- Prior failed attempts with conservative treatment
- Deformity of the foot or forces too great to be managed otherwise
- **Prior successful use of custom orthotics**

Contraindications

- The orthotic limits function & motion, increases pain or disrupts balance

- If the orthotic causes abnormal pressure points that would result in potential injury to the skin, joints and other tissues

- Stress/hairline fracture

- The orthotic cannot provide the correct motion or kinematics required

- When greater stabilization is required than the orthotic can provide

Assessment and examination

1. Observe how the patient sits in your waiting room, how they walk into your office

2. **History taking around the chief concern LOC-QSMAT and ask the patient to bring in an old pair of shoes for evaluation!**

3. Visual inspection of both feet (arch height), ankles, legs, thighs and hips looking for any swelling, redness, scars, deformities, bruising

4. Assessment of AROM, PROM RROM of the ankle and foot – depending on chief concern you may need to assess other joints such as the knee if they are having medial knee pain while walking or running for example. If dorsiflexion is restricted the talus bone might be listed

5. **Evaluate arch height in both a seated and standing position to assess for rigid or supple pes planus**. Feiss line or measurement from the navicular tuberosity to the floor may be used to determine if the navicular has dropped

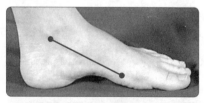

6. Determine limb length and compared bilaterally for structural or functional short leg due to pelvic malposition or muscle imbalances

7. A gait analysis that involves both static and dynamic components

- There are many innovative and diagnostic tools for mapping out gait cycles, determining arch heights and pressure points throughout the foot. For example, the TOG Gait Scan by The Orthotic Group (TOG) aids in analysis of patient biomechanics and helps determine the best course of action for custom orthotic prescription.

- **Clinical tip:** the colorful computer generated images from GaitScan software provide an awesome visual of the patient's gait cycle. This gives the practitioner an easy way to help the patient understand their case and is an excellent educational tool around biomechanical dysfunction and how it might be relating to their dysfunction and pain patterns.

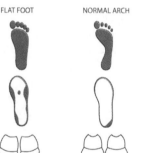

| FLAT FOOT | NORMAL ARCH | HIGH ARCH |

Ask the patient to bring in an old pair of shoes for evaluation

Other options before the advent of technology include using compressive foams, weight bearing and semi weight bearing plaster casting to aid in analysis of foot biomechanics and dysfunction.

More and more insurance companies are moving away from requiring any foams or plaster casting. Insurance companies are recognizing computer and **mechanical imaging systems provide sufficient analysis of gait cycle and correlate that with a proper history**

Application

Once a detailed clinical assessment has be done and a gait analysis has been reviewed custom orthotics can be prescribed. When possible **go for a firm but flexible orthotic that allows the arch to still act as a shock absorber and flex towards the ground with each step**. Certain companies have extremely rigid and solid orthotics which do not allow proper foot kinematics.

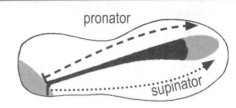

pronator

supinator

The prescription for a custom orthotic should include the following:

- Type of material to be utilized
- History, exam and gait analysis notes
- Depth of heel cup required
- Length of orthotic required: full length, ¾ or ½ length
- Style of design (based on needs of patient: dress shoe, steel toe boot specific or athletic style orthotic)
- Doctors recommendation letter

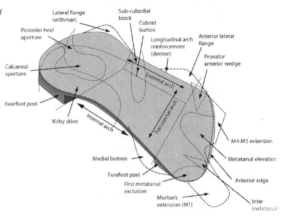

Additional patient information required to provide the lab that builds and creates the custom orthotics:

- Shoe size and width
- Heel height of shoe
- Heel lifts, if required
- Weight, Age
- Activity level & occupation
- Differential diagnosis

Depending on the patient's specific biomechanical limitation and need, various specifications can be included on their custom orthotic:

- Forefoot extensions and top covers
- Rear foot flaring and postings
- Full or ¾ length inserts (to fit into more narrow or tighter footwear)
- Metatarsal pads to support the transverse arch

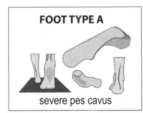

FOOT TYPE A

severe pes cavus

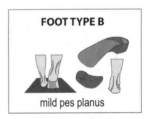

FOOT TYPE B

mild pes planus

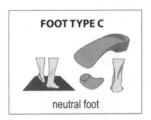

FOOT TYPE C

neutral foot

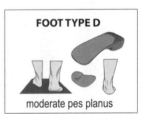

FOOT TYPE D

moderate pes planus

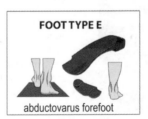

FOOT TYPE E

abductovarus forefoot

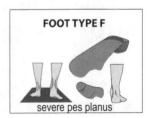

FOOT TYPE F

severe pes planus

The 3 minute orthotic assessment

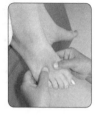

Have the **patient begin seated or supine with the arch in a non weight bearing state**. With 1 finger/thumb, rub with firm pressure between the first, second and third metatarsal heads on both feet to determine if there is any pain or discomfort.

Next, locate the muscle belly of their erector spinae and palpate up and down the entire back with firm pressure to determine if there are any trigger points or discomfort. Finish off the seated exam by muscle testing the latissimus dorsi and triceps long head for any weakness. For detailed examples of how to muscle test these areas please refer to the Muscle Manual or prohealthsys video database.

As the arch is not weight-bearing when seated you will likely note some or all of the following:

* Minimal tenderness between the metatarsal heads (transverse arch maintained in non weight bearing position)

* Minimal trigger points and tenderness in the paraspinal muscles of the back (postural muscles holding well because longitudinal arch is maintained and the ankle remains in neutral)

* Strong triceps long head and latissimus muscle test (extensor weakness not found because foot and ankle positions are maintained and not disrupting the posterior chain)

Next, have your **patient stand in bare feet and repeat the above tests**. If the arch is a significant issue for your patient a spinal muscle extensor weakness pattern will display. You will notice some or all of the following when you retest:

* Significant pain and tenderness between the metatarsal heads on palpation (fallen transverse arch)

* Multiple trigger points and areas of discomfort on palpation of the erectors and paraspinal muscle groups (dropped longitudinal arch and medial rotation at the ankle can travel up posterior chain disrupting neuromuscular patterning)

* Weak latissimus dorsi and triceps long head muscle test

For the final part of the 3 minute exam, **have the patient now stand on a generic pair of orthotics that support the arch of the foot** and ensure the ankle is kept in alignment. Retest all the above areas. If you note less tenderness at the metatarsal heads, strong erectors with minimal trigger points and no issues with their latissimus and triceps long head you have determined their arch drop to be a strong causative factor in kinetic chain balance, stability and performance.

This helps the patient understand what is going on and in under 3 minutes they can see how their arch can affect not just their foot, but entire body as well.

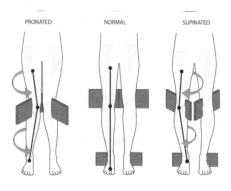

PRONATED   NORMAL   SUPINATED

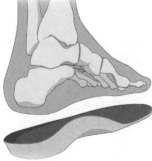

3 minute orthotic assessment summary

1. **Patient seated** palpate foot and spine

2. **Standing bare foot**, palpate foot & spine

3. **Standing with orthotic**, re-assess

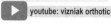
youtube: vizniak orthotic

Appendix

1. How many joints are in the human body? (72)
   A. ~214
   B. ~350
   C. ~456
   D. ~650

2. For an evidence informed practice, which of the factors below must be used to establish clinical expertise? (v)
   A. Evidence, research and experience
   B. Healthcare resources
   C. Client preferences & actions
   D. All of the above

3. In regard to the therapeutic order of assessment and treatment, interactions should progress from _____? (vi)
   A. Least invasive to most invasive
   B. Most invasive to least invasive
   C. Surgical treatment to rehab.
   D. Medications to surgery

4. How many hours per day is the average North American sitting/laying/sleeping? (2)
   A. 10
   B. 15
   C. 20

5. What is the first known written record of joint mobilization? (3)
   A. 7000 BCE Neolithic period
   B. 3000 BCE Egypt
   C. 1700 BCE Chinese Tui Na
   D. 1895 D.D. Palmer

6. According to university academic calendars, what profession has the most training in joint mobilization/manipulation? (5)
   A. Doctor of Chiropractic
   B. Medical Doctor
   C. Doctor of Physical Therapy
   D. Registered Massage Therapist

7. Define the Term 'Subluxation' according to the World Health Organization (7) _____
   _____
   _____

8. Which of the following is a factor that will NOT improve healing? (vii)
   A. Laughter, positive mood & good sleep
   B. Good blood supply
   C. Soft tissue/joint mobilization
   D. Increased age, malnourishment

9. As levers get longer, speed _____ gets and power gets _____? (9)
   A. faster, weaker
   B. slower, weaker
   C. faster, stronger
   D. slower, stronger

10. Which of the following is NOT a force that can act on joints and bones? (12)
    A. Compression
    B. Tension
    C. Shear
    D. Torsion
    E. Teleportation

11. Proteoglycans are hydrophilic? (13)
    A. T
    B. F

12. Examples of **osteokinematic** motions include all of the following except? (14)
    A. Flexion
    B. Abduction
    C. Spin
    D. Pronation

13. Examples of **arthrokinematic** motions include? (14)
    A. Slide (glide)
    B. Spin
    C. Roll
    D. All of the above

14. Concave on convex rule, when a concave surface moves on a convex surface roll and slide occur in the _____ direction? (15)

   A. Same

   B. Opposite

   C. Flexion

   D. All of the above

15. Define closed packed? Open packed? (15)
   A. Closed: _____
   B. Open: _____

16. Which of the following are accessory movements at joints, ie. cannot be performed voluntarily but require muscle relaxation and application of passive movement? (15)

   A. Medial and lateral glides

   B. AP or PA glides

   C. Rotation and distraction

   D. All of the above

17. Which of the following conditions would you consider the most appropriate indication for the use of joint mobilization techniques? (15)

   A. Loss of accessory joint movement due to capsular restriction

   B. Functional immobility: eg paralysis

   C. Joint hypomobility due to osteoarticular blockage

   D. Pain

18. List the types and functions of receptors in joints, and muscles? (16-17)

   Golgi tendon organ: _____

   Muscle spindle: _____

   Joint Mechanoreceptors

      Type 1: _____

      Type 2: _____

      Type 3: _____

      Type 4: _____

19. Pain gates may be closed by _____? (19)

   A. Being in a 'good' mood, positive mind set

   B. Movement, exercise & sleep

   C. Heat, cold, massage, mobilizations

   D. All of the above

20. Outside of bony end-feels - most PROM tissue resistance is due to _____? (20)

   A. Ligaments/capsule

   B. Muscles

   C. Tendons and skin

   D. None of the above

21. Define the grades of mobilization? (21)

   Grade 1: _____

   Grade 2: _____

   Grade 3: _____

   Grade 4: _____

   Grade 5: _____

22. In cases of pain, muscle guarding and spasm, small amplitude, high velocity oscillatory movements may be used to stimulate mechanoreceptors, thus inhibiting the transmission of nociceptive stimuli. (21)

   A. True

   B. False

23. Examples of tissue pull and force vectors include _____? (25)

   A. I-S, S-I

   B. M-L, L-M

   C. P-A, A-P

   D. All of the above

24. Define the potential causes for joint sounds? (26)

   A. Cavitation: _____

   B. Clunk: _____

   C. Crepitus: _____

   D. Snap or Strum: _____

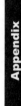

25. Following a cavitation, it takes ~__ minutes for the joint gas bubble to be reabsorbed? (26)

   A. 5

   B. 20

   C. 60

   D. 120

26. Which of the following may be an indications for joint mobilizations? (28)

   A. Symptom reproduction with assessment

   B. Asymmetry in motion, joint play

   C. Both 'A' and 'B'

   D. None of the above

27. Give 5 relative & 5 absolute contraindications for joint mobilization? (30)

   Relative: _____

   Absolute: _____

28. List 3 potential negative side effects of joint mobilization. (31)

   1. _____

   2. _____

   3. _____

29. During informed consent, what is does acronym PAR-Q stand for? (37)

   P. _____

   A. _____

   R. _____

   Q. _____

30. What does the acronym o-HIPMNRS stand for? (46) _____

31. What are the parts of a fracture screen? (47)

   _____

   _____

32. List 3 red flags of serious pathology (48)

   1. _____

   2. _____

   3. _____

33. Which of the following can be used as an outcome marker to evaluate client progression? (50)

   A. ROM and pain scale (0-10)

   B. Medication intake

   C. Activities of daily living

   D. All of the above

34. Which of the following can affect posture (54)

   A. Pain and muscle spasm

   B. Ligament laxity or contracture

   C. Poor habits & anatomical variations

   D. All of the above

35. On lateral view postural assessment, the plumb line should fall through all of the following except _____? (55)

   A. Anterior to lateral malleolus

   B. Greater trochanter

   C. Acromion

   D. EOP (external occipital protuberance)

36. Which of the following is tight/shortened in an upper cross postural syndrome? (58)

   A. Upper trapezius & sub-occipital muscles

   B. Pectoralis major and anterior deltoid

   C. Posterior ligaments of the cervical spine

   D. All of the above

37. A 'knee back gait' may be due to _____. (59)

   A. Quadriceps or gluteal weakness

   B. Cerebral palsy

   C. L5 disc herniation

   D. All of the above

38. The parts of stance phase of the walking gait cycle include all of the following except _____. (61)

   A. Heel strike

   B. Mid stance

   C. Toe off

Appendix

D. Float

39. Define the 0-4 objective tenderness scale. (65)

0 = _____

1 = _____

2 = _____

3 = _____

4 = _____

40. Which of the following may affect ROM? (67)

A. Age and gender

B. Injury & life-style choices

C. Anatomical variation

D. All of the above

41. Which of the following is NOT a pathologic joint end-feel? (68)

A. Muscle spasm

B. Soft tissue stretch

C. Empty

D. Capsular

42. 'Movement against gravity but not against examiner's resistance' defines a ____ muscle strength grading. (71)

A. 5/5

B. 4/5

C. 3/5

D. 2/5

43. To improve goniometer reliability, best practices include which of the following? (75)

A. Using the same goniometer and procedure

B. Using the same examiner

C. Same client positioning

D. All of the above

44. HYPOmobility can start the degenerative process, causes may include which of the following? (76)

A. Injury, inactivity, contracture

B. Loss of coordination/proprioception

C. Muscular and vascular atrophy

D. Thickened joint capsules/ligaments

E. All of the above

45. What is the normal ROM for the sacroiliac joint in flexion/extension? (91)

A. 0-10°

B. 5-15°

C. 10-20°

D. 15-20°

46. What is the normal range for the lumbosacral base angle? (88)

A. 0-10°

B. 26-57°

C. 62-75°

D. 10-25°

47. All of the following help resist sacral nutation except? (89)

A. Posterior SI ligaments

B. Sacrotuberous ligament

C. Sacrospinous ligament

D. Iliolumbar ligaments

48. Sacral nutation increase lumbar lordosis? (93)

A. True

B. False

49. Lumbar disc pressure and injury risk is greatest with _____? (128)

A. Extension

B. Flexion

C. Rotation

D. Both 'B' and 'C'

50. In the cervical spine right rotation and right lateral flexion are coupled motions (occur at the same time)? (211)

A. True

B. False

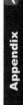

Appendix

C. Flexor pollicis brevis

D. Flexor pollicis longus

51. Which of the following may be signs of vertebral basilar ischemia? (201)

A. Dizziness, Diplopia, Dysarthria Dysphagia, Decrease consciousness

B. Ataxia

C. Nausea, Numbness, Nystagmus

D. All of the above

57. When running ___x body weight goes through the hip joint? (306)

A. 0.3x body weight

B. 2.5x body weight

C. 3x body weight

D. > 4.5x body weight

52. Flexion of thoracic vertebrae is associated with what rib motion? (161)

A. Upward rotation

B. Downward rotation

C. Abduction

D. Both 'B' and 'C'

58. What is considered a 'normal' Q-angle?

A. female 120°, male 60°

B. female 22°, male 18°

C. female 18°, male 22°

D. female 60°, male 120°

53. What is the ratio of scapular to glenohumeral movement during shoulder abduction? (244)

A. 1:2

B. 2:1

C. 120°:60°

D. 60°:120°

59. Traction applied through the long axis of the shaft of the femur will result in distraction at the hip joint.

A. True

B. False

54. What is the tight packed position of the shoulder? (243)

A. maximal abduction & lateral rotation

B. 90° abduction

C. Full elevation

D. None of the above

60. Which of the following ligaments are tight with full knee extension? (329)

A. ACL

B. PCL

C. MCL

D. All of the above

55. The normal carrying angle of the elbow? (275)

A. 5-15°

B. 5-10°

C. 0-10°

D. 60-120°

61. If your client has difficulty everting their foot, it would be important to check the mobility of which of the following joints?

A. Subtalar

B. Calcaneocuboid

C. Talonavicular

D. All of the above should be assessed

56. All of the following tendons that travel through the carpal tunnel except? (289)

A. Flexor digitorum profundus

B. Flexor digitorum superficialis

62. Which of the following bones does not articulate with the cuboid? (349)

A. Fibula

B. Medial cuneiform

C. Calcaneus

D. both A & B

63. Over pronation can cause collapse of the medial longitudinal arch, medial rotation of the tibia and genu valgus. (349)

A. True

B. False

64. Your client presents with restricted talocrural joint plantarflexion, you could glide the talus posteriorly in the mortise to help improve range of motion.

A. True

B. False

65. The talocrural joint is close-packed in dorsiflexion. (348)

A. True

B. False

66. Your client cannot extent their big toe at the MTP joint, it would be important to mobilize the base of the proximal phalanx dorsally. (367)

A. True

B. False

67. What does FITT stand for? (370)

A. Frequency, intensity, type, time

B. Frequency, intention, type, time

C. Fitness, intensity, team, time

D. Frequency, intensity, tailored, thermal

68. When would you use RICE vs METH in a rehab setting? (page X)

A. You should use METH indefinitely regardless of the phase of injury whether it be acute, sub-acute or chronic

B. METH is best following acute injury, particularly the first 6-24 hours. RICE is best for the sub-acute and chronic phases.

C. You should use RICE indefinitely regardless of the phase of injury as it is the best thing for rehab all around

D. RICE is best following acute injury, particularly the first 6-24 hours. METH is best for sub-acute and chronic phases.

69. Common errors in joint mobilizations may include _____? (41)

A. Over gripping by the clinician

B. Poor patient positioning

C. Holding too much tension in the body

D. All of the above

70. Joint mobilization techniques should never be applied to hypermobile joints. (30)

A. True

B. False

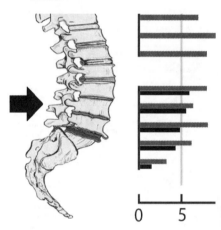

Appendix

Cervicothoracic Regional Exam
☑ Check normal, circle & describe abnormal

Chief complaint & significant history: _____

Patient: _____ date: _____
Insurance: _____

Vital Signs: Height: _____, Weight: _____, Blood Pressure: L _____/_____, R _____/_____, Resp: _____/min, VBI: L _____ R _____

Inspection: ☐ WNL
Development: ☐ good, ☐ fair, ☐ poor
☐ Posture: _____
☐ Skin (bruising, scars): _____
☐ Antalgia: _____
☐ Asymmetry: _____

Observation		L	R
Cervical	Head tilt		
	Head rotation		
	Head carriage (ant. / post.)		
Thoracic	Lordosis (hyper / hypo)		
	High shoulder		
	Scoliosis		
	Kyphosis (hyper / hypo)		
	Adam's sign		

ROM & Joint Play: ☐ WNL

Cervical spine	Active		Passive	
	L	R	L	R
Flexion (50°)				
Extension (60°)				
Lateral flexion (45°)				
Rotation (80°)				
Shoulder	L	R	L	R
Flexion (180°)				
Extension (50°)				
Abduction (180°)				
Adduction (30°)				
Internal rotation (90°)				
External rotation (80°)				
Scapulocostal rhythm				
TMJ				
Depression/elevation				
Lateral deviation				

Palpation: ☐ WNL

Palpation	L	R
Skin (masses, temp)		
Lymph nodes		
Temporalis		
Masseter		
TMJ		
Scalenes		
SCM		
Levator scapulae		
Trapezius/rhomboids		
Suboccipitals		
Posterior c-spine muscles		
Trachea mobility		
Thyroid gland		
Clavicle / thoracic outlet		
Rotator cuff		

Mark on drawing ☐ pain (circle), ☐ spasm (s), ☐ edema (e), ☐ fibrotic (f), ☐ MFTP (x), ☐ ache (a), ☐ burning (b), ☐

Neurologic: ☐ WNL

Sensation ☐ WNL	L	R
Light touch		
Sharp/dull		
Vibration		

Reflexes (0-5) ☐ WNL	L	R
Biceps (C5)(musculocut.)		
Brachioradialis(C6)(radial)		
Triceps (C7)(radial)		

Motor (0-5) ☐ WNL	L	R
Cervical flexion (C1-C2)		
Cervical extension (C2, C3, XI)		
Cervical lat. flexion (C3)		
Cervical rotation (C1-4, XI)		
Trapezius (CN XI)(accessory)		
Deltoid (C5)(axillary)		
Biceps (C6)(musculocut.)		
Triceps (C7, C8)(radial)		
Wrist extensors (C6)(radial)		
Wrist flexors (C7)(med./ulnar)		
Interossei (C8, T1)(ulnar)		

Cranial nerves ☐ WNL	
☐ I (smell)	☐ VII (facial expres)
☐ II (light, vision)	☐ VIII (Weber, Rinne)
☐ III, IV, VI (gaze)	☐ IX, X (ahhh)
☐ V (bite, sensation)	☐ XI (trap/SCM)
☐ V, VII (corneal ref.)	☐ XII (tongue)

Orthopedic: ☐ WNL

Screening	L	R
Valsalva		
Cervical compression		
Max. compression		
Cervical distraction		
Soto Hall		
Jull's test		
Brachial stretch		
Shoulder depression		

	L	R
	C0	
	C1	
	C2	
	C3	
	C4	
	C5	
	C6	
	C7	
	T1	
	T2	
	T3	
	T4	
	T5	
	T6	

TOS	L	R
Eden's		
Wright's		
Adson's		
Roo's		

Additional procedures: ☐ WNL
☐ Abdominal exam: _____
☐ Auscultation (heart, lungs): _____
☐ Ophthalmoscopic exam: _____
☐ Otoscopic exam: _____
☐ Other: _____

DDx: _____

Signature: _____ Date: _____

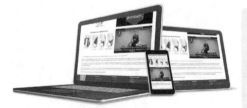

Full sized download & printing for personal & classroom use on website

Video demonstrations at:

prohealthsys.com

prohealthsys

Lumbopelvic Regional Exam

☑ Check normal, circle & describe abnormal

CC & significant history: _____

Patient: _____ date: _____
Insurance: _____ *(dd/mm/yr)*

Fracture screen (tuning fork, percussion, torsion test, 5-step test): □ WNL □ Refer for X-ray: _____

Inspection: □ WNL

Development: □ good, □ fair, □ poor
□ Posture: _____
□ Skin (bruising, scars): _____
□ Swelling: _____
□ Asymmetry: _____

Observation □ WNL	L	R
Antalgia		
Lordosis: hyper, normal, hypo		
Scoliosis		
Postural asymmetry		
Heel walk (L4)		
Toe raises, multiple (S1)		
Squat & rise		
Gait		

Palpation: □ WNL, □ pain (circle), □ spasm (s), □ edema (e), □ fibrotic (f), □ MFTP (x), □ ache (a), □ tingling (t)

Palpation	L	R	Palpation	L	R
Abdomen			Piriformis		
Inguinal lymph nodes			Sacrotuberous lig.		
Skin temperature			Sacroiliac joint		
Pubic symphysis			Sacrospinous lig.		
ASIS iliac crest			Gluteus maximus		
Iliolumbar ligaments			Gluteus medius		
Paraspinal muscles			Quadriceps		
Quadratus lumborum			Gastro-soleus		
Sciatic notch					
PSIS			**Pulses (0-4)**	**L**	**R**
Ischial tuberosities			Femoral pulse		
Hamstrings			Tibial pulse		
TFL			Dorsal pedial		
Greater trochanter					

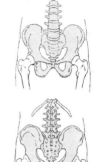

ROM & Joint Play: □ WNL

□ Pain at end ROM: _____
□ Abnormal motion: _____

Lumbar ROM	Active		Passive	
	L	R	L	R
Flexion (60°)				
Extension (25°)				
Lateral flexion (25°)				
Rotation (10°)				

Sacroiliac joint	L	R	L	R
Flex-ext (0-10°)				
Extern/intern (5-10°)				
Lumbopelvic rhythm				

Left	Joint Play	Right
	T12	
	L1	
	L2	
	L3	
	L4	
	L5	
	S1	
	SI	

Neurologic: □ WNL

Sensation, □ WNL	L	R
Light touch		
Sharp/dull		
Vibration		

Reflexes (0-5), □ WNL	L	R
Patellar (L4)		
Hamstring (L5)		
Patellar (S1)		
Babinski		

Motor (0-5), □ WNL	L	R
Abdomen (Beevor's sign)		
Resisted trunk rotation		
Resisted trunk lateral flexion		
Quadriceps (L2-L4)(femoral)		
Iliopsoas (L1-L3)(femoral)		
Tib. anterior (L4-L5)(deep f.)		
Ext. hal. long. (L4-S1)		
Flex. hallicus (L5-S2)		
Fibularis long. (L5-S1)		
Glut. max. (L5-S2)(inf. glut.)		
Hamstring (L4-S1)(sciatic)		
Glut. medius (L4-S1)		

Orthopedic: □ WNL

	L	R
Adam's sign		
Minor's sign		
Belt test		
Neri bowing		
Trendelenburg		
Lat. pelvic shift		
Valsalva		
Bechterew		
Slump test		
Deyerle		
Kemp's test		
Ober's		
Anvil test		
Allis' sign		

	L	R
SLR active/passive		
SLR maximal		
Bragard's		
Goldwait's		
Patrick FABERE		
LaGuerre		
Hip circumduction		
SI compression		
SI distraction		
Thomas/Gaenslen		
Homan's		
Nachlas/Ely/Hibb		
Brudzinski's		
Leg length		

Additional procedures: □ WNL

□ Hip exam: _____
□ Knee exam: _____
□ Abdominal: _____

DDx: _____

Signature: _____ Date: _____

Appendix

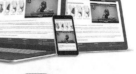

Full sized download & printing for
personal & classroom use on website

Video demonstrations at:

prohealthsys.com

 Printable quizzes   Patient handouts   Stretch & Strengthen   ▶ Video prohealthsys.com

prohealthsys.com

prohealthsys

Lower Body Regional Exam
☑ Check normal, circle & describe abnormal

CC & significant history: _____

Patient: _____ date: _____
Insurance: _____ (dd/mm/yr)

Fracture screen (□ tuning fork, □ percussion, □ torsion test, □ 5-step test): □ **WNL** □ **imaging:** _____

Reflexes: □ **WNL,** □ patellar (L4), □ hamstring (L5), □ Achilles (S1): _____

Lumbosacral:
Inspection □ WNL
- □ Posture:
- □ Skin:
- □ Swelling:
- □ Asymmetry:

Palpation: □ WNL
- □ Soft tissue:
- □ Bone:
- □ Lymph nodes:
- □ Pain:

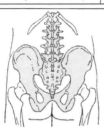

ROM/joint play	L -act.- R	L -pas- R	L -res.- R	Orthoneuro	L	R
Flexion (60°)				Squat & rise		
Extension (25°)				Belt test		
Lateral flexion (25°)				Trendelenburg		
Rotation (10°)				Valsalva		
Sacroiliac joint				Slump test		
Flexion/ext. (0-10°)				Kemp's test		
Extern/int. (5-10°)				SLR active/passive		
Lumbopelvic rhythm				SLR maximal		
				Thomas/Gaenslen		

Hip:
Inspection □ WNL
- □ Posture:
- □ Skin:
- □ Swelling:
- □ Asymmetry:

Palpation: □ WNL
- □ Soft tissue:
- □ Bone:
- □ Femoral pulse:
- □ Pain:

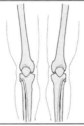

Leg length: L: _____, R: _____

ROM/joint play	L -act.- R	L -pas- R	L -res.- R	Orthoneuro	L	R
Flexion (120°) bent knee				Anvil test		
Flexion (80°-90°) SLR				Patrick FABERE		
Extension (30°)				Laguere		
Abduction (50°)				Scour test		
Adduction (30°)				Telescoping		
Internal rotation (40°)				Ober's		
External rotation (50°)				Ely/Nachlas		
				Hibb's		
				Yoeman's		

Knee:
Inspection □ WNL
- □ Skin:
- □ Swelling:
- □ Asymmetry:

Palpation: □ WNL
- □ Soft tissue:
- □ Bone:
- □ Popliteal pulse:
- □ Pain:

ROM/joint play	L -act.- R	L -pas- R	L -res.- R	Orthoneuro	L	R
Flexion (150°)				Ant./post. drawer		
Extension (0°)				Allis' sign		
Internal rotation				Valgus stress		
External rotation				Varus stress		
Other joint play				Apley compression		
A↔P tibia/femur				Apley distraction		
A↔P tibia/fibula				Lachman's		
Patella joint play				Pat. apprehension		
				Patellar grind		

Ankle/foot:
Inspection □ WNL
- □ Pes planus/cavus:
- □ Skin:
- □ Swelling:
- □ Asymmetry:

Palpation: □ WNL
- □ Soft tissue:
- □ Bone:
- □ Tibial pulse:
- □ Dorsal pedial:
- □ Pain:

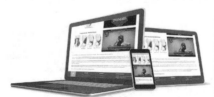

ROM/joint play	L -act.- R	L -pas- R	L -res.- R	Orthoneuro	L	R
Plantarflexion (40°)				Anterior drawer		
Dorsiflexion (20°)				Talar tilt		
Inversion (20°)				Hoffa's sign		
Eversion (10°)				Thompson test		
Other joints				Achilles squeeze		
Toe flexion				Calcaneal squeeze		
Toe extension				Morton's squeeze		
				Buerger's test		
				Tinel's		

Signature: _____ Date: _____

Full sized download & printing for personal & classroom use on website

Video demonstrations at:

prohealthsys.com

 Printable quizzes　　 Patient handouts　　 Stretch & Strengthen　　 Video prohealthsys.com

Appendix

Upper Body Regional Exam
☑ Check normal, circle & describe abnormal

CC & significant history: _____

Patient: _____ date: _____
Insurance: _____ (dd/mm/yr)

Fracture screen (□ tuning fork, □ percussion, □ torsion test): □ WNL, □ Refer for imaging: _____

Reflexes: □ WNL, □ biceps (C5), □ brachioradialis (C6), □ triceps (C7): _____

Cervicothoracic:
Inspection □ WNL
- □ Posture:
- □ Skin:
- □ Swelling:
- □ Asymmetry:

Palpation: □ WNL
- □ Soft tissue:
- □ Bone:
- □ Lymph nodes:
- □ Pain:

C-ROM	L -act.- R	L -pas- R	L -res.- R	Orthoneuro	L	R
Flexion (50°)				Vaslsalva		
Extension (60°)				Cervical compress.		
Lateral flexion (45°)				Max. compression		
Rotation (80°)				Cervical distraction		
Temporomandibular joint				Soto Hall		
Depres./elevation				Shoulder depression		
Lateral deviation				Adson's		
				Wright's		
				Roo's		

Shoulder:
Inspection □ WNL
- □ Posture:
- □ Skin:
- □ Swelling:
- □ Asymmetry:
- □ Step defect:

Palpation: □ WNL
- □ Soft tissue:
- □ Bone:
- □ Brachial pulse:
- □ Pain:

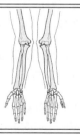

ROM/joint play	L -act.- R	L -pas- R	L -res.- R	Orthoneuro	L	R
Flexion (180°)				Apley sup./inf.		
Extension (50°)				Empty can		
Abduction (180°)				Ant. apprehension		
Adduction (30°)				Faegan's		
Internal rotation (90°)				Hawkins-Kennedy		
External rotation (80°)				Yergason's		
Scapulocostal rhythm:				Speeds		
				Clunk/crank		
				O'Brien		

Elbow:
Inspection □ WNL
- □ Skin:
- □ Swelling:
- □ Asymmetry:

Palpation: □ WNL
- □ Soft tissue:
- □ Bone:
- □ Olecranon bursa:
- □ Pain:

ROM/joint play	L -act.- R	L -pas- R	L -res.- R	Orthoneuro	L	R
Flexion (150°)				Valgus stress		
Extension (0°)				Varus stress		
Supination (90°)				Cozen's		
Pronation (90°)				Mill's		
Other joint play				Book lift test		
Ulnohumeral				Reverse Cozen's		
Radiohumeral				Reverse Mill's		
Proximal radioulnar				Pronator stretch		
				Tinel's (ulnar n.)		

Wrist/hand:
Inspection □ WNL
- □ Skin:
- □ Swelling:
- □ Asymmetry:

Palpation: □ WNL
- □ Soft tissue:
- □ Bone:
- □ Radial pulse:
- □ Ulnar pulse:
- □ Pain:

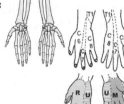

Wrist ROM	L -act.- R	L -pas- R	L -res.- R	Orthoneuro	L	R
Flexion (80°)				Phalen's (median)		
Extension (70°)				Wrist drop (radial)		
Ulnar flexion (30°)				Froment's (ulnar)		
Radial flexion (20°)				Scaphoid fracture		
Finger flex./ext.				Bracelet		
Finger add./abd.				Thumb abd. stress		
Carpal ROM				Thumb grind		
Grip strength				Finklestein's		
				Tinel's at wrist x 2		

This form is a comprehensive checklist of examination procedures. Each item should be utilized as a diagnostic option based on the patient's presenting symptoms and the clinical discretion of the examiner. Every procedure does not have to be performed on every patient. Some procedures may be contraindicated in certain situations. Patient information contained within this form is considered strictly confidential. Reproduction is permitted for personal use, not for resale or redistribution. www.prohealthsys.com ©Professional Health Systems Inc. All rights reserved. "Dedicated to Clinical Excellence."

Signature: _____ Date: _____

Appendix

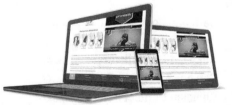

Full sized download & printing for personal & classroom use on website

Video demonstrations at:

prohealthsys.com

Index

Index

Index

(P)	pain	FABQ	Fear-Avoidance Beliefs Questionnaire (FABQ)	OA	osteoarthrosis
(R)	right			OM	osseous manipulation
(L)	left	FID	frequency, intensity, duration	OT	occupational therapist
↑	increase			OTC	over the counter (medication)
↓	decrease	flex	flexion		
→	causes / may indicate or suggest	FMP	functional movement pattern	PA	posterior to anterior
		Fx	fracture	**PAR-Q**	**procedures, alternatives, risk - questions**
(-)	negative	GH	glenohumeral		
(+)	positive	GMMT	general manual muscle testing	PhD	doctor of philosophy
ABCS	AROM, break test, concentric ROM, stretch			PIR	post isometric relaxation
		HA	headache	PFROM	pain free ROM
AC	acromioclavicular joint	HIP-MNRS	history, inspection, palpation - motion, neurovascular screen, referred, special tests	PRICE	protect, rest, ice, compress, elevate
ADL	activity of daily living				
AF	acetabulofemoral joint			PRN	patient return as needed
AIS	adolescent idiopathic scoliosis	HTN	hypertension	PROM	passive range of motion
		Hx	history	pt	patient
AP	anterior to posterior	HVLA	high velocity low amplitude	PT	physical therapist
AROM	active range of motion			PTR	patient to return
AAROM	active assisted range of motion	IAM	instrument assisted mobilization	Px	prognosis
				RA	rheumatoid arthritis
AS	ankylosing spondylitis	IASTM	instrument assisted soft tissue mobilization	RMT	registered massage therapist
ASIS	anterior superior iliac spine				
AVN	avascular necrosis	ICD	international classification of disease	ROF	review of findings
BHK	bachelor of human kinetics			ROM	range of motion
		IMS	intermuscular stimulation	SCFE	slipped capital femoral epiphysis
BP	blood pressure	IVD	intervertebral disc		
cc	chief complaint, chief concern	IVF	intervertebral foramen	SLAP	superior labrum anterior posterior (tear)
		KIS	keep it simple		
CI	contra-indication	LBP	low back pain	SMART	specific, measurable, attainable, realistic, time
CMC	carpometacarpal joint	LLI	leg length inequality		
CPRs	clinical prediction rules	LMP	licensed massage practitioner	SOL	space occupying lesion
CSCS	certified strength & conditioning specialist			SP	spinous process
		LMNL	lower motor neuron lesion	STM	soft tissue manipulation
CT	computed tomography	LOC	loss of consciousness	TBI	traumatic brain injury
CTS	carpal tunnel syndrome	MCP	metacarpophalangeal joint	TENS	transcutaneous electrical nerve stimulation
DC	doctor of chiropractic				
DDx	differential diagnosis	MD	medical doctor	TIA	transient ischemic attack
DIP	distal interphalangeal joint	METH	motion, exercise, traction, heat	TFC	triangular fibrocartilage (ulnar meniscus)
DJD	degenerative joint disease	MFR	myofascial release	TOS	thoracic outlet syndrome
		MFTP	myofascial trigger point	tp	tender point
DN	dry needling	MMT	manual muscle testing	TP, TvP	transverse process
DO	doctor of osteopathy	MRI	magnetic resonance imaging	Tx	treatment
DOI	date of injury			UA	urinalysis
DOMS	delayed onset muscle soreness	MVA	motor vehicle accident	UMNL	upper motor neuron lesion
		NCS	nerve conduction study	US	ultrasound
DTR	deep tendon reflex (muscle stretch reflex)	ND	naturopathic doctor	VAS	visual analog scale (0-10 pain rating)
		NMS	neuromusculoskeletal		
Dx	diagnosis	NRS	numeric rating scale	VRS	verbal rating scale (0-10)
ext	extension/external	NSAID	non-steroidal anti-inflammatory medication	WNL	within normal limits

Index

Joint Mobilization Practical Exam

Student has 15 minutes to complete this exam

Candidate: Printable form on website   /100

grade ___/5 & comment if issue

0	1	2	3	3.5	4	5
unacceptable	poor	developing		acceptable	good	excellent

Proctor: _____

Intro statement, explain procedure & consent.... ___/5
- □ Provides list of relative or absolute CIs (see page 30)   (___/5)

Functional Movement.. ___/10
- □ Start with functional motion   (___/5)
- □ Bilateral comparison   (___/5)

AROM .... ___/10
- □ Bilateral comp. & list of tissue activated & stretched (___/5)
- □ Logical progression, most painful movements last   (___/5)

PROM .... ___/20
- □ Permission to palpate & detailed exam of region   (___/5)
  (list structures below hand - muscle, ligament, nerve, bone, vessel)
- □ Good limb handling & biomechanics   (___/5)
- □ Bilateral comparison painful movements last   (___/5)
- □ End-feel identified   (___/5)

Mobilization #1 _____........ ___/20
- □ Safe limb handling/biomechanics (patient & clinician) (___/5)
- □ Names & uses appropriate contacts   (___/5)
- □ Tissue pull (slack) and vectors effective   (___/5)
- □ Controlled mobilization technique application   (___/5)

Mobilization #2 _____.......... ___/20
- □ Safe limb handling/biomechanics (patient & clinician) (___/5)
- □ Names & uses appropriate contacts   (___/5)
- □ Tissue pull (slack) and vectors effective   (___/5)
- □ Controlled mobilization technique application   (___/5)

Overall .... ___/15
- □ Confidence in procedure & explanation of process   (___/5)
- □ Effective, safe, professional demeanor   (___/5)
- □ Lack of prompting, good flow & time management   (___/5)

Extremity
- PA or AP glides
- ML or LM glide
- IS or SI glide
- Rotational mobes
- Distraction

- □ shoulder
- □ elbow
- □ wrist & hand
- □ hip
- □ knee
- □ ankle/foot

Spinal
- □ SI
  - PI ilium
  - AS ilium
  - Counter-nut sacrum
  - Nutated sacrum
- □ L-spine
  - push pull
  - mammillary push
  - spinous push
  - nutated sacrum
- □ T-spine
  - prone extension
  - supine extension
  - prone rot./side bend
- □ Costal
  - prone costal
  - supine costal
- □ C-spine
  - index pillar
  - thumb pillar
  - occipital

Printable quizzes

Patient handouts

Stretch & Strengthen

Video prohealthsys

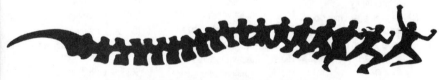

Trusted evidence based resources
In print, in person, and online

Index